D1811059

Patient Safety and Quality in Pediatric Hematology/Oncology and Stem Cell Transplantation

Christopher E. Dandoy • Joanne M. Hilden
Amy L. Billett • Brigitta U. Mueller
Editors

Patient Safety and Quality in Pediatric Hematology/ Oncology and Stem Cell Transplantation

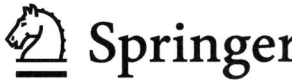 Springer

Editors
Christopher E. Dandoy
Division of Bone Marrow Transplant
and Immune Deficiency
Cincinnati Children's Hospital
Medical Center
Cincinnati, Ohio
USA

Joanne M. Hilden
Center for Cancer and Blood Disorders
Children's Hospital Colorado
Aurora, Colorado
USA

Amy L. Billett
Boston Children's Cancer and Blood
Disorders Center
Dana-Farber
Boston, Massachusetts
USA

Brigitta U. Mueller
Johns Hopkins All Children's Hospital
St. Petersburg, Florida
USA

ISBN 978-3-319-53788-7   ISBN 978-3-319-53790-0   (eBook)
DOI 10.1007/978-3-319-53790-0

Library of Congress Control Number: 2017941078

© Springer International Publishing AG 2017
This work is subject to copyright. All rights are reserved by the Publisher, whether the whole or part of the material is concerned, specifically the rights of translation, reprinting, reuse of illustrations, recitation, broadcasting, reproduction on microfilms or in any other physical way, and transmission or information storage and retrieval, electronic adaptation, computer software, or by similar or dissimilar methodology now known or hereafter developed.
The use of general descriptive names, registered names, trademarks, service marks, etc. in this publication does not imply, even in the absence of a specific statement, that such names are exempt from the relevant protective laws and regulations and therefore free for general use.
The publisher, the authors and the editors are safe to assume that the advice and information in this book are believed to be true and accurate at the date of publication. Neither the publisher nor the authors or the editors give a warranty, express or implied, with respect to the material contained herein or for any errors or omissions that may have been made. The publisher remains neutral with regard to jurisdictional claims in published maps and institutional affiliations.

Printed on acid-free paper

This Springer imprint is published by Springer Nature
The registered company is Springer International Publishing AG
The registered company address is: Gewerbestrasse 11, 6330 Cham, Switzerland

To our patients and their families, who entrust us with the care of their children.
To our families and friends, who provide us with unwavering support.
To our mentors, colleagues, and mentees, who teach us every day.

Foreword

Our systems are too complex to expect merely extraordinary people to perform perfectly 100% of the time. We as leaders must put in place systems to support safe practice.

As I began this book, I was flooded with memories. From the first days of my 50-year career in healthcare, a college student working as a part-time radiology clerk, pediatric hematology and oncology has had a huge impact on me. At Boston Children's Hospital, Division 28 was the inpatient oncology unit, Division 20 was the inpatient research unit for rare hematologic and other illnesses, and the TTC (tumor therapy clinic) was the outpatient center of our partner Children's Cancer Research Foundation (now Dana-Farber Cancer Institute). The children coming to radiology from these places were often desperately sick, yet they demonstrated great courage and resilience and showed us laughter as well as amazing support of those on the journey with them. Their parents appeared suffering and desperate yet somehow were, because they had to be, resolved and engaged. Siblings and grandparents were often dazed yet were there for the child and each other. All held a deep trust in their care team: the expertise and passion of the staff, clinicians, researchers, and so many more, focused on care, caring, hope, and discovery. The team, in turn, seemed to be always supporting the children, huddled in the reading room consulting while pouring through hundreds of films as well as in the clinic, in the lab, and at the bedside morning, noon, and night. They were committed to figuring it out together. They are extraordinary people, indeed, individually and collectively.

Today, 50 years later, after having served as a hospital administrator at Boston Children's Hospital, an executive at Dana-Farber Cancer Institute, a professor at Harvard T.H. Chan School of Public Health, an improvement advisor at IHI (Institute for Healthcare Improvement), and a trustee for the Lahey Health System and Winchester Hospital, my respect for these extraordinary people in the hematology and oncology journey—patients, families, staff, groups, networks, collaboratives, and communities—has deepened enormously. Along with many, I'm forever grateful for the scientific advancement, dramatically better clinical outcomes, and the continuous quality improvement in hematology, oncology, and hematopoietic stem cell transplantation (Hem/Onc/HSCT).

Over the same period, and notably the last 25 years, I confronted the growing and sobering reality of healthcare administrative and clinical practice: adverse outcomes didn't all have to happen. There was significant preventable suffering, harm, tragedy, death, as well as cost waste under all our watches. Circumstances of the tragic overdose that led to the death of Betsy Lehman allowed me, as well as many others, to learn deeply the personal and organizational impacts for all the victims of harm, the patient, family, staff, and community [1]. I discovered that many of our mental models were faulty; things we believed to be true were not. I learned about mindfulness and, as a leader, developed both a preoccupation with failure and a deep understanding of and passion for quality improvement and patient safety. We pursued the respectful management of serious clinical adverse events [2] after they occurred for patients, family members, and staff, with an overarching aim to eliminating their occurrence in the first place. Along the way at my organizations, across the country and around the world, I met many victims of medical error, children and adults, including patients from hematology and oncology, who were seriously harmed due to poor systems, structures, and processes. I've stood on many occasions before and cried with families and staff who were devastated after preventable harm contributed to death. Often, the same people courageously discussed how they could pursue together three questions: what happened, why did it happen, and what can be done to prevent it from happening again. I've learned that we can't expect people, even exceptional people, who suffer from being human and work in complex, often broken, systems to be perfect 100% of the time. To achieve together the outcomes we seek, leadership at every level must put in place the learning, systems, structures, and processes, to support the *right care in the right place at the right time, every time* [3]. This journey applies to everyone, individually and collectively, never worrying alone. I've seen at every level the power and experienced the pride of working in and with high-quality, continuously improving organizations.

This book is edited by a talented expert team—Christopher Dandoy MD, Joanne Hilden MD, Amy Billett MD, and Brigitta Mueller MD—that had a clear vision for systematic continuous improvement in pediatric hematology and oncology and for driving out unintended variation, suffering, harm, tragedy, death, and cost waste. Drawing on the best experience, evidence, and learning from not only pediatrics but the larger healthcare universe, they bring to the text their personal journeys and their clinical/administrative expertise as well as the quality of care journeys of their organizations, Cincinnati Children's Hospital, Boston Children's/Dana-Farber Cancer and Blood Disorders Center, Children's Hospital of Colorado, and Johns Hopkins All Children's Hospital. They are joined by chapter authors with a wide breadth of experience from these and other leading pediatric hematology and oncology services, as well as from healthcare improvement organizations. Many of these writers I've had the privilege of meeting, working with, and learning from through healthcare delivery, in the university classroom, and/or in the improvement setting.

As I read this book, structured in three sections (Introduction to Safety and Quality Improvement, Getting Started, and Quality and Safety Principles Unique to Pediatric Hematology/Oncology/Bone Marrow Transplantation), I noted the breadth and depth of coverage. Content on quality and safety was presented across the care continuum—from detection to posttreatment survivorship and/or care at the end of life—and settings wisely ranging from the home and ambulatory environment to the inpatient service. The content is strong with theories, principles, models, tools, frameworks, examples, case studies, and extensive citation. While many of the citations are well known, I was excited by all the new content I was introduced to. Pediatrics historically has taught us much in the wider healthcare community and specifically about patient- and family-centered care. This teaching and role modeling continues in the text with an emphasis on the patient and family in quality and patient safety. The focus throughout on and learning from collaboration and teamwork at every level (macro, mezzo, micro) is powerful, with the patient and family as essential partners.

As the authors note, patient safety and quality improvement is all about change. For many years, in classrooms at the Harvard T.H. Chan School of Public Health, I've taught a course on leading change. The opening slide on opening day is "Most Change Fails" and the citation is "everyone," referencing the many studies across the industry showing the significant failure rates of change initiatives on execution along with the lack of spread and sustainability. Clinical leaders flooded every classroom with failures they were familiar with. Individuals and organizations are doing "lots of this and that" and are "cooking without a recipe, a framework." To counter that, the authors offer wonderful resources on systematic quality improvement science and methods, implementing evidence-based care, spread, and sustainability. Together they can build a culture of excellence and improvement by making change a foundational habit and not just an epidemic of "projectitis." Throughout the text, they take on the importance of standardized practices while at the same time recognizing unique needs. An important, supportive, and very helpful chapter is the focus on careers in quality improvement and patient safety.

As previously noted, improvement is all about confronting our mental models, the things we believe to be true because *they are!* Many may say "our patients are sicker" suggesting adverse events such as infections in the immunocompromised are inevitable, but the authors through this book, and many others, believed and have experienced that improvement and reduction of harm are possible. Rising to this challenge is essential.

Underscoring the editors' suggestions, readership for this book should be global and include a wide range of clinical and administrative professionals in hematology/oncology, as well as patient and family advisors and other interested parties—it is about them! As an extension of the IHI Getting Boards on Board work [4], I would strongly encourage the text be made available to governance and executive clinical and administrative leadership of organizations with a hematology/pediatric oncology focus for discussion; these leaders are ultimately responsible for the overall culture, quality of care, and leading change. There is much learning in the text that can be applied to pediatrics overall and to the broader quality and safety community.

As with most texts, this isn't just a onetime read but is an essential reference in the journey of individuals and teams to achieve the aims and outcomes we all seek for those we are privileged to partner with, respect, and serve: our patients, families, staff members, groups, and communities.

Again, we owe so much to so many for all they have contributed to improving healthcare quality and patient safety. It has been a privilege to be part of this improvement journey and specifically this text. At the same time, there are many references in the chapters ahead, paraphrasing that, for all that has been done, "We're early in our journey..." and "There is so much more we must do to improve quality and reduce cost."

> To do things differently, we must see things differently. When we see things we didn't see before, we can ask questions we didn't know to ask before. (Nelson [5])

Winchester, MA, USA   James B. Conway

References

1. Conway J, Nathan D, Benz E, Shulman LN, Sallan SE, Ponte PR, et al. Key learning from the Dana-Farber Cancer Institute's 10-year patient safety journey. In: 42nd Annual meeting of American society of clinical oncology educational book, Atlanta, GA, June 2–6, 2006, p. 615–19.
2. Conway J, Federico F, Stewart K, Campbell MJ. Respectful management of serious clinical adverse events. Cambridge: Institute for Healthcare Improvement; 2011.
3. Kaplan G, Lopez MH, McGinnis JM. Transforming health care scheduling and access: getting to now. Washington: Institute of Medicine; 2015. p. 118.
4. Conway MS. Getting boards on board: engaging governing boards in quality and safety. Jt Comm J Qual Patient Saf. 2008;34(4):214–20.
5. Nelson EC, Batalden PB, Godfrey MM, editors. Quality by design: a clinical microsystems approach. Wiley; 2011. p. 260.

Acknowledgments

We gratefully thank the nearly 50 chapter contributors who dedicated their time and efforts in completing this book. Thank you for sharing your knowledge and experience with those who care for pediatric hematology, oncology, and bone marrow transplant patients.

Additionally, we would like to thank the physicians, nurses, care coordinators, and other care providers and staff we interact with each day. Great colleagues are those that understand the importance of being a team; thank you for being by our side.

Finally, thank you to the patients and their families. We appreciate your insights, confidence, trust, and teamwork. We could not do our work without your work.

Contents

Chapter 1
Introduction to Patient Safety and Quality in the Pediatric/Hematology Oncology and Hematopoietic Stem Cell Transplant Practice

Christopher E. Dandoy, Joanne M. Hilden, Amy L. Billett, and Brigitta U. Mueller

A family takes their 4-year-old girl into the hospital for concerns of new bruising and lower extremity pain. The child has been symptomatic for a few weeks, but the symptoms significantly worsened over the past few days. The parents anxiously wait for the lab results to return, not knowing what to expect. The emergency room physician enters the room with a solemn face and explains that their child likely has

C.E. Dandoy (✉)
Department of Bone Marrow Transplant and Immune Deficiency, Cincinnati Children's Hospital Medical Center, Cincinnati, OH 45229, USA

Department of Pediatrics, University of Cincinnati, Cincinnati, OH 45220, USA
e-mail: christopher.dandoy@cchmc.org

J.M. Hilden
Center for Cancer and Blood Disorders, Children's Hospital Colorado, Aurora, CO 80045, USA

Department of Pediatrics, University of Colorado School of Medicine, Aurora, CO 80045, USA
e-mail: Joanne.Hilden@childrenscolorado.org

A.L. Billett
Dana-Farber/Boston Children's Cancer and Blood Disorders Center, Boston, MA 02115, USA

Department of Pediatrics, Harvard Medical School, Boston, MA 02115, USA
e-mail: Amy_Billett@dfci.harvard.edu

B.U. Mueller
Johns Hopkins All Children's Hospital, St. Petersburg, FL 33701, USA

Department of Pediatrics, Johns Hopkins University School of Medicine, Baltimore, MD 21205, USA
e-mail: brigitta.mueller@jhmi.edu

© Springer International Publishing AG 2017
C.E. Dandoy et al. (eds.), *Patient Safety and Quality in Pediatric Hematology/Oncology and Stem Cell Transplantation*, DOI 10.1007/978-3-319-53790-0_1

leukemia and would need to be admitted to the hospital. The words hang in the air, "your child has cancer." The parents do not yet know the massive lifestyle change in store for them. They do not realize the amount of time they will spend in the clinic, in the inpatient unit, and in a waiting room while their child undergoes yet another procedure. They do not know, at this time, the number of medications their child will take on a daily basis for the next several years and how easy it will be to confuse these complicated-sounding medications. There are many long days and sleepless nights ahead for them, but they will do it. They will give their complete trust to the physicians, nurses, pharmacists, and hospital staff to care for their girl.

Years earlier, the leaders and caregivers in the pediatric hematology oncology practice initiated a chemotherapy safety program. They formed a team with physicians, nurses, advanced practice providers, pharmacists, administrative staff and leadership, and patients/families. The established safety guidelines included a standardized process of chemotherapy prescribing, dispensing, administering, documenting, and monitoring. The team initiated oversight of the chemotherapy management practices. They started tracking errors and near misses to understand how to target ongoing improvement. Recommendations for avoiding chemotherapy errors call for standardized approaches, development of policies and procedures for system improvement, and review of errors by interdisciplinary professional staff.

Importantly, the parents can rest assured that their child will be given the right medication, at the right time; they will be engaged in the treatment and the care of their child, and they will learn how to give the proper medications at home.

Standing on the Shoulders of Giants

Advances in Pediatric Oncology

Prior to World War II, children with cancer were treated by surgeons, general practitioners, and pediatricians [1]. Most cancer diagnoses were universally fatal, and treatment was associated with high morbidity and mortality. During World War II, chemotherapy came into being and was applied in lymphoma [2–4] and Wilms tumor [5]. In 1958, multi-agent chemotherapy was shown to improve outcomes [6]. Cures for leukemia were achieved by the addition of central nervous system-directed therapy [7] and then intensification of chemotherapy [8]. In 1986, cure rates for acute leukemia rose above 80% with the inclusion of four-drug induction regimens [9]. Stage IV neuroblastoma went from incurable to curable (>50% 2-year event-free survival) through intensification of chemotherapy and introduction of radiotherapy, autologous stem cell transplant, 13-cis-retinoic acid [10], and immunotherapy [11]. These are but a few examples of the dramatic improvements related to better chemotherapy, better supportive care such as infection prevention, and better risk stratification.

As pediatric cancer is a relatively rare disease, and substantial gains cannot be made without collaboration, clinical collaborative groups began to form. In the mid-1990s, four primary childhood cooperative groups received funding by the National Cancer Institute [12]: two groups, the Children's Cancer Study Group (CCSG) and the Pediatric Oncology Group (POG), studied a diverse array of childhood cancers, while two other groups, the Intergroup Rhabdomyosarcoma Study Group (IRSG) and the National Wilms Tumor Study (NWTS) Group were cancer-specific. In 2000, these four pediatric groups voluntarily merged to create the Children's Oncology Group (COG) [12], which is now the world's largest organization devoted exclusively to pediatric cancer research. Approximately 10,000 children ages 0–14 [13] and approximately 70,000 adolescent and young adults (ages 15–39) are diagnosed with cancer in the United States each year [14], many of whom are cared for in children's hospitals and enrolled in COG studies. The first 3–4 IRS studies lead to steady improvements in outcomes without ever showing that the experimental arm had a better outcome compared to the standard arm. This reflects multiple changes in care delivery including changes in staging, risk assignment, and supportive care in addition to the clinical research questions being asked [15]. In some ways, this clinical research group served as a quality improvement collaborative that standardized care, studied outcomes, shared results with all, and instituted additional changes in care.

Advances in Pediatric Hematology

Some of the most impactful advances in modern medicine have been made through transfusion medicine. In 1969, the feasibility of storing platelets at room temperature, revolutionizing platelet transfusion therapy [16], was a key advancement in successful treatment of leukemia and other malignancies. In 1986, the Prophylactic Penicillin Study (PROPS) found that children should be screened in the neonatal period for sickle cell hemoglobinopathy and that those with sickle cell anemia should receive prophylactic penicillin therapy, thus reducing pneumococcal septicemia rates [17]. Clinical trials over the past 30 years have demonstrated significant advances in improving outcomes in sickle cell disease through the administration of hydroxyurea, limiting episodes of acute chest syndrome and pain crises and decreasing transfusions and overall morbidity and mortality [18–26]. Chelation therapy has proven effective at reducing the toxic effects of chronic transfusion in children with β-thalassemia major [27, 28]. In the late 1950s and much of the 1960s, fresh frozen plasma (FFP) was the primary treatment for hemophilia A and hemophilia B. As only a small amount of factor VIII and factor IX are in each unit of FFP, children and young adults required large volume transfusions and required hospitalizations, oftentimes delaying treatment and gradually leading to chronic joint disease with crippling deformities [29, 30]. The successful cloning of the factor VIII gene in 1984 was a major breakthrough [31], allowing production of recombinant human factor VIII [32, 33] and leading to clinical trials showing efficacy of recombinant factor VIII in hemophilia A patients [34].

Advances in Pediatric Hematopoietic Stem Cell Transplantation (HSCT)

Attempts to treat human patients with supralethal irradiation and marrow grafting were reported by Thomas et al. in 1957 [35]; however, successful transplants in leukemic patients only occurred in HSCT recipients of marrow from an identical twin donor [36, 37]. In the early 1960s, increased pessimism grew in the medical community surrounding HSCT [38], based on poor outcomes. However, by the end of the decade, antibiotic efficacy had improved, transfusion technology had advanced, and more effective cancer agents were developed. In 1968, three patients in the United States and the Netherlands suffering from severe combined immuno-deficiency syndromes successfully underwent HSCT [39–41], and by the 1970s and 1980s, HSCT was utilized on a more frequent basis for difficult-to-treat leukemias [42–45]. Over the next 20 years, advances in antiviral therapies [38], extension of graft selection to umbilical cord blood [46–49], and further understanding of HLA matching [49–52] improved outcomes. Today, over 50,000 individuals undergo HSCT annually as the establishment of registries throughout the world has extended access to stem cell grafts [53–56].

In 1676, in a letter to Robert Hooke, Sir Isaac Newton declared, "if I have seen further, it is only by standing on the shoulders of giants." For the last 50 years, and the centuries before it, thousands of lifetimes have been spent understanding the mechanisms and developing the interventions we utilize in our daily practice. As Newton eluded, we are carried aloft and elevated by the magnitude of the giants before us. Unfortunately, many of the breakthrough discoveries are not applied reliably today, and examples include transcranial Doppler ultrasonography screening for stroke prevention in sickle cell disease and timely antibiotic administration in febrile immunocompromised patients. It is our responsibility and stewardship to ensure our patients receive the right care at the right time, in as safe a manner as possible.

Complexity in Pediatric Hematology, Oncology, and HSCT Healthcare Delivery

In healthcare, complexity can be defined or calculated by the interrelatedness, or influence of system components on each other, inside the system [57].

- *Simple systems* have few components with little interrelatedness. An example of which would be a nurse entering vital signs into the electronic medical record (EMR).
- *Complicated systems* have many components, but low interrelatedness. An example of this would be many nurses and physicians entering data into the EMR, each individual interacting in a limited manner for their specific tasks.
- *Relatively complex* systems have few components with high interrelatedness. Due to the small number of components, they are amendable to change but more difficult to manage or predict. An example of this would be a hematology clinic with a rotation of physicians and nurses. Inside of the group, there may be considerable differences in performance and management of patients between similar teams. These divergences could include variations in protocol compliance and medical errors, showing variable performance between the teams.
- *Complex systems* have many components with high interrelatedness. These systems are challenging to describe, predict, and manage. An example of this would be a hematology oncology unit, with multiple physician providers, rotating residents, dozens of nurses, and multiple patients with a variety of illnesses who are treated on a variety of protocols. Each individual component (i.e., patients, nurses, physicians, residents) of the system is interrelated within and across team members.

The healthcare delivery system is complex. And in addition to providing care in a complex system, our patients are often critically ill, with multi-organ dysfunction, requiring continuous management form different healthcare professionals in multiple settings. Our therapies are not trivial, and the medications and interventions we provide have a narrow therapeutic window; incorrect dosing, timing, or administration can lead to significant morbidity and mortality [58, 59]. Finally, healthcare providers are under significant constraints, attempting to continue to provide safe and equitable healthcare in light of drug shortages, increased documentation requirements, and reduced reimbursement [60]. Healthcare is experiencing increased fragmentation with unintended consequence from care transitions and handoffs [61]. Resident handoffs are more frequent secondary to duty hour regulations, and hospitalists have commonly adopted shift-work-type systems [62]. Hospitalized patients are passed between doctors an average of 15 times during a single five-day hospitalization. If information is omitted or misunderstood, there may be serious clinical consequences [63, 64].

Adding to the complexity is the explosion of new data produced by the brightest minds around the world. Access to the information can be difficult as the volume is so high. Over the past 60 years, Blood has published 125 volumes containing a total of 43,042 original manuscripts, including 2729 clinical trials [65]. In addition, molecular information to diagnose and characterize disease as well as monitor progression or response is increasing, and staying current with the latest advances can be challenging.

Despite these challenges, pediatric hematology/oncology caregivers also have potential strengths that can be leveraged to improve patient safety and quality of care. We are all familiar with standardization of care which is a key component of the many clinical research trials. Team-based approaches are inherent in how we function in both inpatient and outpatient settings. We focus on enhancing the communication skills of our trainees. Thus, we are already enabled with critical skills to maximize patient safety and performance improvement.

Patient Safety

In the past 15 years, there has been a dramatic expansion of efforts focused on improving systems of care and understanding the science of quality and patient safety. The 1999 Institute of Medicine's (IOM) seminal report *To Err is Human: Building a Safer Healthcare System* publicized that approximately 100,000 deaths annually are due to preventable medical errors, at a cost of between $17 and 29 billion [66]. The authors noted that with nearly 33.6 million admissions to hospitals in the United States annually, and with an estimated adverse event rate of 2.9–3.7% of hospitalizations [67, 68], nearly 50,000–100,000 individuals die each year secondary to medical errors [66] (a more recent analysis estimates the number of deaths to be more than 400,000 per year [69]). The IOM report called for a comprehensive effort by healthcare providers, insurers, government officials, and patients and was a catalyst in engaging a broad group of stakeholders in identifying and addressing the reasons why medical errors occur and how they can be prevented. The report brought the issues of medical error and patient safety to the forefront of national concern. A critical component of this process was the acknowledgment that humans, in this case even medical personnel with appropriate training such as physicians, nurses, and other key healthcare personnel, can make errors that could lead to patient harm or death.

Adverse drug events (ADEs) comprise the largest single category of adverse events experienced by hospitalized patients, accounting for about 19 percent of all injuries [70]. The occurrence of ADEs is associated with increased morbidity and mortality [71], prolonged hospitalizations [72], and higher costs of care [73]. A 2007 report from the IOM estimated that between 380,000 and 450,000 preventable ADEs occurred annually in US hospitals [74]. Assuming 400,000 preventable ADEs each year at an incremental hospital cost of $5857 each, the estimated cost of ADEs in 2006 was 3.5 billion US dollars [74].

Pediatric hematology/oncology/hematopoietic stem cell transplant (HSCT) patients are highly susceptible to preventable harm. They usually have central venous catheters exposing them to infectious or thrombotic complications, receive toxic medications, are highly susceptible to healthcare-acquired infection, and are at high risk of home medication errors and non-adherence with oral agents such as chemotherapy, hydroxyurea, and iron chelators. Poor adherence with home medication is of particular concern in patients with cancer, as relapse rates are significantly associated with lower adherence [75]. The IOM defines patient safety as the prevention of harm to patients. Board members, organizations leaders, and frontline staff in healthcare delivery systems have an obligation to prevent harm through the design of systems that account for human fallibility, cultivation of a culture of safety that prevents errors, and learning from the errors that do occur. In *To Err is Human: Building a Safer Health System*, safety was defined as freedom from accidental injury, as this is the primary safety goal from the patient's perspective. The authors note that not all errors result in harm and that errors that do result in harm are called preventable adverse events [66]. The administration of chemotherapy to children and adolescents with cancer is a high-risk process with the potential to cause harm to both patients and nurses if not performed accurately and safely. This process requires strict adherence to established safety guidelines [76].

Quality Improvement

Modern quality improvement (QI), based on the theory and methods developed by Dr. Walter Shewhart and W. Edwards Deming in the 1920s, was originally applied in manufacturing industries in the mid-1900s and occasionally in the healthcare industry [77, 78]. In 2001, the IOM published *Crossing the Quality Chasm: A New Health System for the 21st Century* [79]. After the IOM report, there was a resurgence of QI in healthcare to provide safe, effective care. The IOM defined the six aims for improvement in healthcare: safe, effective, patient-centered, timely, efficient, and equitable (Table 1.1).

While QI has become a widespread method for improving care, its acceptance as a rigorous scientific method has faced challenges. Traditional experimental research designs examine effects of one or two isolated interventions under controlled conditions, where in contrast, QI methods involve multiple sequential changes over time and utilize continuous measurement and analysis. In complex and dynamic systems, QI allows for rapid testing and evaluation of new processes and methods for delivering care and addresses the gaps between the level at which a healthcare system currently functions and the level at which it could function.

Table 1.1 Institute of Medicine's six aims for improvement [79]

Safe	Avoiding injuries to patients from the care that is intended to help them
Effective	Providing services based on scientific knowledge to all who could benefit and refraining from providing services to those not likely to benefit
Patient-centered	Providing care that is respectful of and responsive to individual patient preferences, needs, and values and ensuring that patient values guide all clinical decisions
Timely	Reducing waits and sometimes harmful delays for both those who receive and those who give care
Efficient	Avoiding waste, including waste of equipment, supplies, ideas, and energy
Equitable	Providing care that does not vary in quality because of personal characteristics such as gender, ethnicity, geographic location, and socioeconomic status

Variations in Healthcare: The Good and the Bad

In the 1970s, epidemiologists demonstrated substantial geographic variation in the delivery of healthcare [80, 81]. Over the next few years, geographic variation in patient management was repeated through multiple studies crossing nearly all disciplines. In fact, variation in practice is one of the most consistently documented characteristics of modern medicine and is not explained by case mix, confounding factors, or technical errors [82].

It is not uncommon for healthcare professionals to feel threatened by the effort to reduce variation in practice; however, understanding and addressing this fear can help reduce it [83]. Variation in healthcare delivery adds to costs and may lead to misinterpretation of clinical data. QI efforts can successfully reduce practice variation, without insult to the professional autonomy, dignity, or purpose of the providers [83].

Medical science and technology have advanced at an unprecedented rate during the past 50 years; and for providers there is more to know and more to manage than ever before. In light of these rapid changes, the nation's healthcare delivery system has fallen short in its ability to translate knowledge into practice appropriately. The IOM believes that in the next few years, "90% of clinical decisions will be supported by accurate, timely, and up-to-date clinical information, and will reflect the best available evidence" [84]. Clinical decision support (CDS) provides timely information, usually at the point of care, to help inform decisions about a patient's care. CDS tools and systems help providers by assuming some routine tasks, warning of potential problems, or providing suggestions for the clinical team and patient to consider. Oftentimes, CDS directs the provider to provide evidence-based care to their patients, but allows for justifiable deviations to ensure provider autonomy. CDS can be used on a variety of platforms (such as the Internet, personal computers, electronic medical record networks, handheld devices, or written materials) [85–87].

> Alone we can do so little; together we can do so much
>
> —Helen Keller

Through collaboration, the COG has improved the outcomes of pediatric oncology patients at a rate that far exceed that which could be done through individual hospitals working alone. Through collaboration, the Working to Improve Sickle Cell Healthcare (WISCH) group is improving sickle cell disease (SCD) screening and follow-up for those who have tested positive and improving care across the life span for individuals with SCD. The goal of the collaborative was to address quality of care through development and implementation of evidence-based guidelines and measurement of healthcare quality by ongoing quality improvement initiatives. Through the consortium, they have improved pain management for SCD patients both at home [88] and in the emergency department [89]; and they are improving the transition of care from the pediatric to adult setting [90].

Through the Children's Hospital Association (CHA), 32 pediatric hematology oncology and bone marrow transplant units implemented standardized central line care to prevent central line-associated bloodstream infections (CLABSIs). Through the collaboration and shared learnings, the multicenter team reduced CLABSI rates across all centers by 27%, accounting for nearly 100 infections per year and many patient lives [91].

When possible, we should collaborate in patient safety and quality. It is imperative that we share our learnings with others, so that we can learn from each other. Much like the scientific discoveries that broke down barriers in pediatric hematology, oncology, and bone marrow transplant care, we too have an obligation to work together to improve the care of all children.

Book Structure

This book is structured in three sections.

Section 1

"Introduction to Safety and Quality Improvement" provides an introduction to the concepts of quality improvement and patient safety (Chap. 1). Chapter 2 provides an overview of the Model for Improvement, Lean, and Six Sigma and provides an overview of high-reliability organizations. Chapter 3 reviews patient safety, an introduction to human factors and creating a culture of safety and quality.

Section 2

"Getting Started" will provide the healthcare provider and team with the tools required to improve the quality of care in their practice. Chapter 4 provides the basics of team composition and emphasizes patient and family inclusion in healthcare delivery. In Chap. 5, the basics of improvement science methods are covered, including the Plan-Do-Study-Act cycle, identification of key drivers, and how to overcome barriers to implementation. Chapters 6 and 7 provide a comprehensive overview of data collection and improvement measurement, as well as mechanisms to maintain sustainability of the project proposal and spread, respectively. In Chap. 8, we provide an in-depth review of patient safety, including safety reporting systems, communication after adverse events, and root cause analysis with a specific focus on pediatric hematology oncology and stem cell transplant. Finally, we review mechanisms to implement evidence-based practices (Chap. 9).

Section 3

"Quality and Safety Principles Unique to Pediatric Hematology/Oncology/Bone Marrow Transplantation" provides a more granular review of specific topics that are important to our patient population. We review chemotherapy administration safety in the inpatient setting (Chap. 10), healthcare-associated infections (Chap. 11), catheter-related thrombus (Chap. 12), and blood product administration safety (Chap. 13). Home medication compliance and safety is a looming issue that is gathering focus, and Chap. 14 reviews the latest research, as well as evidence and measurement supporting quality improvement efforts. We provide a specific focus on pediatric oncology practices such as antibiotic stewardship, safe handoffs, and timely antibiotic administration in febrile immunocompromised patients (Chap. 15). Chapter 16 reviews practices focused on the population with nonmalignant hematology diseases, such as those with sickle cell disease or hemophilia. We discuss the specific issues involving bone marrow transplant patients in Chap. 17 and focus on quality and safety in palliative care (Chap. 18). Finally, in Chap. 19, we review mechanisms for providers to incorporate quality improvement and safety into their practice.

How to Use This Book

This book is for pediatric hematology and oncology physicians, advanced practice providers, nurses and unit leaders caring for pediatric hematology oncology/stem cell transplant patients, fellows and residents in training, pharmacists, and healthcare administrators hoping to make improvements in their practice and/or their organization. The contributors of this text include physicians, pharmacists, nurses, and quality improvement leaders. All chapters are written by experts in their fields and include the most up-to-date scientific and clinical information. The book provides a concise, yet comprehensive, summary of quality improvements and the safety issues of pediatric hematology patients. This book can be used by those with basic or advanced quality improvement of safety knowledge and will provide a foundation for those who build their practices. It is our hope that the tools described in this book can be used to improve the quality and provide safer care to our patients.

References

1. Wolff JA. History of pediatric oncology. Pediatr Hematol Oncol. 1991;8(2):89–91.
2. Gilman A, Philips FS. The biological actions and therapeutic applications of the B-chloroethyl amines and sulfides. Science. 1946;103(2675):409–15.
3. Goodman LS, Wintrobe MM. Nitrogen mustard therapy; use of methyl-bis (beta-chloroethyl) amine hydrochloride and tris (beta-chloroethyl) amine hydrochloride for Hodgkin's disease,

lymphosarcoma, leukemia and certain allied and miscellaneous disorders. J Am Med Assoc. 1946;132:126–32.

4. Farber S, Diamond LK. Temporary remissions in acute leukemia in children produced by folic acid antagonist, 4-aminopteroyl-glutamic acid. N Engl J Med. 1948;238(23):787–93.

5. Farber S, D'Angio G, Evans A, Mitus A. Clinical studies on actinomycin D with special reference to Wilms' tumor in children. Ann N Y Acad Sci. 1960;89:421–5.

6. Frei E, Holland JF, Schneiderman MA, et al. A comparative study of two regimens of combination chemotherapy in acute leukemia. Blood. 1958;13(12):1126–48.

7. Aur RJ, Simone J, Hustu HO, et al. Central nervous system therapy and combination chemotherapy of childhood lymphocytic leukemia. Blood. 1971;37(3):272–81.

8. Link MP, Goorin AM, Miser AW, et al. The effect of adjuvant chemotherapy on relapse-free survival in patients with osteosarcoma of the extremity. N Engl J Med. 1986;314(25):1600–6.

9. Clavell LA, Gelber RD, Cohen HJ, et al. Four-agent induction and intensive asparaginase therapy for treatment of childhood acute lymphoblastic leukemia. N Engl J Med. 1986;315(11):657–63.

10. Matthay KK, Villablanca JG, Seeger RC, et al. Treatment of high-risk neuroblastoma with intensive chemotherapy, radiotherapy, autologous bone marrow transplantation, and 13-cis-retinoic acid. Children's cancer group. N Engl J Med. 1999;341(16):1165–73.

11. Yu AL, Gilman AL, Ozkaynak MF, et al. Anti-GD2 antibody with GM-CSF, interleukin-2, and isotretinoin for neuroblastoma. N Engl J Med. 2010;363(14):1324–34.

12. O'Leary M, Krailo M, Anderson JR, Reaman GH. Group CsO. Progress in childhood cancer: 50 years of research collaboration, a report from the Children's oncology group. Semin Oncol. 2008;35(5):484–93.

13. American Cancer Society: Cancer Facts and Figures. 2015. http://www.cancer.org/acs/groups/content/@editorial/documents/document/acspc-044552.pdf. Accessed 19 Sept 2016.

14. Keegan TH, Ries LA, Barr RD, et al. Comparison of cancer survival trends in the United States of adolescents and young adults with those in children and older adults. Cancer. 2016;122(7):1009–16.

15. Maurer HM, Beltangady M, Gehan EA, et al. The intergroup Rhabdomyosarcoma study-I. A final report. Cancer. 1988;61(2):209–20.

16. Murphy S, Gardner FH. Effect of storage temperature on maintenance of platelet viability--deleterious effect of refrigerated storage. N Engl J Med. 1969;280(20):1094–8.

17. Gaston MH, Verter JI, Woods G, et al. Prophylaxis with oral penicillin in children with sickle cell anemia. A randomized trial. N Engl J Med. 1986;314(25):1593–9.

18. Charache S, Terrin ML, Moore RD, et al. Effect of hydroxyurea on the frequency of painful crises in sickle cell anemia. Investigators of the multicenter study of hydroxyurea in sickle cell anemia. N Engl J Med. 1995;332(20):1317–22.

19. Charache S, Barton FB, Moore RD, et al. Hydroxyurea and sickle cell anemia. Clinical utility of a myelosuppressive "switching" agent. The multicenter study of hydroxyurea in sickle cell anemia. Medicine. 1996;75(6):300–26.

20. Kinney TR, Helms RW, O'Branski EE, et al. Safety of hydroxyurea in children with sickle cell anemia: results of the HUG-KIDS study, a phase I/II trial. Pediatric Hydroxyurea Group Blood. 1999;94(5):1550–4.

21. Wang WC, Wynn LW, Rogers ZR, Scott JP, Lane PA, Ware RE. A two-year pilot trial of hydroxyurea in very young children with sickle-cell anemia. J Pediatr. 2001;139(6):790–6.

22. Zimmerman SA, Schultz WH, Davis JS, et al. Sustained long-term hematologic efficacy of hydroxyurea at maximum tolerated dose in children with sickle cell disease. Blood. 2004;103(6):2039–45.

23. Hankins JS, Ware RE, Rogers ZR, et al. Long-term hydroxyurea therapy for infants with sickle cell anemia: the HUSOFT extension study. Blood. 2005;106(7):2269–75.

24. Voskaridou E, Tsetsos G, Tsoutsias A, Spyropoulou E, Christoulas D, Terpos E. Pulmonary hypertension in patients with sickle cell/β thalassemia: incidence and correlation with serum N-terminal pro-brain natriuretic peptide concentrations. Haematologica. 2007;92(6):738–43.

25. Pashankar FD, Carbonella J, Bazzy-Asaad A, Friedman A. Prevalence and risk factors of elevated pulmonary artery pressures in children with sickle cell disease. Pediatrics. 2008;121(4):777–82.
26. Wang WC, Ware RE, Miller ST, et al. Hydroxycarbamide in very young children with sickle-cell anaemia: a multicentre, randomised, controlled trial (BABY HUG). Lancet. 2011;377(9778):1663–72.
27. Ehlers KH, Giardina PJ, Lesser ML, Engle MA, Hilgartner MW. Prolonged survival in patients with beta-thalassemia major treated with deferoxamine. J Pediatr. 1991;118(4 Pt 1):540–5.
28. Propper RD, Cooper B, Rufo RR, et al. Continuous subcutaneous administration of deferoxamine in patients with iron overload. N Engl J Med. 1977;297(8):418–23.
29. Kulkarni R, Soucie JM. Pediatric hemophilia: a review. Semin Thromb Hemost. 2011;37(7):737–44.
30. Bolton-Maggs PH, Pasi KJ. Haemophilias A and B. Lancet. 2003;361(9371):1801–9.
31. Gitschier J, Wood WI, Goralka TM, et al. Characterization of the human factor VIII gene. Nature. 1984;312(5992):326–30.
32. Wood WI, Capon DJ, Simonsen CC, et al. Expression of active human factor VIII from recombinant DNA clones. Nature. 1984;312(5992):330–7.
33. Eaton DL, Hass PE, Riddle L, et al. Characterization of recombinant human factor VIII. J Biol Chem. 1987;262(7):3285–90.
34. Lusher JM, Arkin S, Abildgaard CF, Schwartz RS. Recombinant factor VIII for the treatment of previously untreated patients with hemophilia A. Safety, efficacy, and development of inhibitors. Kogenate previously untreated patient study group. N Engl J Med. 1993;328(7):453–9.
35. Thomas ED, Lochte HL, Lu WC, Ferrebee JW. Intravenous infusion of bone marrow in patients receiving radiation and chemotherapy. N Engl J Med. 1957;257(11):491–6.
36. Thomas ED, Lochte HL, Cannon JH, Sahler OD. Supralethal whole body irradiation and isologous marrow transplantation in man. J Clin Invest. 1959;38:1709–16.
37. Thomas ED, Lochte HL, Ferrebee JW. Irradiation of the entire body and marrow transplantation: some observations and comments. Blood. 1959;14(1):1–23.
38. Thomas ED. Landmarks in the development of hematopoietic cell transplantation. World J Surg. 2000;24(7):815–8.
39. Bach FH, Albertini RJ, Joo P, Anderson JL, Bortin MM. Bone-marrow transplantation in a patient with the Wiskott-Aldrich syndrome. Lancet. 1968;2(7583):1364–6.
40. De Koning J, Van Bekkum DW, Dicke KA, Dooren LJ, Rádl J, Van Rood JJ. Transplantation of bone-marrow cells and fetal thymus in an infant with lymphopenic immunological deficiency. Lancet. 1969;1(7608):1223–7.
41. Gatti RA, Meuwissen HJ, Allen HD, Hong R, Good RA. Immunological reconstitution of sex-linked lymphopenic immunological deficiency. Lancet. 1968;2(7583):1366–9.
42. Thomas ED, Buckner CD, Clift RA, et al. Marrow transplantation for acute nonlymphoblastic leukemia in first remission. N Engl J Med. 1979;301(11):597–9.
43. Thomas ED, Sanders JE, Flournoy N, et al. Marrow transplantation for patients with acute lymphoblastic leukemia in remission. Blood. 1979;54(2):468–76.
44. Fefer A, Cheever MA, Thomas ED, et al. Bone marrow transplantation for refractory acute leukemia in 34 patients with identical twins. Blood. 1981;57(3):421–30.
45. Thomas ED, Sanders JE, Flournoy N, et al. Marrow transplantation for patients with acute lymphoblastic leukemia: a long-term follow-up. Blood. 1983;62(5):1139–41.
46. Broxmeyer HE, Douglas GW, Hangoc G, et al. Human umbilical cord blood as a potential source of transplantable hematopoietic stem/progenitor cells. Proc Natl Acad Sci U S A. 1989;86(10):3828–32.
47. Gluckman E, Broxmeyer HA, Auerbach AD, et al. Hematopoietic reconstitution in a patient with Fanconi's anemia by means of umbilical-cord blood from an HLA-identical sibling. N Engl J Med. 1989;321(17):1174–8.
48. Broxmeyer HE, Gluckman E, Auerbach A, et al. Human umbilical cord blood: a clinically useful source of transplantable hematopoietic stem/progenitor cells. Int J Cell Cloning. 1990;8(Suppl 1):76–89. discussion 89-91

49. Kohli-Kumar M, Shahidi NT, Broxmeyer HE, et al. Haemopoietic stem/progenitor cell transplant in Fanconi anaemia using HLA-matched sibling umbilical cord blood cells. Br J Haematol. 1993;85(2):419–22.
50. Malkki M, Single R, Carrington M, Thomson G, Petersdorf E. MHC microsatellite diversity and linkage disequilibrium among common HLA-A, HLA-B, DRB1 haplotypes: implications for unrelated donor hematopoietic transplantation and disease association studies. Tissue Antigens. 2005;66(2):114–24.
51. Petersdorf EW, Gooley TA, Malkki M, et al. HLA-C expression levels define permissible mismatches in hematopoietic cell transplantation. Blood. 2014;124(26):3996–4003.
52. Petersdorf EW, Malkki M, O'hUigin C, et al. High HLA-DP expression and graft-versus-host disease. N Engl J Med. 2015;373(7):599–609.
53. Ruutu T, Barosi G, Benjamin RJ, et al. Diagnostic criteria for hematopoietic stem cell transplant-associated microangiopathy: results of a consensus process by an international working group. Haematologica. 2007;92(1):95–100.
54. Gratwohl A, Baldomero H, Aljurf M, et al. Hematopoietic stem cell transplantation: a global perspective. JAMA. 2010;303(16):1617–24.
55. Niederwieser D, Baldomero H, Szer J, et al. Hematopoietic stem cell transplantation activity worldwide in 2012 and a SWOT analysis of the worldwide network for blood and marrow transplantation group including the global survey. Bone Marrow Transplant. 2016;51(6):778–85.
56. Yoshimi A, Baldomero H, Horowitz M, et al. Global use of peripheral blood vs bone marrow as source of stem cells for allogeneic transplantation in patients with bone marrow failure. JAMA. 2016;315(2):198–200.
57. Kannampallil TG, Schauer GF, Cohen T, Patel VL. Considering complexity in healthcare systems. J Biomed Inform. 2011;44(6):943–7.
58. Fernandez CV, Esau R, Hamilton D, Fitzsimmons B, Pritchard S. Intrathecal vincristine: an analysis of reasons for recurrent fatal chemotherapeutic error with recommendations for prevention. J Pediatr Hematol Oncol. 1998;20(6):587–90.
59. Hennipman B, de Vries E, Bökkerink JP, Ball LM, Veerman AJ. Intrathecal vincristine: 3 fatal cases and a review of the literature. J Pediatr Hematol Oncol. 2009;31(11):816–9.
60. Smith RB, Dynan L, Fairbrother G, Chabi G, Simpson L. Medicaid, hospital financial stress, and the incidence of adverse medical events for children. Health Serv Res. 2012;47(4):1621–41.
61. Himmelstein DU, Jun M, Busse R, et al. A comparison of hospital administrative costs in eight nations: US costs exceed all others by far. Health Aff. 2014;33(9):1586–94.
62. Nasca TJ, Day SH, Amis ES, Force ADHT. The new recommendations on duty hours from the ACGME task force. N Engl J Med. 2010;363(2):e3.
63. Jagsi R, Kitch BT, Weinstein DF, Campbell EG, Hutter M, Weissman JS. Residents report on adverse events and their causes. Arch Intern Med. 2005;165(22):2607–13.
64. Sutcliffe KM, Lewton E, Rosenthal MM. Communication failures: an insidious contributor to medical mishaps. Acad Med. 2004;79(2):186–94.
65. Coller BS. Blood at 70: its roots in the history of hematology and its birth. Blood. 2015;126(24):2548–60.
66. Kohn L, Corrigan J, Donaldson M. To err is human: building a safer health care system. Washington DC: National Academy of Sciences; 2000.
67. Thomas EJ, Studdert DM, Burstin HR, et al. Incidence and types of adverse events and negligent care in Utah and Colorado. Med Care. 2000;38(3):261–71.
68. Studdert DM, Thomas EJ, Burstin HR, Zbar BI, Orav EJ, Brennan TA. Negligent care and malpractice claiming behavior in Utah and Colorado. Med Care. 2000;38(3):250–60.
69. James JT. A new, evidence-based estimate of patient harms associated with hospital care. J Patient Saf. 2013;9(3):122–8.
70. Leape LL, Brennan TA, Laird N, et al. The nature of adverse events in hospitalized patients. Results of the Harvard medical practice study II. N Engl J Med. 1991;324(6):377–84.
71. Phillips DP, Christenfeld N, Glynn LM. Increase in US medication-error deaths between 1983 and 1993. Lancet. 1998;351(9103):643–4.

72. Fanikos J, Cina JL, Baroletti S, Fiumara K, Matta L, Goldhaber SZ. Adverse drug events in hospitalized cardiac patients. Am J Cardiol. 2007;100(9):1465–9.
73. Classen DC, Pestotnik SL, Evans RS, Lloyd JF, Burke JP. Adverse drug events in hospitalized patients. Excess length of stay, extra costs, and attributable mortality. JAMA. 1997;277(4):301–6.
74. Aspen P, Walcott J, Bootman J, Cronenwett L. Preventing medication errors: quality chasm series. Washington DC: The National Academic Press; 2007.
75. Bhatia S, Landier W, Shangguan M, et al. Nonadherence to oral mercaptopurine and risk of relapse in Hispanic and non-Hispanic white children with acute lymphoblastic leukemia: a report from the children's oncclogy group. J Clin Oncol. 2012;30(17):2094–101.
76. Looper K, Winchester K, Robinson D, et al. Best practices for chemotherapy Administration in Pediatric Oncology: quality and safety process improvements (2015). J Pediatr Oncol Nurs. 2016;33(3):165–72.
77. Berwick DM. A primer on leading the improvement of systems. BMJ. 1996;312(7031):619–22.
78. Varkey P, Reller MK, Resar RK. Basics of quality improvement in health care. Mayo Clin Proc. 2007;82(6):735–9.
79. Crossing the Quality Chasm. A new health system for the 21st Century. Washington DC: National Academy of Sciences; 2001.
80. Wennberg J. Gittelsohn. Small area variations in health care delivery. Science. 1973;182(4117):1102–8.
81. Vayda E. A comparison of surgical rates in Canada and in England and Wales. N Engl J Med. 1973;289(23):1224–9.
82. Margo CE. Quality care and practice variation: the roles of practice guidelines and public profiles. Surv Ophthalmol. 2004;49(3):359–71.
83. Berwick DM. Controlling variation in health care: a consultation from Walter Shewhart. Med Care. 1991;29(12):1212–25.
84. Yong P, Olsen L, McGinnis M. Value in healthcare: accounting for cost, quality, safety, outcomes, and innovation: workshop summary (2010). Washington, DC: The National Academies Press; 2010.
85. Romano MJ, Stafford RS. Electronic health records and clinical decision support systems: impact on national ambulatory care quality. Arch Intern Med. 2011;171(10):897–903.
86. Kukhareva PV, Kawamoto K, Shields DE, et al. Clinical decision support-based quality measurement (CDS-QM) framework: prototype implementation, evaluation, and future directions. AMIA Annu Symp Proc. 2014;2014:825–34.
87. Patel TA, Puppala M, Ogunti RO, et al. Correlating mammographic and pathologic findings in clinical decision support using natural language processing and data mining methods. Cancer. 2016;123:114–21.
88. Crosby LE, Simmons K, Kaiser P, et al. Using quality improvement methods to implement an electronic medical record (EMR) supported individualized home pain management plan for children with sickle cell disease. J Clin Outcomes Manag. 2014;21(5):210–7.
89. Treadwell MJ, Bell M, Leibovich SA, et al. A quality improvement initiative to improve emergency Department Care for Pediatric Patients with sickle cell disease. J Clin Outcomes Manag. 2014;21(2):62–70.
90. Frost JR, Cherry RK, Oyeku SO, et al. Improving sickle cell transitions of care through health information technology. Am J Prev Med. 2016;51(1 Suppl 1):S17–23.
91. Bundy DG, Gaur AH, Billett AL, He B, Colantuoni EA, Miller MR. Preventing CLABSIs among pediatric hematology/oncology inpatients: National Collaborative Results. Pediatrics. 2014;134(6):e1678–85.

Chapter 2
Science of Improvement

Michael A. Rosen and Sallie J. Weaver

Introduction

Healthcare is in the midst of a large-scale transformation and modernization effort. A wide range of stakeholders including regulators, payers, and consumers all demand higher levels of value and transparency in care delivery performance. Quality improvement (QI) methods are one of the key approaches to achieving the new and elevated performance expectations for healthcare delivery systems. QI in healthcare is defined broadly as "the combined and unceasing efforts of everyone—healthcare professionals, patients and their families, researchers, payers, planners and educators—to make the changes that will lead to better patient outcomes (health), better system performance (care) and better professional development" [1, p. 2]. While the pressures exerted on healthcare systems for improved value are new, the application of QI methods are not. Researchers and practitioners have applied a broad range of QI methods for decades [2] and have achieved mixed results [3–5]. In this decades-long experience with QI, the field has learned much about the critical components of effectiveness.

This chapter provides an overview of state of the science and practice of quality improvement in healthcare. First, we describe the fundamental models and exemplar methods of QI in healthcare. There are many techniques, but they can all be organized using a common set of knowledge systems or domains. We describe these systems and discuss how common-structured approaches to QI in healthcare address these varied knowledge domains. Second, we draw insights and guiding principles from the area of high-reliability organizing. This area of scholarship seeks to understand

M.A. Rosen (✉) • S.J. Weaver
Department of Anesthesiology and Critical Care Medicine, Armstrong Institute for Patient Safety and Quality, Johns Hopkins University School of Medicine,
750 E. Pratt Street, 15th Floor, Baltimore, MD 21202, USA
e-mail: mrosen44@jhmi.edu; sjweaver@jhu.edu

© Springer International Publishing AG 2017
C.E. Dandoy et al. (eds.), *Patient Safety and Quality in Pediatric Hematology/Oncology and Stem Cell Transplantation*, DOI 10.1007/978-3-319-53790-0_2

resilient performance in high-risk, yet highly safe, industries. Ultimately, QI is organizational change. Arguably, few organizations are as complex, interdependent, and difficult to change as healthcare organizations. QI models and methods offer tools that can facilitate change and continuous learning when used mindfully.

Quality Improvement Models and Methods

Quality improvement efforts draw on a broad range of methods to achieve better outcomes. However, the use of "systems thinking, data analysis, and [multidisciplinary] teams" [6, p. 203] underlies most QI approaches. The diversity of what is considered QI, and how it is conducted, creates challenges in large-scale assessments of its effectiveness [7, 8] as well as confusion among practitioners about where to begin. In this section, we review the variety of "knowledge systems" that underlie QI in healthcare, discuss common structured approaches that draw from these systems, and review a general set of values that characterize effective QI implementation.

The Knowledge Systems of Quality Improvement

The breadth and depth of theories, strategies, and tools employed in QI in healthcare can be overwhelming. Underlying this complexity, however, are several core domains of knowledge that must be integrated to achieve improved outcomes. Batalden and Davidoff [1] provide a useful framework for understanding the types of work involved in QI in healthcare. Specifically, they define five core "knowledge systems." Each of these knowledge systems described below focuses on different problems and employs different methods. Ultimately, successful QI requires integration across these knowledge systems. Figure 2.1 depicts the relationships between each knowledge systems of QI.

First, *generalizable scientific evidence* is derived from empirical studies of interventions and ultimately the distillation of this evidence into clinical guidelines. This knowledge system seeks to control for contextual factors in analysis in order to generate an understanding what therapies or other interventions are most effective overall. It is the evidence behind evidence-based medicine. However, generating evidence and creating guidelines are necessary but insufficient to produce change or improved care [3]. Second, *particular context awareness* involves generating knowledge about the elements of a specific implementation setting or work context. This includes systematically collecting and analyzing information about local care processes, structural constraints of an organization (e.g., staffing, information technology infrastructure, resource constraints), and local history (e.g., exposure to interventions in the past, personal relationships) that may impact QI efforts. This knowledge system provides insight into what changes may be required to enable a specific organization to achieve its desired outcomes. Third, *performance measurement* provides the

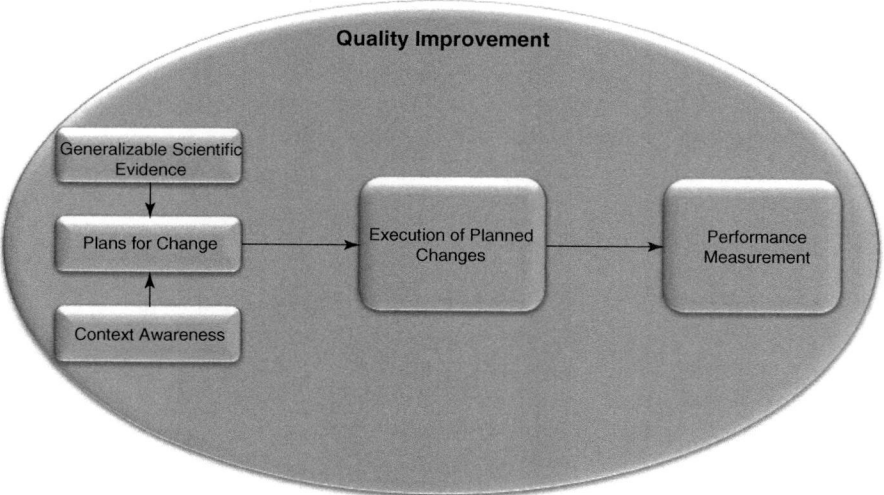

Fig. 2.1 Relationships between the five knowledge systems of QI (adapted from Batalden and Davidoff [1])

means of determining whether or not, or the degree to which, QI efforts are effective at improving targeted outcomes. Effectively measuring quality in healthcare is extraordinarily challenging [9], but progress is being made, and methods are maturing [10]. However, measuring performance alone does not improve performance [11]. Fourth, *plans for change* employs the breadth of systems-based improvement strategies for changing how care is delivered ranging from radical reengineering of systems and technology to training or passive information provision. This knowledge system provides a means to adapt clinical evidence to the local work system—to enable care providers to "do the right thing" (e.g., adhere to clinical guidelines) as reliably as possible. However, designing interventions and system fixes does not improve performance if these changes are not adopted by the organization. Fifth, *execution of planned changes* includes both understanding local barriers and facilitators of change as well as general frameworks for managing change in complex organizations. This knowledge system reviews improvement as organizational change, and as such seeks to connect to the people within a system, understand their perspective, and introduce QI changes consistent with their values and priorities. This is achieved through structured change management approaches.

Structured Approaches to QI in Healthcare

The five knowledge systems of QI in healthcare encompass an impressive breadth of activity. Working within any one of these domains requires deep expertise, and integrating across them truly requires an interdisciplinary team effort. Structured approaches to conducting QI help these teams navigate this process. These approaches provide a set of conceptual and practical tools or steps that QI teams can follow and help to ensure that each knowledge system is incorporated into the QI effort. Below, we briefly review four structured approaches used in healthcare and discuss how they are related to the five knowledge systems.

Translating Evidence into Practice (TRIP)

Translating evidence into practice (TRIP) is a four-step method including (1) *summarizing the evidence* (i.e., identifying the most effective interventions and converting them in to behavioral specifications at the bedside), (2) *identifying local barriers to implementation* (i.e., employing multiple methods to determine "ground truth" of interventions in practice), (3) measuring performance, and (4) *ensuring all patients receive the interventions* [12]. The fourth step involves a series of activities to *engage* staff (i.e., establish the need and value of the program), *educate* staff on the interventions and evidence behind them, *execute* on the plan through design of an intervention toolkit adapted to local needs, and *evaluate* the impact of the intervention. The TRIP model addresses all five knowledge systems of QI. It provides a high-level framework for navigating the full spectrum of QI activities. Compared to other structured approaches, it places unique emphasis on moving from the available evidence to actionable and usable guidance at the bedside. However, large portions of the clinical care knowledge base are underspecified and will likely remain so for some time [13]. Therefore, not all QI efforts will focus on adopting evidence-based guidelines.

Plan-Do-Study-Act (PDSA) Cycle

PDSA is a widely used approach designed to create rapid cycles of improvement in healthcare through "small tests of change" [14]. Specifically, PDSA application begins with an investigation or framing of the problem followed by (1) *planning* an intervention, implementation, and evaluation; (2) implementing (*doing*) the intervention and evaluation plan; (3) *studying* the effects of the intervention by analyzing the evaluation data; and (4) *acting* based on what was learned (i.e., revisit early phases of PDSA, modify intervention, implement fully, or abandon project). This process allows for moving from general ideas to concrete solutions by rapidly and iteratively generating knowledge about what is working in a given situation as well as how it might be modified to be more effective. While conceptually simple, PDSA is sophisticated and can be challenging to implement [15]. It has become a framework that underlies many QI programs. Because of its emphasis on adapting general ideas or solutions to local contexts and use of measurement and evaluation, PDSA integrates across context awareness, plans for change, and measurement knowledge systems.

Lean Thinking

Lean thinking is a principled problem-solving approach that seeks to reduce waste, synchronize workflows, and optimize efficiency and resource management [16]. The application of lean thinking does not follow a prescriptive set of steps, but is guided by a set of principles outlining how work processes should be designed. Specifically, lean principles emphasize (1) articulating the things that create value from the customer's perspective, (2) identifying all of the steps that lead to this value (i.e., the "value stream"), (3) making those steps across the value stream flow efficiently, (4) producing what the customer "pulls" just in time, and (5) continuously removing waste in work processes [17]. As evidenced by the language of these principles, lean thinking is rooted in manufacturing, specifically the Toyota Motor company following World War II [18]. As such, it does not address the generalizable evidence knowledge system, nor does it address organizational change [19]. However, it is a powerful tool for context awareness (i.e., understanding how local processes work) and planning change (i.e., designing new, more efficient, work processes).

Six Sigma

Six sigma is a quality management approach originally formulated by Bill Smith of Motorola in the mid-1980s. The name six sigma refers to the statistical notion that a process should be designed to result in only 3.4 defects (anything that could result in customer dissatisfaction) per one million opportunities, that is, six sigmas (standard deviations) above the mean of a normally distributed process. The six sigma process is built upon total quality management's plan-do-check-act cycle and is implemented via two specific methodologies. The first, DMAIC, consists of five steps: (1) define the goals of the project and customer deliverables, (2) measure key aspects of the current process, (3) determine the root causes of defects in the current process, (4) improve the process by eliminating these defects, and (5) "control" the process so that any future deviations do not end up in full-fledged defects. The second methodology, define-measure-analyze-design-verify (DMADV), is recommended for use in situations where a new process or product is being developed. Like lean, six sigma does not address the evidence-based or change management-related knowledge systems of QI. However, quantitative data and metrics are at the heart of the approach which aligns six sigma nicely with the measurement knowledge system of QI.

Habits of Quality Improvement

The models and frameworks above are offered as reference points to help navigate the range of QI approaches and activities. There is no one correct way to conduct QI. Different methods can be combined in ways that suit the needs of a given project. But, the likelihood of success for any QI effort increases with the degree to which the five knowledge systems are employed and integrated. In support of this "full-spectrum" use of QI, Plesk [6] articulates a set of four habits or routine patterns of thought and action in an organization that enable effective QI. First, organizations should cultivate the habit of viewing clinical practice as a complex process that cuts across traditional boundaries of disciplines or physical location. Second, organizations should build a habit of evidence-based practice, seeking to capitalize on the existing knowledge base of what works. Third, organizations should reinforce the habit of collaborative learning, openness, curiosity, and sharing. Fourth, organizations must develop a habit of change. These habits nicely summarize key behaviors for quality improvement. Table 2.1 summarizes these values and specific strategies used to enact them. In the following section, these ideas will be expanded upon and refined by learning from a special class of organizations.

Table 2.1 The habits enabling effective quality improvement in healthcare (Adapted from Plesk [6])

Habit	Definition and supporting practices
View clinical practice as a process	Healthcare outcomes are the product of complex and interdependent work processes. Organizations that are effective at QI can see past an individual- or discipline-focused approach and focus on how work is managed by all staff and how patients and families are involved. A wide range of process description tools can be employed to map and understand work. These include flow charts, hierarchical task analysis, fault trees. failure mode and effects analysis, and work diagrams
Use of evidence-based practice	Much of quality improvement efforts involve moving care delivery processes closer to standards and guidelines of what is known to work. There is a hierarchy of the quantity and quality of evidence available for different practices, and certainly some key decisions must be made in the absence of good evidence. Effective organizations are sensitive to the strength of evidence around their interventions. Guidelines for professional societies and government agencies can help to pull together evidence. Leading practices may be found in systematic reviews and single studies in the academic literature
Learn collaboratively	There will never be a randomized controlled trial for every component of a quality improvement program. Effective organizations are eager to learn from and with others to fill the inevitable gaps in the literature. Internal structures for sharing project status and lessons learned as well as participation in external collaboratives can help to gain practical wisdom to complement evidence-based guidelines
Change mindfully	Any improvement requires something to be done differently. Organizations continuously improving are continuously changing, and change is not easy. Effective organizations have a mindful approach to change that uses a structured approach, attends to pacing (avoiding change fatigue), and is inclusive throughout—conducting change *with* all stakeholders, not *to* them

High-Reliability Organizations

Research exploring organizations that operate in high-risk environments under extreme conditions yet are able to sustain low rates of errors or harm over time offers a great deal of insight for improvement efforts in healthcare. Originally defined by organizational scholars Karlene Roberts, Todd LaPorte, and Gene Rochlin as "high-reliability organizations" (HROs), these organizations, units, and teams master the ability to remain adaptive, anticipate the unexpected, and produce reliably safe outcomes despite significant risk inherent in the work they do and/or the context in which work is done [20]. Subsequently Kathleen Sutcliffe and Karl Weick revealed that these organizations sustained safe outcomes and high performance through processes of collective mindfulness, adaptation, and resilience, what they call mindful organizing [21, 22]. This collective body of evidence reflects much of what is known about HROs, how they organize, how they function, and how they learn. HROs are notable given their capacity to operate in complex, high-risk environments, where the impact of error can be catastrophic; yet they are able to learn from, adapt to, and utilize this complexity to their advantage. Furthermore, these organizations are better able to mitigate major errors through mindful management of near misses, unexpected outcomes, and minor errors. Nuclear submarines [23], the US naval aircraft carrier fleet [20], electrical grid operators [24], wildland firefighting incident command systems, and some healthcare teams [25, 26] are examples of HROs cited in existing literature. These "ultrasafe" groups, teams, and organizations achieve reliably safe outcomes by building the necessary social-relational foundations (e.g., a climate of mutual respect and trust, an understanding of key interdependencies and interconnections), and they actively organize their work with safety in mind [27].

The Pathway to Reliably Safe Outcomes Involves Three Key Components

The pathway to reliably safe outcomes involves (1) practicing the habits of mindful organizing, (2) reliability-enhancing work practices, and (3) actions that enable, enact, and elaborate a culture of safety. Weick and Sutcliffe's theory and research demonstrate that reliable outcomes (e.g., safety, quality) over time are the result of several social and cognitive habits that are focused on (1) uncovering and correcting unintended consequences and (2) adapting appropriately particularly at early stages when the signals foreshadowing an undesirable outcome or incident might be "weak" [21, 28]. These key processes and assumptions help high performers to (1) identify weak signals of the potential for undesirable outcomes early, (2) anticipate the need to adapt their efforts, and (3) recover quickly when the unexpected or unintended outcomes do occur. These processes are referred to as the habits of mindful organizing because they reflect the fact that high reliability is really an ongoing process of actively organizing for safety, rather than a terminal destination or achievement [27]. Table 2.2 summarizes these key habits and defines them in detail.

These key habits reflect one of the central findings about HROs that initially may seem counterintuitive. While we tend to associate the idea of reliability with the image of highly standardized procedures, routines, or algorithms and think of "high reliability" as synonymous with high levels of compliance, this is not, in fact, the way HROs think about reliability. The underlying theory and the large number of studies examining HROs clearly demonstrate that *reliable outcomes* are actually the product of relatively flexible procedures [21, 28]. The findings underscore that the team members that work in and make up HROs are able to adapt and act in resilient ways that keep relatively minor glitches from turning into major catastrophes. They are able to create reliably safe outcomes because they share habits and mindsets that are vital for detecting and correcting minor unintended issues that can snowball into serious adverse events. In this sense, high reliability is really about creating a sense of collective mindfulness during daily care and mindful approaches to continuous improvement.

Organizations, units, and teams focused solely on efficiency tend to prioritize stability and inflexible routines in order to "get things done." However, the theory and studies of HROs argue that, in reality, there is inherent variation in any standardized routine due to environmental, situational, and social influences that inevitably impact how even the most highly structured routine unfolds at different times across different team members for different patients. Therefore, the idea that reliability is synonymous with inflexible routines and rote compliance with highly prescriptive procedures is erroneous. The lessons from studies of HROs underscore that approaches to improvement that rely highly on re-education on complex, prescriptive routines, standardization of procedures, and scripts are insufficient means of mitigating serious errors [20, 26]. Rather they point to developing and strengthening the habits of mindful organizing outlined in Table 2.3 as critical components of impactful, sustainable improvement in patient safety and care quality.

These habits alone, however, are not the only hallmarks of HROs. Team members must have the resources, as well as both peer and leadership support, to act on the concerns or weak signals in order for mindfulness to translate into reliable, safe outcomes. HROs combine the habits of mindful organizing with organizational practices and structures that support these habits. Selecting and mentoring for interpersonal skills and investing in skill building and training opportunities that foster an orientation toward continuous learning are examples of these "reliability-enhancing work practices" identified by Tim Vogus and Dawn Iacobucci. In their study of over 1600 registered nurses working in 95 nursing units, they found that these work practices were related to significantly fewer medication errors and patient falls [29]. Specifically, they found that these work practices impacted these outcomes by improving the use of some of the key habits listed in Table 2.2.

HROs also develop strong cultures of safety [23] and collective accountability for addressing system issues that contribute to undesirable outcomes [30]. Borrowing from Edgar Schein [31], a leading scholar on organizational culture, patient safety culture refers to one specific aspect of an organization's culture that can be defined as a:

Table 2.2 The habits of highly reliable organizing (adapted from Weick and Sutcliffe [21, 26, 28])

Habit	Definition
Be preoccupied with failure: Do not be tricked into complacency by your success	Errors, glitches, and unexpected circumstances are considered an inevitable component of operations, but they do not have to end with catastrophic outcomes. Pay close attention to weak signals; encourage yourself and others to identify potential symptoms of system malfunctioning early. Approach previous successes and situations or cases that "look just like that previous one" with a healthy dose of skepticism to avoid over confidence and complacency. Invest time and effort in imagining potential mistakes, glitches, or imperfect circumstances. Think about or simulate potential failure pathways to learn about the broad range of "weak signals" that might suggest the potential for an undesirable outcome
Be reluctant to simplify interpretations: Embrace complexity	Preserve details. Openly identify your assumptions, heuristics, categories, and cognitive biases in an effort to limit the tunnel vision unintentionally created by the assumptions and labels we apply in our minds. In negotiations and decisions, focus on points of divergence versus convergence in order to detect anomalies and to elicit unique information
Be sensitive to operations: Be real about what is actually happening, and resist the urge to focus only on information that confirms your hypotheses	Foster a deep situational awareness that reflects objective observations of actual work processes, rather than intentions or formal procedures. "See…what we are actually doing, regardless of what we are supposed to do based on intentions, designs, or plans" (2007, p. 59). Value and evaluate near misses. Do not interpret them as confirmation that that current approaches or operations are sufficient to mitigate error. Near misses are often the result of luck and pure statistical probability. Interpret them as cues indicating potential system failures that need to be addressed in order to prevent complacency
Commit to resilience: Anticipate, but know we cannot anticipate everything; improvisation and action under unexpected circumstances	Accept the inevitability of the unexpected and commit to absorb changes, persist, actively participate in improving the system, and continuously incorporate lessons learned from these inevitable glitches, workarounds, and unintended outcomes. Support creative thinking, improvisation within reason, use of ad hoc networks, and a healthy skepticism about the applicability of past practice to the current scenario
Deference to expertise: Defer to your experts doing the work on the front line	Open traditional hierarchical structures of command and decision-making to all organizational team members, especially during crisis situations. Push decision-making authority down and outward to frontline team members doing the work. Consider how structure and routines may be fluid. Decoupling vital decisions from higher-ranking positions far removed from frontline operations improves the efficiency of critical decisions and expands the variety of expertise available to make sense of cues that might suggest the potential for unintended consequences

(continued)

Table 2.2 (continued)

Habit	Definition
Interact heedfully: Pay attention to what is happening upstream and downstream	Pay attention to interdependencies and interconnections between people, departments, and other organizations where your patients may be receiving care. Help yourself and others to see your work as part of and a critical contribution to the larger shared, collective goals your team, group, or organization is working toward
Foster a climate of trust and respect: Improving the system means listening and learning with humility	Listen humbly and respectfully when others bring forward concerns or "gut feelings" that something may not be right, even if they have difficulty articulating the details. Do not discount disconfirming information or unique information or perspectives that differ from the majority opinion or the perceptions of the majority about a particular situation, patient, loved one, or team member. Share novel or disconfirming information when you have it respectfully.

Table 2.3 Components of the 3 E's model of enabling, enacting, and elaborating a culture of safety (adapted from Vogus, Sutcliffe, Weick [32])

Component	Description
Enabling	Leaders enable safer practices through • Directing attention to safety • Creating contexts where staff feel safe to speak up and act in ways that improve safety
Enacting	Frontline staff enact a safety culture through • Highlighting and accurately representing emerging threats to safety • Mobilize resources to resolve threats
Elaborating	Leaders and staff implement practices that • Rigorously reflect on safety outcomes • Use feedback to modify enabling practices and enacting processes

...system of [shared knowledge, beliefs,] meaning, and symbols [related to patient safety] that shape how an organization's members interpret their experience and act on an ongoing basis. [32, p. 62]

The related, yet distinct, concept of patient safety climate refers to perceptions of the more observable aspects of culture like patient safety practices, procedures, policies, and the actions of leaders and peers related to patient safety that are shared by members of a given group (e.g., unit, department, profession, or organization) [33]. Culture and climate influence a broad range of issues, including (1) what cues or signals the members of an organization, profession, department, unit, or team view as indicators of potential harm, (2) their willingness to speak up about potential issues or opportunities for improvement (also known as a sense of psychological safety [34]), (3) and their orientation toward improvement of work and motivation to engage in it.

The broad range of evidence examining culture and climate demonstrate that formal and informal leaders play critical roles in shaping them over time [35, 36]. Formal leaders include group members with formal leadership titles, such as supervisors, unit or department managers, department or committee chairs, medical directors, nursing directors, and administrative executive leaders. Informal leaders refer to group members that may not have formal leadership titles, but hold informal power through seniority, tenure, expertise, or relational trust. As shown in Table 2.3, Tim Vogus' "3 E's" to patient safety culture framework [32] emphasizes that formal and informal leaders can help to enable a strong culture of safety by drawing attention to safety-relevant aspects of their unit, department, or organization's culture. Leaders can direct attention to safety and quality by role modeling and acting in ways that demonstrate that safety comes first in situations where it may compete with other priorities like throughput. Additionally, leaders can direct attention toward safety by actively participating in and investing their time in safety-related activities and discussions with non-leadership team members. They can also enable a strong culture of safety by making it safe to speak up and act and creating or maintaining forums where threats to safety or quality are identified and discussed proactively. These formal and informal leader actions send strong signals about the extent to which safety, quality, and continuous improvement are valued, expected, and rewarded. This sets the tone and begins to establish the context necessary for translating the idea or belief that safety and improvement are important into daily practice.

The framework emphasizes that these enabling conditions are necessary in order for frontline care providers to effectively enact a culture of safety in their daily practice. Specifically, the framework suggests identifying and disclosing glitches, errors, near misses, or undesirable outcomes, as well as problem-solving and mobilizing resources to resolve such issues as key behaviors that reflect safety culture in practice. Finally, the framework underlines that organizations, units, and teams can continue to elaborate and evolve their culture through reflective learning practices, specifically by investing time in constructive reflection on outcomes and near misses and by using feedback or lessons learned from this reflection to modify the enabling practices and enacting processes previously described. Constructive reflection can take many forms, from formal presentations to informal discussions about defect, errors, or undesirable outcomes. Debriefings and after-action reviews [37–39], advanced versions of mortality and morbidity conferences structured as patient-centered learning discussions [40], and the learning from defects process that is part of the Comprehensive Unit-Based Safety Program (CUSP) [41] are all examples of processes and tools that can help facilitate this type of constructive, learning-oriented reflection and the integration of lessons learned.

High Reliability Is a Continual Process of "Actively Organizing for Safety" [27]

Overall, the theory and evidence about HROs teach us that reliably safe outcomes require attention and mindful work. It also underscores that the idea of high reliability is a continuous practice, not something to be achieved or checked off a checklist. There are tools available to help understand where your team or organization may currently lie in terms of the habits, work practices, and cultural elements that are the hallmarks of HROs. For example, the Safety Organizing Scale [42] and several short self-assessments which appear in the first and second editions of the seminal book on HROs, *Managing the Unexpected* [26], can be useful.

Conclusions

Firm grounding in the theoretical foundations and science of improvement is critical for improvement practitioners. This chapter synthesized core definitions of continuous improvement and described key models of improvement from the patient safety, care quality, and organizational sciences. We also summarized insights from the science concerning high-reliability organizations (HROs) that excel at maintaining extremely low rates of error or harm despite operating in high-risk environments by building strong practices of mindful organizing. We summarized practical principles for high-reliability organizing and what we know from the science about how leaders, both formal and informal, contribute to the context and practice of improvement.

References

1. Batalden PB, Davidoff F. What is "quality improvement" and how can it transform healthcare? Qual Saf Health Care. 2007;16(1):2–3.
2. James BC, Savitz LA. How intermountain trimmed health care costs through robust quality improvement efforts. Health Aff. 2011;30(6):1185–91.
3. Shojania KG, Grimshaw JM. Evidence-based quality improvement: the state of the science. Health Aff. 2005;24(1):138–50.
4. Schouten LMT, Hulscher MEJL, van Everdingen JJE, Huijsman R, Grol RPTM. Evidence for the impact of quality improvement collaboratives: systematic review. BMJ. 2008;336(7659): 1491–4.
5. Kaplan HC, Brady PW, Dritz MC, Hooper DK, Linam WM, Froehle CM, et al. The influence of context on quality improvement success in health care: a systematic review of the literature. Milbank Q. 2010;88(4):500–59.
6. Plsek PE, Blumenthal D, Carlin E, Carlson R, Nordin J, Heckman M, et al. Quality improvement methods in clinical medicine. Pediatrics. 1999;103(1 Suppl E):203–14.
7. Balasubramanian BA, Cohen DJ, Davis MM, Gunn R, Dickinson LM, Miller WL, et al. Learning evaluation: blending quality improvement and implementation research methods to study healthcare innovations. Implement Sci. 2015;10:31.
8. Harvey G, Wensing M. Methods for evaluation of small scale quality improvement projects. Qual Saf Health Care. 2003;12(3):210–4.
9. Jha A, Pronovost P. Toward a safer health care system: the critical need to improve measurement. JAMA. 2016;315:1831.
10. Cohen ME, Liu Y, Ko CY, Hall BL. Improved surgical outcomes for ACS NSQIP hospitals over time: evaluation of hospital cohorts with up to 8 years of participation. Ann Surg. 2016;263(2):267–73.
11. Berwick DM. Measuring surgical outcomes for improvement: was Codman wrong? JAMA. 2015;313(5):469–70.

12. Pronovost PJ, Berenholtz SM, Needham DM. Translating evidence into practice: a model for large scale knowledge translation. BMJ. 2008;337:a1714.
13. Rosen MA, Pronovost PJ. Advancing the use of checklists for evaluating performance in health care. Acad Med. 2014;89(7):963–5.
14. Taylor MJ, McNicholas C, Nicolay C, Darzi A, Bell D, Reed JE. Systematic review of the application of the plan-do-study-act method to improve quality in healthcare. BMJ Qual Saf. 2014;23(4):290–8.
15. Reed JE, Card AJ. The problem with plan-do-study-act cycles. BMJ Qual Saf. 2016;25(3):147–52.
16. Wickramasinghe N, Al-Hakim L, Gonzalez C, Tan J. Lean thinking for healthcare. New York, NY: Springer; 2014.
17. Womack JP, Jones DT. Lean thinking: banish waste and create wealth in your corporation. New York, NY: Simon and Schuster; 2010.
18. Ohno T. Toyota production system: beyond large-scale production. Portland, OR: Productivity, Inc.; 1988.
19. Andersen H, Røvik KA, Ingebrigtsen T. Lean thinking in hospitals: is there a cure for the absence of evidence? a systematic review of reviews. BMJ Open. 2014;4(1):e003873.
20. Rochlin GI, LaPorte TR, Roberts KH. The self-designing high-reliability organization: aircraft carrier flight operations at sea. Nav War Coll Rev. 1987;(Autum):76–90.
21. Weick KE, Sutcliffe KM, Obstfeld D. Organizing for high reliability: processes of collective mindfulness. In: Sutton RS, Staw BM, editors. Research in organizational behavior, vol. 1. Greenwich, CT: JAI Press; 1990. p. 81–123.
22. Sutcliffe KM. High reliability organizations (HROs). Best Pract Res Clin Anaesthesiol. 2011;25(2):133–44.
23. Bierly PE. Culture and high reliability organizations: the case of the nuclear submarine. J Manage. 1995;21(4):639–56.
24. Christianson MK, Sutcliffe KM, Miller MA, Iwashyna TJ. Becoming a high reliability organization. Crit Care. 2011 Jan;15(6):314.
25. Edmondson AC. Learning from failure in health care: frequent opportunities, pervasive barriers. Qual Saf Health Care. 2004;13(Suppl 2):ii3–9.
26. Weick KE, Sutcliffe KM. Managing the unexpected. 2nd ed. San Francisco, CA: Jossey-Bass; 2007.
27. Sutcliffe KM, Paine L, Pronovost PJ. Re-examining high reliability: actively organising for safety. BMJ Qual Saf. 2016;26(3):248–251.
28. Weick KE, Sutcliffe KM. Managing the unexpected. 3rd ed. Hoboken, NJ: Wiley; 2015.
29. Vogus TJ, Iacobucci D. Creating highly reliable health care: how reliability-enhancing work practices affect patient safety in hospitals. ILR Rev. 2016;7:0019793916642759.
30. Weaver SJ, Che X-X, Pronovost PJ, Goeschel CA, Kosel KC, Rosen MA. Improving patient safety and care quality: a multiteam system perspective. InPushing the boundaries: Multiteam systems in research and practice 2014 Sep; 24 (pp. 35–60). Emerald Group Publishing Limited.
31. Schein EH. Organizational culture and leadership. 4th ed. Hoboken, NJ: Jossey-Bass; 2010.
32. Vogus TJ, Sutcliffe KM, Weick KE. Doing no harm: enabling, enacting, and elaborating a culture of safety in health care. Acad Manag Perspect. 2010;24:60–77.
33. Zohar D, Luria G. A multilevel model of safety climate: cross-level relationships between organization and group-level climates. J Appl Psychol. 2005;90(4):616–28.
34. Nembhard IM, Edmondson ACMYC. Making it safe: the effects of leader inclusiveness and professional status on psychological safety and improvement efforts in health care teams. J Organ Behav. 2006;27(7):941–66.
35. Zohar D. Thirty years of safety climate research: reflections and future directions. Accid Anal Prev. 2010;42(5):1517–22.
36. Weaver SJ, Lubomksi LH, Wilson RRF, Pfoh ER, Martinez KA, Dy SM, et al. Promoting a culture of safety as a patient safety strategy: a systematic review. Ann Intern Med. 2013;158(5 Pt 2):369–74.

37. Paull DE, Mazzia LM, Wood SD, Theis MS, Robinson LD, Carney B, et al. Briefing guide study: preoperative briefing and postoperative debriefing checklists in the veterans health administration medical team training program. Am J Surg. 2010;200(5):620–3.
38. Vashdi DR, Bamberger PA, Erez M, Weiss-Meilik A. Briefing-debriefing: using a reflexive organizational learning model from the military to enhance the performance of surgical teams. Hum Resour Manag. 2007;46(1):115–42.
39. Makary MA, Mukherjee A, Sexton JB, Syin D, Goodrich E, Hartmann E, et al. Operating room briefings and wrong-site surgery. J Am Coll Surg. 2007;204(2):236–43.
40. Berenholtz SM, Hartsell TL, Pronovost PJ. Learning from defects to enhance morbidity and mortality conferences. Am J Med Qual. 2009;24(3):192–5.
41. Agency for Healthcare Research and Quality. AHRQ CUSP Toolkit: Learn from Defects Tool [Internet]. 2012 [cited 2016 Mar 1]. Available from: http://www.ahrq.gov/professionals/education/curriculum-tools/cusptoolkit/toolkit/learndefects.html.
42. Vogus TJ, Sutcliffe KM. The safety organizing scale: development and validation of a behavioral measure of safety culture in hospital nursing units. Med Care. 2007;45(1):46–54.

Chapter 3
Introduction to Patient Safety

Frank Federico and Amy L. Billett

Understanding and improving patient safety in healthcare have been a focus in the United Stated since the early 1990s. Despite more than 20 years of effort, harm from healthcare remains high leading to over 400,000 deaths and over $1 trillion in costs in the United States annually. Much work remains to be done to understand the risks and mitigation strategies for care in the ambulatory setting and in the patient's home. Errors in healthcare, as in other industries, are primarily due to the faulty systems, processes, and conditions that lead people to make mistakes or fail to prevent them. Improving safety in healthcare requires a framework that addresses such topics as leadership, governance, teamwork and communication, culture, effective error-prevention strategies embedded in the care systems, and patient/family engagement in care, care design, and organizational structures. Improving safety must be embedded in an organization's approach to patient care, rather than a set of safety improvement projects. A wide range of publicly available tools can be used by organizations to improve safety. We do not yet have effective strategies to address patient safety across the entire continuum of care from the home, to the clinic, and to the hospital. Eliminating harm will require multiple groups acting in concert across the entire spectrum of healthcare.

F. Federico
Institute for Healthcare Improvement, Cambridge, MA, USA
e-mail: ffederico@IHI.org

A.L. Billett (✉)
Dana-Farber/Boston Children's Cancer and Blood Disorders Center, Harvard Medical School, Boston, MA 02115, USA
e-mail: Amy_Billett@dfci.harvard.edu

© Springer International Publishing AG 2017
C.E. Dandoy et al. (eds.), *Patient Safety and Quality in Pediatric Hematology/Oncology and Stem Cell Transplantation*, DOI 10.1007/978-3-319-53790-0_3

Introduction to Patient Safety

History of the Patient Safety Movement

Many consider the publication of the Harvard Medical Practice Study in the New England Journal of Medicine in 1991 the true beginning of the modern patient safety movement [1]. The study examined 30,000 records from hospitals in New York State in 1984 and found that 3.7% of all hospitalizations included an adverse event caused by medical treatment. More than two-thirds of the adverse events were considered preventable. Of the approximately 2.7 million discharges in New York State in 1984, they estimated there were 98,609 adverse events, including 13,451 deaths. Total costs of these adverse events were estimated at $4 billion [2].

Public attention became focused on medical error after a series of publicly reported events including Betsy Lehman's death, a Boston Globe health reporter, from a fourfold chemotherapy overdose at Dana-Farber Cancer Institute in 1994, the death of Ben Kolb at Martin Memorial Hospital from a tenfold overdose of epinephrine during routine surgery in 1996, the death of Jose Eric Martinez at Memorial Hermann Hospital in Texas from a tenfold overdose of digoxin that was almost intercepted three different times, and multiple episodes of wrong-site surgery [3–5]. Multiple newly formed and existing organizations began to focus on error prevention and improving the quality of care including the Institute for Healthcare Improvement (IHI), the Institute for Safe Medication Practices (ISMP), the Joint Commission for the Accreditation of Healthcare Organizations (JCAHO, now TJC), the National Patient Safety Foundation (NPSF), and the National Quality Forum.

By 1999, the IOM report *To Err Is Human* reported that there were as many as 98,000 preventable deaths/year in US hospitals, far exceeding the number of deaths from motor vehicle accidents, breast cancer, and AIDS [6]. The total costs of medical error including lost income and disability were estimated at $17 to $19 billion. The IOM report laid out a comprehensive strategy including government, healthcare providers, industry, and consumers to reduce preventable medical errors. A key conclusion of the report was that the majority of medical errors do not result from individual recklessness but "are caused by faulty systems, processes, and conditions that lead people to make mistakes or fail to prevent them." In 2001, Congress appropriated $50 M annually to the Agency for Healthcare Research and Quality (AHRQ) for patient safety research but cut that funding only 3 years later. Hospitals began to focus on changes to improve the safety of their patients. Research in error prevention and patient safety grew steadily.

Current State of Patient Safety

Despite all of these efforts and the focus on improving safety, harm from healthcare that is intended to help is still too common. It is estimated that medical errors are the third leading cause of death in the United States with over 400,000 deaths annually and costs over $1 trillion [7–9]. Recent studies show harm in 13–33% of all hospital admissions, with 44–63% of events categorized as preventable, 2% leading to permanent injury, and 1.5% resulting in to death [10–12]. Similar rates have been reported in pediatrics [13].

Pediatric-Specific Patient Safety Risks

Pediatric healthcare has unique risks. Pediatric patients may be particularly vulnerable to medication errors due to the need for weight-based dosing with weights ranging from <1 kg to >100 kg, medications formulated and packaged primarily for adult dosing, lack of pediatric-specific indications, healthcare settings primarily built around the needs of adults, and immature hepatic and renal function in newborns [14]. Compared to adults, children have a higher risk of inpatient potential adverse drug events and a higher rate of prescription errors [15, 16]. The widespread use of liquid medications which require conversion from ingredient amounts (in mg) to volumes (in ml) and the choice between multiple concentrations also increases risk.

Many pediatric patients have limited communication skills. If the wrong wrist band is placed on a child, can he or she speak up? Some pediatric early warning systems thus assign an extra risk point to a child without a parent or other adult at the bedside who can speak up on behalf of the child [17]. The wide range of normal vital signs in pediatrics, where a heart rate of 50 can be the appropriate resting heart rate for a teenage athlete or an indication for cardiopulmonary resuscitation in a newborn, can make the recognition of abnormal vital signs difficult. Chlorhexidine gluconate, a common antibacterial solution used to prevent infections, can cause harm in preterm infants [18].

Pediatric Hematology/Oncology Patient Safety Risks

Pediatric hematology/oncology has additional safety risks. The narrow therapeutic index of many chemotherapy drugs may increase the impact of any dosing errors in both adult and pediatric oncology. Of 310 pediatric chemotherapy errors, 85% reached the patient and 16% required additional monitoring or a therapeutic intervention [19]. Although clinical research studies have led to the many major advances in pediatric cancer outcomes, the research studies themselves may cause safety risks with conflicting information about chemotherapy agents both between protocols and within the same protocol [20]. Despite standardization of the protocol document layout and road maps by the Children's Oncology Group (COG), the treatment regimens remain highly complex with varying dosing rules, modifications for specific disease characteristics, and modifications for specific side effects that may vary during different treatment phases. Advances in precision medicine are creating a virtual explosion in the amount of information that must be synthesized in order to make optimal treatment decisions, and the complexity of the reports increases the risk of misinterpretation.

But the risks are not just associated with the use of chemotherapy. Since most children do not have an extensive past medical history, the first discovery of children at risk of bleeding may be unmasked by routine pediatric surgical care. Challenges with venous access in young children with both cancer and blood disorders lead to the increased use of implanted central venous catheters both in the hospital and at home with the attendant risk of infection. Fixed tablet sizes for many key medications make it difficult to achieve child-appropriate dosing. In short, the potential safety risks in pediatric hematology/oncology are many.

Patient Safety Across the Care Continuum

The vast majority of patient safety research has focused on the inpatient setting. Limited research in the ambulatory setting has generally focused on such issues as medication safety, diagnostic errors, office-based surgery and anesthesia, and communication. The generalizability of the results is in question given the limited number of research sites, usually only in primary care and often with electronic health records. Intervention research has been remarkably rare [21]. Still less is known about safety in the patient's home, including care delivered either by trained healthcare professionals or, more frequently, by the patient and/or the patient's family. Implementation of line care bundles to prevent central line-associated blood stream infections (CLABSI) has been effective in reducing CLABSI in pediatric hematology/oncology inpatients [22]. However, the vast majority of days at risk for a CLABSI occur when the patient is at home with the central line. These infections are twice as common in outpatients and cost $35,000 per episode, but little attention has been focused on ambulatory prevention until the ongoing efforts of the Children's Hospital Association Childhood Cancer and Blood Disorders Network [23, 24]. Line removal, another key prevention strategy in the inpatient setting, is rarely appropriate for pediatric hematology/oncology patients whose care is dependent on a central line for months to years at a time. Medication errors in the outpatient and home setting are more common in pediatric than adult visits with at least one medication error detected at each pediatric visit [25]. Little is known about how to prevent such error.

Errors in Healthcare

Error Definition

Errors in healthcare are common, although not all lead to harm. The model developed for medication error can be applied more broadly to healthcare errors in general [26].

- *Medical error* is the failure of a planned action to be completed as intended or the use of a wrong plan to achieve an aim. Medical error results from either an act of commission (doing something wrong) or an act of omission (failing to do the right thing) and may lead to an undesirable outcome or a significant potential for an undesirable outcome. Most medical errors do not result in harm and have no potential to cause harm.

- An *adverse event* is an injury resulting from medical care rather than from the underlying disease or patient condition. Examples include graft-versus-host disease, myelosuppression from chemotherapy, and anaphylaxis from penicillin. An adverse event is an undesired outcome of care but does not imply error, negligence, or poor quality of care.
- A *preventable adverse event* occurs when the harm is the result of an error or system design flaw. Anaphylaxis to penicillin which was ordered and administered despite a known allergy to penicillin is a preventable adverse event.
- A *potential adverse event* is an error with potential to harm. Some potential adverse events are intercepted before they reach the patient, such as when a pharmacist intercepts the order for penicillin in a patient with a known allergy. Still other potential errors reach the patient but do not cause harm. Potential adverse events are also called *near misses*.

The overall frequency of adverse events in pediatrics is not known, but medication errors are common. In the first large-scale study of pediatric medication errors and events, medication errors were made in 5.7% of all orders and impacted 55% of admitted patients. Potential adverse events occurred in 1.1% of orders and impacted 10% of admitted patients. Preventable adverse events occurred in only 0.05% of orders and impacted 0.5% of patients [15].

Error Causation

Human Factors

We know that errors are common, and we know the conditions that contribute to errors. Human factors engineering, the study of the interaction between individuals, individuals and machines, and individuals and the environment, helps us to understand the human condition that contributes to errors. In any process, errors can occur at the "sharp end" when a human being involved in the process makes an "active" mistake. In general, these errors are not deliberate. Errors can be classified by Rasmussen's three levels of performance. [27] *Skill-based mistakes, slips and lapses,* involved stored patterns of preprogrammed instructions that are applied incorrectly leading to the final action not matching what was intended. Examples include a skilled driver stepping on the brake instead of the clutch or forgetting to sign an order after writing it. *Rule-based mistakes* occur in the setting of familiar problems that the person usually addressed by application of stored rules. The action does not match the intention because the wrong rule is applied and thus does not achieve the desired result. An example is applying the rule "order prophylactic antiemetics for chemotherapy" when ordering vincristine which is not emetogenic. *Knowledge-based mistakes* usually occur in novel situations when the actions must be planned but fail because of knowledge deficits. An example is an intern who orders fresh frozen plasma (FFP) to treat a prolonged PTT in a patient with severe hemophilia who is admitted for observation after minor surgery. In this case, the appropriate treatment, factor was given prior to surgery, and the prolonged PPT is a manifestation of the underlying disease. There is no reason to treat the prolonged PPT, and, if the patient was bleeding, FFP would have been the wrong treatment. A *violation*, as described further below, occurs when there is deliberate deviation from an accepted protocol or standard of care.

Contributing factors to human error include conditions such as fatigue, illness, distractions, and stress (Table 3.1). When we investigate adverse events and design countermeasures to minimize the opportunity for recurrence, we must consider human factors and develop processes that address the human condition to minimize the opportunity for errors. The patient safety movement has embraced the need to understand and incorporate human factors as a key part of improvement. Some organizations are now hiring engineers, former pilots, and other system designers to join improvement teams. In addition, we recommend that organizations, at the very least, help staff learn about the conditions and contributing factors and use that understanding to develop countermeasures.

As technology continues to advance and more and more electronic tools become available, it is necessary to understand how humans interact with the technology. Many errors occur when the interface between humans and machines is poorly designed. An example of well-designed technology is the smartphone. The developers purposely designed the phone to be easy to use right out of the box. The icons are easily recognized, and the features are intuitive. In *The Design of Everyday Things, (Basics Books 2013)*, Donald Norman offers an easy way to understand the impact of poor design on human actions. The author describes the use of affordances, the design of a device, or an environment that helps a user perceive how to perform an action. An example is the design of handles or doors: a bar implies a

Table 3.1 Factors contributing to human error	Fatigue
	Lack of sleep
	Illness
	Drugs or alcohol
	Boredom, frustration
	Cognitive shortcuts
	Fear
	Stress
	Shift of work
	Reliance on memory
	Reliance on vigilance
	Interruptions and distractions
	Noise
	Heat
	Clutter
	Motion
	Lighting
	Too many handoffs
	Unnatural workflow
	Procedures or devices designed in an accident prone fashion

push is needed to open a door versus a handle implies a pull is needed. Proper design of processes and equipment must be taken into account when making improvements. The Food and Drug Administration (FDA) offers advice on how to incorporate human factors into the design of equipment [28].

System Design

A system is a number of processes or steps that interact with each other to achieve a desired outcome. James Reason uses this definition to describe the difference between active and latent errors. Latent errors are those errors that result from poor system design [29]. The common approach to managing errors was to train and educate individuals and/or to punish, driven by the expectation that individuals will execute flawlessly. What we have learned, however, is that errors are common. Even the best-trained individual will find himself or herself in a position to make an error. Disciplining or removing the individual who made the error does not prevent someone else from making the error again if the contributing factors are part of the system. Reason referred to these as latent errors: errors just waiting to happen. The cause of latent errors includes poor design, situations where staff is constantly distracted, complex protocols, policies that do not support evidence-based practices, and pressures from management and others that cause individuals to take shortcuts.

Reason Swiss Cheese Model

Many times there are a series of steps in the process that are intended to block an error from reaching the patient. Reason likened these barriers to slices of *Swiss cheese* (Fig. 3.1). The holes represent flaws in the system that may go undetected until an event occurs. The more layers and the smaller the holes in each layer, the higher the chance of blocking an error. However, there are times when all of the holes line up, and the error reaches a patient. Efforts to address error reduction should focus on strengthening the design and the defenses of the system so that the opportunity for error is minimized and likewise is the opportunity for any errors to reach a patient.

Normalization of Deviance (Amalberti)

Amalberti and colleagues introduced us to the concepts of violations and migration, and they provide a framework to understand and manage them [30]. Violations are deliberate deviations from standard protocols which may result in bad or good results. Bad results are when a patient is harmed. Good results are when the protocol is violated because of its complexity and the outcome for the patient is good. The problem is that unless someone is harmed, these violations are seldom acknowledged or tracked and in fact sometimes encouraged and accepted and they become the norm. Managers build systems and processes in which they anticipate clinicians

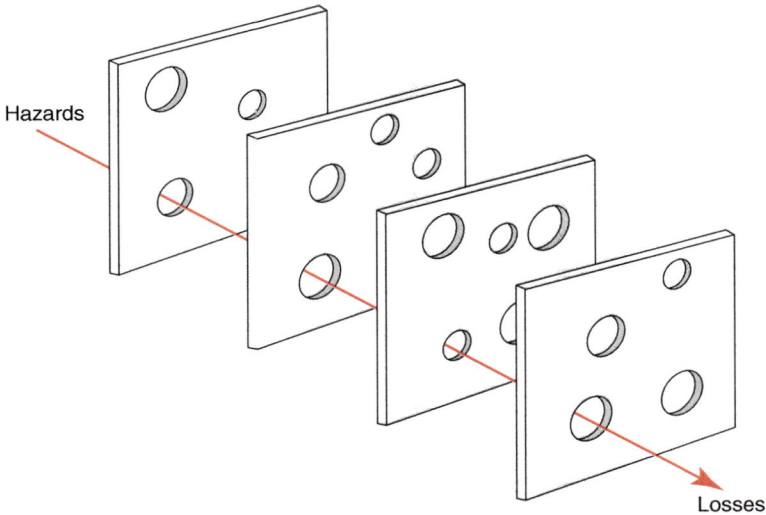

Fig. 3.1 Reason Swiss Cheese Model for Error

and staff to work, expecting operations in a safe space. Because of a myriad of external pressures or complexity of the procedures, individuals will migrate away from the safe space to the point where they may not be following the protocols just to complete tasks as expected. Amalberti calls this phenomenon migration to an illegal normal space. That is the area where many in healthcare function everyday. The systems and processes put undue pressure on clinicians, resulting in work-arounds and violations. The further someone drifts from this safe space, the greater the chance of serious harm. Managers are usually not aware of the staff performing in this space until something bad happens and there is an investigation. Staff is not likely to inform managers that they are performing in the illegal normal space because they fear being punished. It is the responsibility of managers to understand staff performance and the pressures that may be forcing individuals to perform in this space. Corrections must be made to the processes in the safe space so that people can use processes as designed.

How Often Do Errors Occur?

How often errors occur remains an unknown, and different error measurement strategies lead to very different results [12]. Mandated reporting by federal and state agencies, as well as nongovernmental groups such as the Joint Commission, may be useful to identify a subset of serious adverse events, particularly so-called "never" events such as wrong-site surgery. Another approach such as adjusted hospital mortality rates also measures safety at the very crude level of only extreme events. This measure is even less useful in pediatrics where the overall mortality ratio is lower and variation between hospitals is hard to measure [31]. Other sources of error detection range from regional or national malpractice claim data to mortality and morbidity conferences within a specific program. Many healthcare organizations utilize internal safety event reporting systems to measure safety within their own systems. Even in an organization with a very strong safety culture, such reporting will miss many events. At the other end of the spectrum, direct observation finds a higher rate of error than chart review, but both are extremely expensive and impractical to use outside of a research setting [32]. Automated review of discharge codes to detect adverse events has been shown to have relevance for pediatrics [33, 34]. The Institute for Healthcare Improvement (IHI) Global Trigger Tool detects adverse events at a rate nearly ten times the rate of the AHRQ Patient Safety Indicators [12]. A modified pediatric system has also been developed [35]. We have very limited tools to measure harm in ambulatory care and in the patient's home or to measure preventable harm and potential adverse events in all settings.

How to Make Healthcare Safer

Learning from Other Industries

We often hear that aviation and healthcare have much in common. However, there are differences in that in the aviation industry, the teams involved consist of a smaller group of individuals, the norms and processes to operate a plane have been standardized and provide customization-based well-evaluated and practiced activities, and the equipment has been tested and will not react differently because of individual variation. Healthcare on the other hand involves a team with many players, best practices exist but may have to be individualized based on the patient, there is more than one way to achieve the same result, and individual autonomy has been allowed. So why the comparisons? [36]. John Nance in *Why Hospitals Should Fly* describes how a fictitious hospital can take the lessons learned in the aviation industry to help a hospital achieve the same kind of reliability found in the aviation industry [37, 38].

The comparisons between healthcare and aviation serve to help understand what should be in place to ensure that we provide the safest care possible for patients. Although there are many routines in healthcare that have been standardized, healthcare providers also encounter highly unpredictable situations which require rapid responses on a daily basis. Emergencies and departures from routine practices are unusual and to be avoided in other high-risk industries. In healthcare it is not uncommon to encounter a patient with an unknown diagnosis, where the disease may be masked or may be complicated by comorbidities.

High-risk industries have developed a culture in which individuals share a common vision and work together as teams, communicate clearly and frequently, have flattened the hierarchy, see any defect as an opportunity to improve, and have developed a learning system so that any improvements are shared with all who need to know. In healthcare, we identify these characteristics in a safety culture in which there is little tolerance for poor practice and staff are uniformly conscientious and careful. [38].

Framework for Preventing Error/Maximizing Safety

An Institutional Response to Patient Safety

In March of 1995, the leaders of the Dana Farber Cancer Institute (DFCI) and many others around the country woke to this headline:

Big Doses of Chemotherapy Drug Killed Patient, Hurt 2d. The two patients, one a reporter for the Boston Globe, received a fourfold overdose of chemotherapy which caused life ending damage to their hearts. The normal reaction at the time was to find out who was involved and discipline or dismiss them from employment so that they could not hurt someone else at the institution. During the investigation by a number of agencies including The Joint Commission, Boards of Registration in Medicine, Nursing and Pharmacy, and the Department of Public Health, it became evident that the clinical team involved included very capable and experienced individuals. The investigation also identified numerous deficiencies, including protocol violations, ineffective drug error reporting, and oversight of quality assurance by hospital leaders.

The response from DFCI leadership included the following:

- New rules were adopted mandating close supervision of physicians in fellowship training.
- Nurses were required to double-check high-dose chemotherapy orders and to complete specialized training in new treatment protocols.
- Interdisciplinary clinical teams reviewed new protocols and reported adverse events and drug toxicities.
- A trustee-level quality committee was reorganized and strengthened.
- Discussions were begun regarding the transfer of inpatient beds to nearby Brigham and Women's Hospital.

However, as important as these changes were to decrease the opportunity for error, the leaders of the organization under Chief Operating Officer James Conway learned that other more profound changes contributed to improving safety.

First was the adoption of a systems approach and design to prevent errors. Understanding the contribution of human factors contribution to the error, DFCI worked to design systems to prevent errors including the development of protocols and templates for chemotherapy ordering, as well as implementing technology to assist in the process. The application of the principles of standardization and simplification was critical to this change.

- Safety was no longer to be viewed as someone else's problem. All clinical staff and leaders, up the Board, had a responsibility and accountability to ensure safe practices.
- DFCI developed a learning system through which staff and others collected and analyzed information from reporting systems, pharmacy interventions, and safety rounds. This analysis helped to identify opportunities for improvement.

- DFCI began the process of engaging patients in advisory councils that provided patients' view of the system and what kind of improvements would help them be safer.

  The staff at DFCI adopted the approach that cancer care is very risky because of the condition of the patients and the medication used. As a result, the clinicians and leaders adopted a relentless pursuit of constantly improving. They recognized that mistakes will happen even in the best designed systems, and it is the responsibility of all the staff to identify these errors, mitigate their impact, disclose to patients, and provide support to the clinicians involved.

In order to achieve long-lasting improvements in safety, it is necessary to change the paradigm from improving safety as a project to improving safety as a part of the organization's work in all ways, at all times. The second is to use a framework that provides the skeleton upon which all of the work can be added. There are two overarching components under which a set of elements must be in place and depend on each other: a learning system and culture [39].

Common to each is the role of *leadership*. It is the responsibility of leaders at all levels of the organization to develop an environment of teamwork, psychological safety, and respect. *Psychological safety* is an environment where people feel free to speak up, are respected, and are accepted [40]. *Accountability* is ensuring that individuals know their roles and are held to a standard of acting and in a safe way will receive the appropriate training to act in that way and will be judged fairly. *Teamwork and communication* are key building blocks to ensuring safe care. Healthcare providers develop a shared understanding, anticipate needs and problems, and have agreed methods to manage these as well as conflict situations. Empirical evidence from high-risk industries has been demonstrated to produce high-quality results [41]. *Negotiation skills* to be able to gain genuine agreement on matters of importance to team members, patients, and families are critical components of safety. *Continuous learning* refers to the organization's commitment to collect and learn from defects and reflect on what changes are necessary to improve [42]. *Improvement and measurement*: in order to improve the processes we work in, organizations must adopt an improvement method which applies the appropriate techniques to the issues to be addressed in order to improve processes and outcomes. Measurement is a critical part of testing and implementing changes; measures tell a team whether the changes they are making actually lead to improvement. *Reliability* refers to the application of processes to ensure continued failure-free operations over time in which patients receive evidence-based care. *Transparency* refers to respectfully sharing data and information with staff and patients and families.

The patient safety movement urged us to move away from a culture of blame to a blame-free culture. The pendulum swung too far from one extreme to the other. Over time, we came to realize that we must act in a manner that is a balance between blame and blame-free, a balance between safety and accountability [43]. The biggest challenge in adopting this culture is the implementation across the entire organization. There are several guides available: James Reasons Decision Tree for Unsafe Acts Culpability [29], David Marx Just Culture [44, 45], and the Fair Evaluation and Response Chart [46].

The *Manchester Patient Safety Framework (MaPSaF)* is a tool to help National Health Service (NHS) organizations and healthcare teams in the UK and assess their progress in developing a *safety culture* [47]. The framework can be applied in the acute care, ambulatory, mental health, and ambulance settings. The Agency for Healthcare Research and Quality (AHRQ) sponsored the development of patient safety culture assessment tools for hospitals, nursing homes, ambulatory outpatient medical offices, community pharmacies, and ambulatory surgery centers [48]. Similar to the Manchester tool, organizations can assess the present state of the culture, identify where there are differences, identify strengths and opportunities for improvement, and conduct internal and external comparisons.

In order to change a culture, it is necessary to match strategy and culture. The ingrained attitudes and practices may be such that any new strategy will be at odds with the prevailing culture. In order to build a different culture, one must act in the new way that is desired. By matching the actions with the beliefs, over time attitudes will change and along with the culture.

Deming offered advice on improvement in his 14-point philosophy [49]. He included items such as make the vision clear. Slogans are great and may be memorable but may not clearly indicate the direction and what is expected of staff. He also added that organizations should continuously improve their processes and systems. This is the kind of change that will impact the culture of an organization. The phrase "Act your way into believing" comes to mind.

Governance

Healthcare board members, senior executives, and physician leaders play key roles in patient safety. Patient safety depends on effective governance with highly engaged executive leadership teams working with highly engaged boards [50, 51]. Ensuring safe and harm-free care is a board responsibility, not one that is delegated to the executive leadership team. Table 3.2 illustrates Conway's six key steps for boards

Table 3.2 Six key steps for boards

Setting specific, public, and transparent aims to reduce harm
Getting data and hearing stories that put a "human face" on harm data
Establishing and monitoring system-level measures to understand how the organization is achieving its aim(s)
Changing the environment, policies, and culture, to maintain an environment that is respectful, fair, and just for patients, families, and staff
Learning, starting with the board. Ensure the board and the staff are educated and knowledgeable about such topics as patient safety, leadership in patient safety, and strategies for improvement
Establishing executive accountability for clear quality improvement targets

[52]. Empirical studies have shown that boards demonstrating effective patient safety leadership have positive impacts on their organization's safety performance and that boards that review and track their organization's performance have better quality outcomes [53]. Although ensuring high-quality, safe care was already clearly within the fiduciary responsibility of hospital boards, the Affordable Care Act of 2010 emphasized that responsibility still further.

Teamwork and Communication

Teamwork and communication are critical to healthcare delivery, which depends on multiple individuals and systems. Communication failure is a major contributing factor in 70% of sentinel events [54]. Multiple reviews have shown that various aspects of team function contribute to team performance [55–57]. Effective teamwork has been shown to be a critical ingredient in multiple aspects of patient safety including the reduction of safety events, increasing safety culture, improving communication, improving staff satisfaction, and decreasing staff turnover [58]. There has been increasing recognition that patients and families can and should be core members of healthcare teams in addition to staff. Bedside multidisciplinary rounds and bedside report include patients and families in the care team. Inclusion of patients and families in other teams, such as process improvement or safety teams, is necessary to ensure that patient-centered care is designed *with* patients and families not *for* them.

High functioning teams have a common purpose, a shared mental model of the situation and the goals, effective communication, a common understanding of how each team member can contribute to the outcome, mutual trust with good cohesion and respect among team members, effective leadership, good situational awareness, and the ability to resolve conflicts. All members of the team participate in the work, and all feel comfortable speaking up regardless of rank or role. Leadership within a team is clear but flexible, and the same individual does not always serve in the leadership role. Conflicts can be raised and resolved. Teams emphasize "we" and "us" not "I" and "me."

Effective strategies to improve teamwork focus on the cognitive and interpersonal skills needed to manage a process within a system rather than specific technical knowledge and skills. Team training focuses on facilitating human interaction and provides opportunities to practice and develop the necessary skills [57]. The principles of team training began with crew resource management (CRM) in the aviation industry and were first applied in healthcare in the 1990s [59]. TeamSTEPPS™ is a team training program developed by AHRQ specifically for use in healthcare [60].

Specific communication strategies facilitate team function. Structured *briefings* are opportunities to increase situational awareness, set a common goal, share information, and improve teamwork. *De-briefings* after an event, a simulation, or routine patient care provide an opportunity for teams to assess their own performance and identify opportunities for improvement. Planned and unplanned *huddles* help reestablish situational awareness and review existing plans and assess the need to adjust the plan.

Communication is critical to team function but can be impeded by perceptions of hierarchy, gender, culture, and many other factors. Key elements of effective communication include clarifying the problem and gathering relevant data, concisely describing the problem, actively listening to the response, and asserting concerns if needed [61]. Specific communication strategies that have been used in healthcare, such as SBAR, Call-out, Check-Back, two-challenge rule, DESC, and CUS, are designed to minimize conflict and the impact of hierarchy and maximize effective information transfer. Specific communication strategies to support handoffs, such as IPASS, maximize transfer of complex information including synthesis by the receiver [13].

A clinical example of SBAR communication from an experienced nurse

Situation	Dr. Smith, I am calling about Mary Jones who has a fever and a new oxygen requirement
Background	She is a 12-year-old girl with sickle cell disease, admitted for vaso-occlusive pain crisis. Her pain control is poor despite PCA. Her oxygen saturation is usually 96%
Assessment	Her oxygen saturation is now 90% despite 1 L by nasal cannula, and her fever is 39. I am concerned that she is developing acute chest syndrome
Recommendation	I think you need to order a CXR and blood culture and come see her right away

Addressing Human Error

You cannot change the human condition, but you can change the conditions under which people work.

—Dr. James Reason [29].

Since errors result from a combination of system design and the fallible human beings who work within those systems, the key to error prevention is proactively addressing those issues. Human factors is the "scientific discipline concerned with the understanding of interactions among humans and other elements of a system, and the profession that applies theories, principles, data and methods to design in order to optimize human well–being and overall system performance" [62]. If the system is designed to make it easier for people to do their jobs well, while accounting for their fallibilities, the overall system performance will improve. When analyzed thoughtfully, however, few systems in healthcare are actually designed to achieve the desired results. This frequently leads to *work-arounds*, consistent bypassing of policies or procedures by frontline workers, which then creates additional opportunities for error. Adding to this complexity is the tendency of many healthcare organizations to react to an event by adding a new step to an existing process rather than asking how that process should be changed or simplified.

Table 3.3 illustrates error-prevention strategies in order of effectiveness for creating lasting change to decrease errors. The most powerful strategies focus on the systems in which individuals operate. They are usually the hardest to implement. The next most effective strategies still target the systems but also depend on human vigilance and memory. The least effective strategies are usually the easiest to implement but rely entirely on human vigilance. Human factors engineering is critical to designing effective error-prevention strategies that account for our underlying human fallibilities. Usability testing involves testing the systems and equipment under real-world conditions to identify potential problems and unintended consequences of system design. The goal is to build a system that is "mistake proof," facilitates correct actions, prevents simple errors, and mitigates the negative impact of errors that due occur.

Fail-safes or forcing functions and constraints are among the most powerful and effective error-prevention strategies. True fail-safes, such as a microwave that will not start with the door open, are relatively rare in healthcare. Constraints that make it more difficult to do the wrong thing are more common. Preparation of vinca alkaloids in mini-bags makes administration via a spinal needle almost impossible. Many healthcare organizations have policies limiting chemotherapy prescribing to designated physicians. A computer-order entry system that only allows the designated physicians to order chemotherapy ensures that policy is actual practice. Reminders and checklists have gained widespread use in healthcare to prompt spe-

Table 3.3 Error-prevention strategies

Most reliable	Forcing functions *Example: removal of potassium from floor stock to prevent inadvertent potassium bolus*
	Constraints *Example: creation of a portable bone marrow kit with a breakaway lock to ensure needed supplies are available*
	Computerization and automation *Example: smart infusion pumps*
	Human-machine redundancy *Example: combine bedside visual checking and bar code checking of medications*
Somewhat reliable	Checklists *Example: checklist for initial evaluation of new diagnosis aplastic anemia*
	Reminders *Example: allergy alerts in electronic order entry*
	Standardization *Example: standardized antibiotic algorithms for fever and neutropenia*
	Planned pause points for self-check or double check *Example: surgical safety checklist review prior to the start of a procedure*
Least reliable	Rules, policies, and standard operating procedures
	Education and training
Unreliable	"Do better next time"
	"Be more vigilant"

cific steps to be followed in a specific order. Implementation of a surgical safety checklist has been shown to reduce surgical deaths, but it remains unclear if it is the checklist itself or the culture changes induced by use of the checklist that improved outcomes [63]. Checklists, however, are only helpful if they are used in a meaningful way, not just a rote performance.

Patient and Family Engagement

Patients are at the center of healthcare. In a 5-day retreat at a Salzburg Seminar, a group of 64 individuals from 29 countries adopted the guiding principle of "nothing about me without me." The intent was to switch how clinicians thought about care from a biomedicine (it is all about the care we deliver) to an infomedicine (patients and healthcare workers are informed, and there is shared decision making and governance) [64]. Thus was started a movement to engage patients in deciding about their care, developing "quality contracts" that served as building blocks for quality measurement which could be aggregated and recognize the individuality of patient. As Susan Edgman-Levitan notes: "Typically, the most important "experts"—ordinary people managing their health—are left out of the discussion and treated as objects *of* care, rather than partners *in* care" [65]. There are three ways to engage patients. The first is in their own care. When planning treatment, it is important to understand the patient's goals and desires. Opportunities to incorporate patient and family preferences into pediatric hematology/oncology include such decisions as when to start prophylactic factor in severe hemophilia, choosing between surgery and radiation for local control in Ewing's sarcoma, and many decisions in palliative care. The second way is to engage patient and/or family members in improvement teams. Any efforts to improve systems should include those who will be most affected by the improvement. Although there is little empirical data that this approach has resulted in more significant improvement, patient satisfaction has increased, and systems are designed with more consideration for the patient's condition and needs. In "Engaging Patients in Team-Based Redesign," Davis et al. describe different approaches used by the improvement teams to engage patients. The results were positive changes in staff attitudes for partnering with patients and higher patient satisfaction scores than nonparticipating teams [65]. The third way in which patients and or families can be engaged is to establish patient and family advisory councils and include patients on governance committees. In this model, patients and families are partnered with healthcare providers to provide guidance on how to improve the patient and family experience. AHRQ and others offer getting started toolkits [66].

Responding to an Event

As noted, there are many errors in healthcare, and most do not cause harm. However, when an error contributes to patient harm, the impact of that event is felt by patients and families. That impact may be physical, such as damage to an organ; psychological, such as fear of continuing treatment; and emotional for family members. There may be financial loss for the patient and family as well.

Responding to an adverse event requires that clinicians first ensure that harm to the patient is limited or do what is necessary to mitigate the harm. The organization should then begin an investigation into the factors that contributed to the error that resulted in harm. The most common method of investigation is the root cause(s) analysis (RCA) [67]. Adapted from other industries, the RCA involves examining the event in depth and identifying the root causes. The emphasis is on causes because there is always more than one cause. While the investigation is ongoing, there should be ongoing communication with patient and/or family to provide support and share as much as possible. There is a moral and, in some cases, legal requirement that there will be full disclosure to patients and families, as well as an apology and appropriate compensation if warranted. Research at the University of Michigan reports a decrease in claims when there is disclosure to patients and families [68]. The organization must also provide psychological support for clinicians [69]. As the contributing factors to the event are identified, the organization must use this information to improve and strengthen systems and processes to minimize the opportunity for such an error to occur again. In the spirit of improving care for all patients, sharing lessons learned with the healthcare community will be useful to help other organizations work to prevent similar errors.

Supporting Involved Clinicians: The "Second Victim(s)"

Clinicians are impacted as well. Dr. Albert Wu coined the term "the second victim" for clinicians involved in a serious event [70]. These individuals can suffer from physical and cognitive/emotional symptoms. The physical symptoms can include fatigue, insomnia, backache, and nausea. The emotional range experienced is anger, fear, stress, isolation, anxiety, rumination over the event, loss of interest in their work, burnout, and depression. At its most severe, there is post-traumatic stress, self-medication with alcohol and other drugs, and suicidal ideation [70–72]. It is important to note that this is not limited to the clinicians "responsible" for the error itself. All involved are at risk for such impact.

Institutions have the responsibility to put in place support systems for all involved clinicians. The successful programs have included both individual peer-to-peer support and support for teams [73]. Consider the difference between these two quotes from affected individuals, the first receiving no such institutional support, and the second benefitting from a peer-to-peer program: (1) "Twenty years later I still find myself angry at the lack of institutional support. There has to be more than getting a handout on PTSD." (2) "Words cannot express how effective and outstanding this program has been. I truly do not believe I could have dealt (and continue to deal) with this tragedy without knowing that caring people/physicians do exist and do understand and do not judge. The most important aspect to me has been the understanding part which is very difficult to find. I could go on and on about the positives of this system." Plews-Ogan et al. have shown that such support can help clinicians to not only avoid the array of negative outcomes described above but can give the experience an element of positivity: they become experts in prevention methodology, they improve teamwork, and they find themselves able to teach about the issue [72].

Leading Edge of Patient Safety

In a thought-provoking exercise, eight thought leaders imagined patient safety in 2025. [74] Their perspectives cover wide ranging topics such as the true embedding of safety culture throughout all of healthcare, the design of the healthcare system, the design of the physical design of healthcare environments, technology that supports both personal health records and a multitude of smart devices, truly patient-centered care with fully activated and engaged patients and families, comprehensive strategies to use simulation to maximize patient safety, and the elimination of risk associated with transitions. All shared, however, that no one change alone could truly improve safety. Commenting on this exercise, Dixon-Woods and Pronovost observed, "While these visions include new approaches and definitions for the concept of transitions in care (for example, admission and discharge), they fail to provide a specific vision for patient safety across the entire continuum of care from the patient's home to the clinic to the hospital. Eliminating harm from health care cannot be achieved by any single health care organization but requires the multiple groups acting in concert across the entire spectrum of health care including payors, regulators, manufacturers" [75].

References

1. Brennan TA, et al. Incidence of adverse events and negligence in hospitalized patients. Results of the Harvard medical practice study I. N Engl J Med. 1991;324(6):370–6.
2. Johnson WG, et al. The economic consequences of medical injuries. Implications for a no-fault insurance plan. JAMA. 1992;267(18):2487–92.
3. Knox RA. Doctor's orders killed cancer patient. In: Boston globe; 1995.
4. Hatlie M. Examining errors in healthcare: developing a prevention, education and research agenda. California: Annenberg Center for Health Sciences at Eienhower; 1996.
5. Belkin L. How can we save the next victim? In: New York times; 1997.
6. Khon LT, Corrigan JM, Donaldons MS. To err is human: building a safer health care system. Washington DC: National Academic Press; 2000.
7. Barriga F, et al. Hematopoietic stem cell transplantation: clinical use and perspectives. Biol Res. 2012;45:307–16.
8. Andel C, et al. The economics of health care quality and medical errors. J Health Care Finance. 2012;39(1):39–50.
9. Van Den Bos J, et al. The $17.1 billion problem: the annual cost of measurable medical errors. Health Aff (Millwood). 2011;30(4):596–603.

10. Landrigan CP, et al. Temporal trends in rates of patient harm resulting from medical care. N Engl J Med. 2010;363(22):2124–34.
11. Levinson D Adverse events in hospitals: national incidence among medicare beneficiaries. 2010 October 5. 2016. Available from: https://oig.hhs.gov/oei/reports/oei-06-09-00090.pdf.
12. Classen DC, et al. 'global trigger tool' shows that adverse events in hospitals may be ten times greater than previously measured. Health Aff (Millwood). 2011;30(4):581–9.
13. Starmer AJ, Sectish TC, Simon DW, Keohane C, ME MS, Chung EY, Yoon CS, Lipsitz SR, Wassner AJ, Harper MB, Landrigan CP. Rates of medical errors and preventable adverse events among hospitalized children following implementation of a resident handoff bundle. JAMA. 2013;310(21):2262–70.
14. Miller MR, et al. Medication errors in paediatric care: a systematic review of epidemiology and an evaluation of evidence supporting reduction strategy recommendations. Qual Saf Health Care. 2007;16(2):116–26.
15. Kaushal R, et al. Medication errors and adverse drug events in pediatric inpatients. JAMA. 2001;285(16):2114–20.
16. Kaushal R, et al. Medication errors in paediatric outpatients. Qual Saf Health Care. 2010;19(6):e30.
17. Kleinman M, Romano J. Children's hospital Boston early warning score: early detection + early intervention = better outcomes. 2010.
18. Chapman AK, Aucott S, Milstone AM. Safety of chlorhexidine gluconate used for skin antisepsis in the preterm infant. J Perinatol. 2012;32(1):4–9.
19. Rinke ML, et al. Characteristics of pediatric chemotherapy medication errors in a national error reporting database. Cancer. 2007;110(1):186–95.
20. Sievers TD, et al. Variation in administration of cyclophosphamide and mesna in the treatment of childhood malignancies. J Pediatr Oncol Nurs. 2001;18(1):37–45.
21. Lorincz CY, Drazen E, Sokol PE, Neerukonda KV, Metzger J, Toepp MC, Maul L, Classen DC, Wynia MK. Research in ambulatory patient safety 2000–2010: a 10-year review. Illinois, USA: American Medical Association; 2011.
22. Bundy DG, Gaur AH, Billet AL, He B, Colantuoni EA, Miller MR. Preventing CLABSIs among pediatric hematology/oncology inpatients: natrional collaborative results. Pediatrics. 2014;134(6):1678–85.
23. Hord JD, et al. Central line associated blood stream infections in pediatric hematology/oncology patients with different types of central lines. Pediatr Blood Cancer. 2016;63(9):1603–7.
24. Wong Quiles CI, et al. Health care institutional charges associated with ambulatory bloodstream infections in pediatric oncology and stem cell transplant patients. Pediatr Blood Cancer. 2016;64(2):324–9.
25. Walsh KE, Dodd KS, Seetharaman K, Roblin DW, Herrinton LJ, Von Worley A, Usmani GN, Baer D, Gurwitz JH. Medication errors among adults and children with cancer in the outpatient setting. J Clin Oncol. 2009;27(6):891–6.
26. Gandhi TK, Seger DL, Bates DW. Identifying drug safety issues: from research to practice. Int J Qual Health Care. 2000;12(1):69–76.
27. Rasmussen J. Skill, rules, knowledge: signals, signs and symbols and other distinctions in human performance models. IEEE Trans Syst Man Cybern. 1983;13(3):257–66.
28. Sawyer, D. Do it by design: an introduction to human factors in medical devices. 2 Oct 1996 2016. Available from: http://www.fda.gov/downloads/medicaldevices/deviceregulationand-guidance/guidancedocuments/ucm095061.pdf.
29. Reason J. Managing the risks of organizational accidents. Burlington, VT: Ashgate Publishing Company; 1997.
30. Amalberti R, et al. Violations and migrations in health care: a framework for understanding and management. Qual Saf Health Care. 2006;15(Suppl 1):i66–71.
31. Feudtner C, et al. Statistical uncertainty of mortality rates and rankings for children's hospitals. Pediatrics. 2011;128(4):e966–72.

32. Brennan TA, et al. Accidental deaths, saved lives, and improved quality. N Engl J Med. 2005;353(13):1405–9.
33. Zhan C, Miller MR. Administrative data based patient safety research: a critical review. Qual Saf Health Care. 2003;12(Suppl 2):ii58–63.
34. Sedman A, et al. Relevance of the agency for healthcare research and quality patient safety indicators for children's hospitals. Pediatrics. 2005;115(1):135–45.
35. Landrigan CP, et al. Performance of the global assessment of pediatric patient safety (GAPPS) tool. Pediatrics. 2016;137(6): e20154076
36. Chassin M, Loeb J. High-reliability health care: getting there from here. Milt Q. 2013;91(3):459–90.
37. Nance J. Why hospitals should fly: the ultimate flight plan to patient safety and quality care. Bozeman, MT: Second River Healthcare Press; 2008.
38. Vincent C, editor. Patient safety. 2nd ed. Hoboken, NJ: John Wily & Sons; 2010.
39. The essential guide for patient safety officers. 3rd Ed.. Forthcoming 2017, Oakbrook Terrace, IL: Joint Commission Resources.
40. Edmondson A. Psychological safety and learning behavior in work teams. Adm Sci Q. 1999;44(4):350–83.
41. Clements D, Dault M, Priest A. Effective teamwork in healthcare: research and reality. Healthc Pap. 2007;7:26–34.
42. Leonard M, Frankel A, Federico F, Frush K, Haraden C, editors. The essential guide for patient safety officers. 2nd ed. Oakbrook Terrace, IL: Joint Commission Resources; 2013.
43. Dekker S. Just culture: balancing safety and accountability. Burlington, VT: Ashgate Publishing; 2007.
44. Frankel A, et al. Essential guide for patient safety officers. 2nd ed. Oakbrook Terrace, IL: Joint Commission Resources; 2012.
45. Marx D. Patient safety and the "just culture": a primer for health care executives. Columbia University: New York; 2001.
46. Leonard MW, Frankel A. The path to safe and reliable healthcare. Patient Educ Couns. 2010;80(3):288–92.
47. Nezelof C, Basset F, Diebold N. Histiocytosis X: a differentiated histiocytic process. Pathol Biol (Paris). 1975;23(6):499.
48. Surveys on patient safety culture. 2016 October 11. 2016. Available from: http://www.ahrq.gov/professionals/quality-patient-safety/patientsafetyculture/index.html
49. Deming W. Out of the crisis. Cambridge, MA: Massachusetts Institute of Technology, Center for Advanced Engineering Study; 1986.
50. Muscari A, et al. Non-cardiac determinants of NT-proBNP levels in the elderly: relevance of haematocrit and hepatic steatosis. Eur J Heart Fail. 2006;8(5):468–76.
51. Goeschel CA, Wachter RM, Pronovost PJ. Responsibility for quality improvement and patient safety: hospital board and medical staff leadership challenges. Chest. 2010;138(1):171–8.
52. Conway J. Getting boards on board: engaging governing boards in quality and safety. Joint Commission J Qual Patient Saf. 2008;34(4):214–20.
53. Millar R, et al. Hospital board oversight of quality and patient safety: a narrative review and synthesis of recent empirical research. Milt Q. 2013;91(4):738–70.
54. Jaïs X, et al. Splenectomy and chronic thromboembolic pulmonary hypertension. Thorax. 2005;60(12):1031–4.
55. Manser T. Teamwork and patient safety in dynamic domains of healthcare: a review of the literature. Acta Anaesthesiol Scand. 2009;53(2):143–51.
56. Baker D, et al. Medical teamwork and patient safety: the evidence-based relation. 2005. Available from: http://www.ahrq.gov/research/findings/final-reports/medteam/index.html.
57. Weaver SJ, Rosen M. Making health care safer II: an updated critical analysis of the evidence for patient safety practices. Rockville, MD: Agency for Healthcare Research and Quality; 2013.
58. O'Daniel M, Rosenstein A. Professional communication and team collaboration, in patient safety and quality: an evidence-based handbook for nurses. Rockville, MD: Agency for Healthcare Research and Quality; 2008.

59. Howard SK, et al. Anesthesia crisis resource management training: teaching anesthesiologists to handle critical incidents. Aviat Space Environ Med. 1992;63(9):763–70.
60. TeamSTEPPS: Strategies and tools to enhance performance and patient safety, U.D.o.H.H. Services, Editor. Agency for Healthcare Research and Quality: Rockville, MD; 2016.
61. Leonard M, Graham S, Bonacum D. The human factor: the critical importance of effective teamwork and communication in providing safe care. Qual Saf Health Care. 2004:85–90.
62. Suri H, et al. Pulmonary langerhans cell histiocytosis. Orphanet J Rare Dis. 2012;7(1):16.
63. Haynes AB, et al. Changes in safety attitude and relationship to decreased postoperative morbidity and mortality following implementation of a checklist-based surgical safety intervention. BMJ Qual Saf. 2011;20(1):102–7.
64. Delbanco T, et al. Healthcare in a land called PeoplePower: nothing about me without me. Health Expect. 2001;4(3):144–50.
65. Davis S, et al. Implementation science workshop: engaging patients in team-based practice redesign – critical reflections on program design. J Gen Intern Med. 2016;31(6):688–95.
66. Working with patient and families as advisors implementation handbook. 2013. October 2, 2016; Available from: http://www.ahrq.gov/professionals/systems/hospital/engagingfamilies/strategy1/index.html.
67. RCA2 improving root cause analyses and actions to prevent harm. 2015, National Patient Safety Foundation: Boston, MA.
68. Boothman R, Imhoff S, Campbell DJ. Nurturing a culture of patient safety and achieving lower malpractice risk through disclosure: lessons learned and future directions. Front Health Serv Manag. 2012;28(3):13–28.
69. Conway J, et al. Respectful management of serious clinical adverse events. 2nd Ed. IHI Innovation Series white Paper. 2011. Available from: http://www.ihi.org/resources/pages/ihiwhitepapers/respectfulmanagementseriousclinicalaeswhitepaper.aspx.
70. Wu A. Medical error: the second victim. BMJ. 2000;320(7237):726–7.
71. Harrison R, et al. Emotion and coping in the aftermath of medical error: a cross-country exploration. J Patient Saf. 2015;11(1):28–35.
72. Plews-Ogan M, et al. Wisdom in medicine: what helps physicians after a medical error? Acad Med. 2016;91(2):233–41.
73. Shapiro J, Galowitz P. Peer support for clinicians: a programmatic approach. Acad Med. 2016;91(9):1200–4.
74. Henriksen K, et al. Envisioning patient safety in the year 2025: eight perspectives. In: Henriksen K, et al., editors. Advances in patient safety: new directions and alternative approaches, vol. 1. Rockville, MD: Agency for Healthcare Research and Quality; 2008.
75. Dixon-Woods M, Pronovost PJ. Patient safety and the problem of many hands. BMJ Qual Saf. 2016;25(7):485–8.

Chapter 4
Teamwork and Collaboration

Melissa Sundberg, Raina Paul, and George R. Verghese

Introduction

Successful quality improvement (QI) endeavors are achieved through working in collaboration with all stakeholders involved in the process. Optimal teamwork allows project members from frontline staff to team leaders to have a voice and contribute potential ideas. Development and collaboration between all team members will enhance the success of projects through idea sharing, problem solving, and creation of a shared work culture.

Creating a Quality Improvement Infrastructure to Support Successful Teams

Appropriately developing staff, resources, and institutional support is an integral, but often overlooked, component of ensuring quality improvement activities are successful. Having dedicated staff and resources for global quality improvement efforts can enhance long-term success rather than creating new leadership and teams

M. Sundberg, MD, MPH (✉)
Division of Emergency Medicine, Boston Children's Hospital, Harvard Medical School, Boston, MA, USA
e-mail: melissa.sundberg@childrens.harvard.edu

R. Paul, MD, MPH
Division of Emergency Medicine, Ann and Robert Lurie Children's Hospital, Feinberg School of Medicine Northwestern University, Chicago, IL, USA
e-mail: rpaul@luriechildrens.org

G.R. Verghese, MD, MBA
Division of Cardiology, Ann and Robert Lurie Children's Hospital, Feinberg School of Medicine Northwestern University, Chicago, IL, USA
e-mail: gverghese@luriechildrens.org

© Springer International Publishing AG 2017
C.E. Dandoy et al. (eds.), *Patient Safety and Quality in Pediatric Hematology/ Oncology and Stem Cell Transplantation*, DOI 10.1007/978-3-319-53790-0_4

for individual quality improvement projects. The main components of creating a sustainable infrastructure are outlined below with appropriate consideration given to differing resources available between institutions.

A permanent set of individual(s) trained specifically in QI methodology can provide a base for an effective team. Baseline knowledge of tools for improving care include but are not limited to those related to formal barriers assessment, gap analyses, reliability science as it informs interventions, and run/control chart analytics discussed in more depth later in the chapter. Not every team member will need to have this depth of knowledge, but each should understand the goals, mission, and aim of the project with a basic understanding of the chosen quality improvement framework. There are external resources to aid in this knowledge and further support efforts if there are a lack of internal resources initially; however, it is recommended that building a strong, consistent foundational base is optimal. Leadership of the organization should assist in framing the quality improvement agenda, aligning incentives, and ensuring the overall strategy is consistent with the global vision and mission [1]. Leadership support embedded within institutional QI infrastructure can improve overall performance of an organization and patient outcomes and therefore should not be underestimated. The presence of a knowledgeable point person to communicate goals of QI initiatives, successes, and barriers to organizational leadership is also essential for success.

Although team members with in-depth QI methodology knowledge are integral, managers, trainees, and other frontline staff are also essential. A broad integration of all team members from varying levels and departments in the organization is essential in developing a comprehensive assessment of barriers [2]. Obtaining "buy-in" from frontline staff by providing education regarding the importance of quality improvement and its role in improving patient outcomes and increased patient and provider satisfaction is an important first step. Education regarding quality specific language and control chart interpretation is also crucial in disseminating real-time results [3]. Interdisciplinary communication and teamwork empowers all members and contributes to the culture of safety, thus enhancing sustainability and improving patient care and provider retention. The interaction between leadership and frontline staff should include opportunities for feedback, ongoing monitoring of initiatives, frequent updates, review of barriers using applications of QI tools, as well as dedication by leadership to time for training and educational efforts for all staff. Communicating results for critical indicators and measures across the organization as well as beyond the organization can lead to enhanced success and team engagement.

Although support from leadership and educated team members are essential for developing successful QI initiatives, resources dedicated to creating a culture that supports continuous process change play an important role in creating an environment that supports critical self-evaluation and continuous improvement [2]. This type of resourcing includes financial support for training, purchasing technology and equipment, testing changes, as well as protected time to allow team members to actively participate in the change processes. Statistical support with a working knowledge of improvement science including the generation of control charts is a major advantage to allow real-time evaluation of a process.

Employing a Team-Based Approach: Importance of Teams

Teamwork is essential for the success for quality improvement endeavors in healthcare settings. Although an individual may find an opportunity for improvement, healthcare is a "team sport" in which patients and families, providers, and staff at many levels contribute to both process and outcome. The team effort is integral to QI as healthcare delivery is complex and no one member of a system understands all aspects of a process. A team consisting of all stakeholders allows for perspectives from all levels of care to be reviewed and discussed. Although these members of the core team will meet on a regular basis, these same members should find opportunities to seek guidance and feedback from external team members. As each member brings individual and solicited perspective and ideas to the discussion, it allows the entire team to consider unique contributions of all potential components from a care process of achieving change. Additionally, the involvement of a multidisciplinary team will add to the sustainability of the quality improvement efforts as all members will be invested within the process from the outset.

Team Composition

Once a quality improvement opportunity has been identified and a global infrastructure created, establishing a team to lead improvement actions will build commitment, generate ideas, and coordinate tasks. Teamwork is now well understood to be essential in providing high-quality and safe patient care throughout medicine [4]. In healthcare improvement, working alone is rarely effective, and having a multidisciplinary team allows for individuals at all levels of the care system to be involved in identifying and implementing the best approach to solving the challenge.

In developing a team for an improvement project, one should consider characteristics of an effective team as well as team dynamics. In general, teams should have clear goals and tasks consisting of members with experience and skills in line with the goal. Consideration for building a team should include patient and family representatives. Patient and families are an integral part of the team striving to meet the needs and expectations of the patient in conjunction with the improvement team. Their critical role will be described in more detail later in the chapter.

In general, the Institute for Healthcare Improvement (IHI) states that teams should include, although are not limited to, the following [1]:

Clinical leadership: Understanding of the clinical care process globally, at the divisional level, is integral to how the change will affect clinical care. This individual should have the authority to test and implement change and problem solve issues on a global scale [2].

Technical expertise: Understanding of the clinical process or area where the change will be occurring. This includes frontline staff [3].

Day-to-day leadership or operational lead: This individual is the lead for quality improvement teams ensuring completion of data collection, analysis, and change implementation [4].

Project lead or executive lead: An individual who serves as a link between the team implementing the work and senior leadership [5].

Team members most affected by implementation decisions are usually those who can also provide the most accurate information regarding the impact of these decisions. Improved teamwork and communication by frontline caregivers are often required to make the changes that lead to improved patient outcomes. The knowledge of direct operations lies with those working directly in care areas, and their membership is fundamental for change. In general, trainees, attending physicians, advanced practice providers, nurses, pharmacists, laboratory staff, interpreter services, as well as patients and families should all have membership within a successful team depending on the project (Fig. 4.1).

An alternative structure for team formation in healthcare quality improvement shares some characteristics with the above-proposed composition but may be more comprehensive with respect to the ultimate goal of successful improvement project implementation in an organization. This relatively simple yet effective project team structure proposed by healthcare quality improvement pioneer Brent James has proved successful in practical experience for many [6]. He identifies three major roles within teams: team members, team leader, and team facilitator (Fig. 4.2). First, team members should be drawn from the frontlines of the work process that is trying to be improved. These individuals have fundamental knowledge of the process and understand the intricacies of how work gets done on a day-to-day basis. And as Deming said, in quality improvement, we ought to "organize everything around value-added high-priority work processes" [7]. In addition to providing that

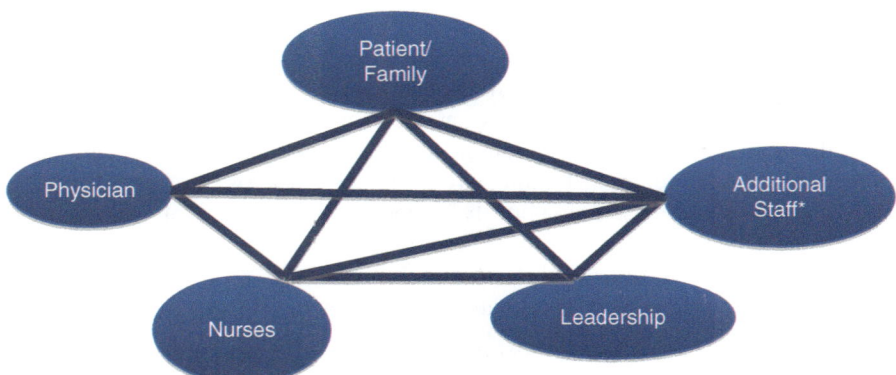

Fig. 4.1 QI team members should include all members throughout the spectrum of the care process and allow for facile communication between all members. **Additional staff*: advanced practice providers, pharmacists, laboratory, interpreters, social work, child life, paramedics, environmental services, engineering, etc

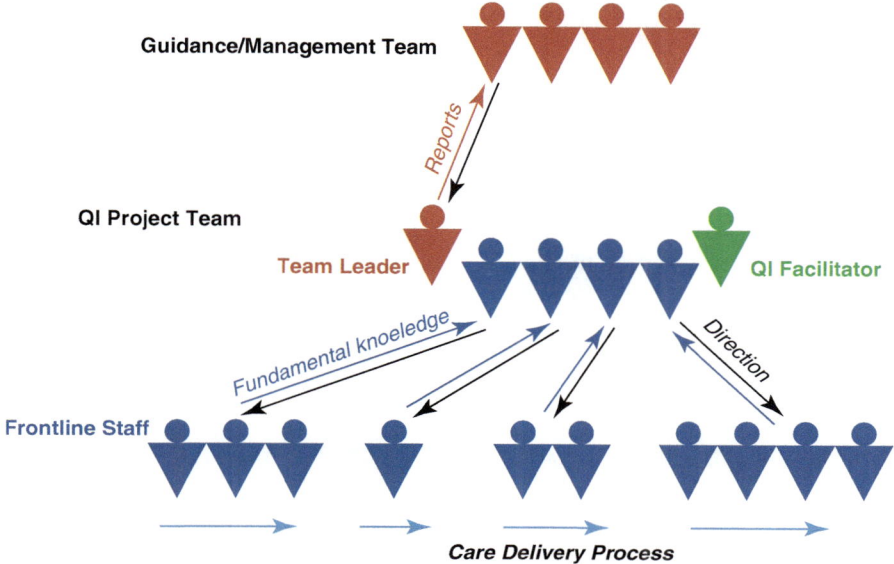

Fig. 4.2 Brent James' teams model. Adapted with permission from Dr. Brent James, Intermountain Healthcare, Institute for Healthcare Delivery Research, 2009

fundamental knowledge, a key role of these team members is to communicate the team's output back to their non-team member frontline counterparts. The advantage of this structure is that a peer is keeping the frontline informed about the decisions being made by the team and they can solicit further feedback or refinements from other frontline staff engaged in a similar part of the process throughout the project. This approach makes a critical difference when implementing or scaling efforts. Given these responsibilities, identifying frontline staff up with robust leadership and organizational skills is critical.

In James' model, an improvement team should also have a team leader. Often this individual may be a member of a guidance or more senior management team. They typically set the agenda, record team activities, and report back to senior leadership or executive sponsors. Similar to how the frontline team members communicate back to their frontline peers, team leaders should communicate with their management peers to keep them informed of the project and solicit feedback from the beginning. As a result, when the team presents their final recommendations, senior leadership can implement their findings quickly and effectively with little resistance or rework required from the team. James goes as far to say that senior management has a duty to implement the teams' recommendations "as is" since they have been kept informed of the teams' activities and had plenty of opportunity to offer feedback or constructive critique. Though some may disagree, Dr. James also makes the point that record keeping and the details of the team's output should be performed by the team leader (not delegated to another individual on the team or to administrative support), as ultimately in this structure, the team leader needs to be able to accurately and fully communicate the team findings throughout the process to senior leadership.

The final role in the basic structure of an improvement team is that of a QI facilitator. Not all teams need a facilitator but it can be helpful in many situations. The role of the facilitator according to James is primarily to keep the team "healthy" rather than attempt to improve the actual problem the team has been assigned. It is the facilitator's responsibility to ensure the team is healthy enough to focus on truly following through on the specific aim the team is committed to improving. Team health can be defined in terms of the components listed under the team dynamics section below that define an effective team—safety, inclusivity, openness, and consensus-seeking. One approach to facilitate this is to establish "ground rules" from the start of how team members will conduct themselves in their interactions inside and outside of the team. For example, a team may choose upfront that once they have achieved consensus that the team speaks with "one voice" to others outside of the team. Similarly, if team members don't voice dissent, this is will be considered akin to assent. Additionally, the facilitator also should have expertise in the QI tools described above and can assist the team leader and the group in the application of formal QI concepts.

Stages of Team Formation

The development of teams focused on implementation and continuous evaluation of strategy within and external to the team can improve the overall outcome of the results [8]. Although teams were once considered to be static in nature, as goals are defined and projects evaluated with time, they can be dynamic, reflecting changes in resources and priorities [9, 10]. One cannot expect a team to work optimally when it first comes together. Forming a successful team takes time to allow members to progress through a series of well-characterized stages. The model described by Bruce Tuckerman in 1965 established a theory of group dynamics that can be integral to understanding these stages of team development. There are four recognizable stages: forming, storming, norming, and performing [11] (Table 4.1). As a group is

Table 4.1 Bruce W. Tuckman's stages of team development

Stage	
Forming	The team is developing and learning about goals and direction usually with excitement and eagerness. As this stage is focused on direction primarily by the team leader, goal setting productivity may be low
Storming	Team members' excitement wanes; they push the boundaries of others with frustrations, conflicts, and disagreements
Norming	Although there are differences among team members, these differences are accepted with the ability to move on as a team
Performing	The team now has a shared vision and goal, and individuals have more autonomy in decision-making

formed, team members will act independently, will be motivated, and will act politely and courteously toward others. However, as the team may not be informed of the goals and objectives, some individuals may also be anxious and fearful. As the team progresses, the next stage of storming may develop; other teams may progress to norming without this stage. While in the storming stage, members feel compelled to voice their opinions, which may be positive or negative, pushing against the boundaries and resisting quality improvement strategies proposed by other members. During this stage, it can be difficult to move toward the group's goals, but with time and strong leadership, one can move to the next phase of norming. In this stage, individuals start to resolve their differences, appreciate the input and skills of their colleagues, as well as respect leadership. At this time, team members know one another, are able to socialize, ask for help, and provide constructive criticism leading to a stronger team and progress toward the goal. As norming is established, a team's hard work without friction leads to the performing stage and, in turn, achievement of the team's goals. It is important to consider these stages as a team is being established, as recognition of the stage of a team can allow for knowledge as to how the team may progress especially from storming to norming, allowing time for the dynamics to develop through the stage without failures and dissolution of the team.

Although it is important to consider internal team dynamics for successful progress toward a goal, several recent studies have shown that how much a team's members interact with individuals outside the team boundaries can also be an important factor in team performance [12]. Other members outside a team can influence the behaviors, expectations, and motivations that team members bring back to the group and thus should be given appropriate consideration [11].

Team Dynamics

After successful development of a team, how individuals work within the team is integral to obtaining the desired outcome. Dr. Brent James again has identified a number of features of effective QI teams [6]. He asserts that teams do not just happen but rather require thoughtful planning, leadership, and organization. He draws in part from work written about communities by psychiatrist and author M. Scott Peck to note four qualities of effective teams: *safety, inclusivity, openness, and consensus-seeking. Safety* means that members are free to offer ideas without personal attack. Ideas stand on their own; critique of an idea is not a personal attack on the individual it came from, and future ideas should not be judged within the context of prior ideas. *Inclusivity* means examining ideas from different viewpoints. If current team members do not have the relevant fundamental knowledge for a particular aspect of the project, the team should be dynamic enough to bring the appropriate experts into the team on an ad hoc basis. A related concept is that of groupthink, popularized in the 1970s by social psychologist Irving Janis in his discussion of foreign policy as cited by Hart [13]. In this psychosocial phenomenon, dissenting opinions are ostracized, and group members shun confrontation or personal doubts which leads to a distorted view of reality, unjustified optimism, and ultimately poor decisions. Many involved in teams (including these authors) have discovered that one way to curtail this is for a group leader to intentionally and explicitly raise counterpoints or alternative strategies for the purposes of holistic discussion. The feature of *openness* refers to counteracting hierarchy or dominance based on authority within a group. Finally, James notes that if the aforementioned are present, consensus-seeking, the final characteristic, can occur. *Consensus-seeking* is a fundamental tenet of teams, and it is this characteristic that truly differentiates teams from other group structures. Dr. James defines consensus as finding a solution that is acceptable enough that all members can support it and that no member opposes it. He adds that consensus is neither a unanimous opinion nor a majority vote and does not mean that everyone is completely satisfied. That said, once consensus is reached, all team members should support it, particularly in interactions outside of the team.

Ungerleider and Ungerleider, leaders in team dynamics in healthcare and in particular the complex setting of pediatric cardiac care, have described another set of related but more specific features of team dynamics they have identified as the "Seven Practices of the Highly Resonant Teams" [14]. They argue that attention to the intra- and interpersonal factors that create teamwork can result in substantial improvements in quality and outcomes. They remind us that medical knowledge, skills, and judgement alone are likely not enough to achieve high standards of quality and safety in healthcare. These seven practices are built upon a foundation of psychological safety—a space free of judgment, ridicule, and blame as well as attunement, a reflective quality described as mindful sensitivity for the individual's self, for others on the team, and for the context of the present situation. *Mindful integration* focuses on the ability to manage one's own needs and the needs of others within the context and demands of the team. This awareness and ability to manage self, others, and the current situation or environment has also been described as emotional intelligence. Mindfully integrated communication requires that team members are consistently aware of the competing demands of these three elements and find a way to nonjudgmentally value each or risk creating one of several negative cultures depending on which is discounted. The second feature of highly resonant teams is that teams must *invite learning*. The ability to create an environment where it is safe to struggle and learn from failures, where failures are viewed as opportunities to explore and discover rather than being ashamed of, increases the chances of identifying new solutions. Challenging team members to learn and ask questions, even when the answers are not immediately apparent, is part of this element of high resonance teams. The third principle, referred to as the *push-up button*, stresses the importance creating team environments that promote positivity. They cite recent research on creating teams indicating that *how* we communicate is far more important than *what* we communicate. For example, several studies reveal that high-performing teams have a greater amount of positive compared to negative elements and emotions because negativity can have a more powerful influence than positivity, and therefore it takes more positivity to counterbalance the negative. Although there has to be space for conflict and imperfection, the elevation and support among team members must outweigh this for continued success. *Creating*

Table 4.2 Seven practices of highly resonant teams	Mindful integration
	Invite learning
	Push-up button
	Creating systems with outcomes in mind
	Be flexible and stable
	Shared accountability
	Good upstander

systems with outcomes in mind is the fourth principle that includes creating systems for establishing psychological safety. Teams that demonstrate this fourth practice also need to have clarity surrounding the outcomes that they desire including identifying the drivers of those outcomes. The fifth principle focuses on the ability to *be flexible and stable*. Though at first glance these two features may seem mutually exclusive, they are not and rather are requisites for healthy team growth. Resonant teams strive toward a balanced approach to rules. When a team can identify their core values and principles, they can then transform their rules into guidelines but then simultaneously understand the exceptions to their rules that can "create energy and growth, consistency without rigidity, flexibility with stability." The sixth principle is centered upon *shared accountability*. This practice promotes acceptance of an outcome *and* recognition that it belongs to the entire time—the team wins and loses together. Lastly, the seventh principle of highly resonant teams encourages team members to speak up by being a *good upstander* when they see other members being treated unfairly. This is particularly relevant for teams improving patient safety in that concerns are taken seriously and evaluated objectively, regardless of the "role" of the person on the team (Table 4.2).

Quality improvement success can be seen with team member integration and a structure and an environment conducive to all members having the ability to contribute openly. Knowledge of the team dynamics and its evolution as a project progresses can be pivotal to the success of a quality improvement effort.

Novel Approaches and Progression of Teams Within a Quality Improvement Framework

The dynamic nature of a team includes its members during the various stages of progression during a QI project. For example, a clinical team typically forms initially with physicians, nurses, pharmacists, patients, and other members as the stakeholder barriers are explored. This group of larger members may disband or suspend work to form subgroups consisting of other smaller numbers but more directed toward a specific goal. For example, in determining that a barrier to expeditious delivery of antibiotics for sepsis patients is stemming from delay in pharmacy distribution, a subgroup could consist of just pharmacy and floor nurses that deliver that antibiotic.

Like other teams in the new era of business, in QI efforts, successful teams often display this rapid formation/dissolution life cycle referred to by Professor Amy Edmondson as "teaming" [9]. She refers to this as "teamwork on the fly: a pickup basketball game rather than plays run by a team that has trained as a unit for years. When companies or health care organizations need to accomplish something that has not been done before, and might not be done again, traditional team structures are not practical. It is just not possible to identify the right skills and knowledge in advance and to trust that circumstances will not change. Under those conditions, a leader's emphasis has to shift from composing and managing teams to inspiring and enabling teaming" [15]. In consideration of this, teaming still relies on recognizing and clarifying interdependence, establishing trust, and exploring ways to coordinate efforts. Unlike the "core" team, there is no time to build a foundation of familiarity, but rather, members must develop and use new capabilities for sharing crucial knowledge quickly. Edmondson notes that teaming does not happen spontaneously, rather it takes leadership. In healthcare environments, she suggests three tasks that promote teaming: frame the work, make it safe, and build facilitating structure. Historically in healthcare a common frame has been that individual expertise, provided by separate experts, will lead to optimal health outcomes. Rather, leaders interested in teaming need to reframe healthcare delivery as a complex system that is critically dependent on the interdependence of work rather than simply individual expertise—in other words, how does what I do for this patient fit into the larger context of their care? Next, leaders can promote psychological safety by asking questions thereby modeling curiosity and inviting others to speak up. Finally, building facilitating structures such as systematic communication methods like SBAR (situation, background, assessment, recommendation) or redesigning facilities to force cross-disciplinary collaboration aids in creating the environment and context for teaming [16]. Teaming will not always be applicable for all quality improvement work. For some projects, traditional stable teams of individuals who have learned to work well together over time will make more sense; however, as healthcare reimbursement transforms toward value over the coming years, novel and innovative approaches to care delivery are likely to be increasingly utilized, and improvement science teams will need to be at the forefront to ensure optimal outcomes while reducing cost.

Regardless of the approach, a team must also understand the progression of workflow from barrier assessment to measurement development, to interventions, and then analysis. There are several guides and techniques to achieve this, including but not limited to key driver diagrams, workflow mapping, and PDSA (plan, do, study, act) cycles depending on the preferred QI framework [17, 18]. In the development of a QI plan, it is integral to begin with a vision statement, description of the structure of the program, membership, meeting schedule, as well as a list of the improvement goals or priorities that adhere to the goals of a specific, measurable, achievable, relevant, and time-bound (SMART) aim [18]. Once the aim is developed, barriers should be assessed and organized using key driver diagrams, fishbone diagrams, and process maps. Outcome, process, and balancing measures should be assigned to all key drivers within the driver diagram. Interventions should be prioritized using tools such as the PICK chart or Pareto mapping and should follow the principles of reliability science. Measures should then be tracked using ongoing time-series analysis including run and statistical process control charts. If teams understand that every QI project follows this flow, they will be less apt to perceive that the process is slow or disorganized and will be more willing to contribute to the task at hand.

Knowing When a Stage Is Complete

In quality improvement initiatives, it is important to understand the objectives of a project that are be defined through a SMART aim, driver diagram, or other tools described above. It is integral to understand when moving through the Model for of Improvement (e.g., as one QI framework) when a stage is complete and one can move to the next phase. It is important to set predefined checkpoints with tests upon implementation of whether or not each object has been met. Predefined end points ("exit criteria") with criteria that must be met before completing the process must be established early and be part of the project goals [19]. At times the stages may overlap as PDSA cycles are iterative in nature. This allows for alignment of the end product and expectations of the team working together.

Sustaining improvements after completion of QI initiatives is often challenging. As such, QI initiatives should not be seen as stop-and-go initiatives but as a system that may need continued small improvements. In turn, there should be continuing, although likely less frequent, touch points at a control level to evaluate continued system improvement after the team has navigated to other more active initiatives.

Shared Decision-Making

Collaboration and teamwork moves beyond the relationship between practitioners to that between practitioners and their patients and families, represented as the "voice of the customer." Shared decision-making (SDM) and patient- and family-centered care are a key component of change for improved quality and safety in healthcare [20]. Patient-centered care is respectful of and responsive to individual patient preferences, need, and values, ensuring that clinicians and patients are working together to produce the best possible outcomes. SDM stresses the importance of better understanding the experience of illness and addressing patients' needs within the healthcare system. By including patients within a QI team, the "voice of the customer" becomes forefront. Patient-centered care was stressed within the Institute of Medicine report of Crossing the Quality Chasm, as one of the fundamental approaches to improving the quality of US healthcare. Further investigations and studies have continued to support the importance of SDM in creating sustainable QI successes [21].

The Agency for Healthcare Research and Quality (AHRQ) presents one framework for approaching shared decision-making [22]. In this model, there are five steps to achieving patient and family participation and understanding, SHARE:

Step 1: **S**eek your patient's participation.
Step 2: **H**elp your patient explore and compare treatment options.
Step 3: **A**ssess your patient's values and preferences.
Step 4: **R**each a decision with your patient.
Step 5: **E**valuate your patient's decision.

This model allows for a transparent presentation of all risks and benefits for procedures and treatments and allows the patient to own the decision to proceed within a context of informed understanding.

Although a comprehensive review of shared decision-making and patient- and family-centered care is beyond the scope of this chapter, the concept of patient and family involvement is critical to the discussions surrounding effective improvement teams. As emphasized above, teamwork and collaboration in healthcare quality improvement requires input from not only frontline staff but also patients and families. Recently, this notion of patient- and family-centered care has been conceptualized as the "coproduction" of healthcare [23]. The concept stems from economics in the 1960s as the new service-related economy (retail, banking, education) required a different framework from the old industrial economy (manufacturing and agriculture). In services (unlike products), creating value requires the combined input of companies and customers. Companies often seek focus groups or structured input in the design of products, but the actual product is not truly dependent on them. In the delivery of healthcare, however, the creation of health outcomes in many cases is completely dependent on the dual input of healthcare professional and the patient or family—i.e., health outcomes are coproduced. In general pediatric cardiac care, for example, we can describe the etiology and management of syncope to a patient or family, but they ultimately decide how much water they will drink, how much salt to take in, or whether or not they will perform maneuvers we recommend when they experience prodromal symptoms, and without this, optimal outcomes cannot be achieved. Dr. Maren Batalden (daughter of healthcare QI leader Paul Batalden) describes the power and opportunity of coproduction as helping her see healthcare delivery not as a process in which value is made by health professionals and *pushed* out to patients, but one where value is created by patients with help *pulled* form health professionals [24].

An excellent example of this concept in pediatric healthcare is coproduction within "learning networks." The oldest and most established of these is the learning network for children and adolescents with inflammatory bowel disease (IBD) called ImproveCareNow. This over 70-site network has increased the clinical remission rate for patients with IBD from 60 to 79% in large part through coproduction of care. By example, patients, families, and healthcare professionals have together cocreated tools such as electronic pre-visit planning templates and population management algorithms, self-management support handbooks and shared decision-making tools, parent disease management binders, adolescent transition materials, handbooks for newly diagnosed families, and a mobile app to track symptoms, plan a visit, or test ideas about how to improve symptoms [23].

In pediatric cardiology, a similar learning network exists called the National Pediatric Cardiology Quality Improvement Collaborative (NPC-QIC) in which coproduction with parents has also been used since early in its inception, in part based on the positive experience of the IBD network. In NPC-QIC, parents are engaged in all aspects of the collaborative including leadership, research, workgroups, and committees. At semiannual learning session, parents are strongly represented (anecdotally, at a recent session one of the authors attended in 2016, there were over 60 parents in attendance), and together with their medical teams, they share information across the collaborative to further develop and spread best clinical practices for a population of patients (hypoplastic left heart syndrome or HLHS) where there is little definitive evidence-based care [25].

In addition to cocreating various tools and resources for new parents with a baby with HLHS, another specific example of coproduction of care has been the "Research Explained" series in which clinicians and parents summarize the results of key articles in the medical literature related to HLHS. This was initiated by a parent group that recognized that some families were discussing research articles online and drawing conclusions from abstracts for their child. Out of concern that their conclusions of the medical research were not always accurate, the "Research Explained" write-up was cocreated [24]. Additionally, academic work itself has been published in the medical literature with parents as first authors on important topics like supporting transparency of outcomes among congenital heart disease centers (in which the working group is made up of equal numbers of parents and clinicians) or even as coauthors of more traditional medical research that have come out of the collaborative [26, 27].

Though the concept of patient and family engagement has been discussed and utilized to a varying degree for many years, the expanded concept of coproduction is less widely recognized. Implementing robust future collaboration with patients and families using similar approaches is likely to become increasingly common and intertwined in care delivery and ultimately improve patient outcomes across pediatric healthcare.

Conclusion

Teamwork and collaboration is particularly important in quality improvement work. Healthcare systems are complex, and improving them requires extensive knowledge of how each piece fits into delivering optimal patient care, and no one individual can understand this. Optimizing teamwork and collaboration across organizations, while including patients and families, will likely be increasingly essential to improvement efforts as healthcare reform rapidly moves us toward value-based care.

References

1. Wagner EH, Austin BT, Davis C, Hindmarsh M, Schaefer J, Bonomi A. Improving chronic illness care: translating evidence into action. Health Aff. 2001;20(6):64–78. doi:10.1377/hlthaff.20.6.64.
2. Silow-Carroll S, Alteras T, Meyer JA. Hospital quality improvement: strategies and lessons from U.S. hospitals. Quality. New York: The Commonwealth Fund pub 1009. http://www.commonwealthfund.org/Publications/Fund-Reports/2007/Apr/Hospital-Quality-Improvement--Strategies-and-Lessons-From-U-S--Hospitals.aspx (2007).
3. Hughes RG. Section VI: tools for quality improvement and patient safety. Patient Saf Qual Evid Handb Nurses. 2008:1–39.
4. Leonard M. The human factor: the critical importance of effective teamwork and communication in providing safe care. Qual Saf Heal Care. 2004;13 Suppl 1:i85–i90. doi:10.1136/qshc.2004.010033.
5. Langley GL, Moen R, Nolan KM, Nolan TW, Norman CL, Provost LP. The improvement guide: a practical approach to enhancing organizational performance. 2nd ed. San Francisco: Jossey-Bass Publishers; 2009.
6. James BC, Foss J. Features of effective teams (video lecture). Salt Lake City: Intermountain Healthcare Institute for Healthcare Delivery Research; 2009.
7. Nelson EC, Batalden PB, Lazar JS, eds. Practice-based learning and improvement: a clinical improvement action guide. 2nd ed. Oakbrook Terrance, IL: Joint Commission Resources, Inc; 2007.
8. Bleakley A, Boyden J, Hobbs A, Walsh L, Allard J. Improving teamwork climate in operating theatres: the shift from multiprofessionalismto interprofessionalism. J Interprof Care. 2006;20(5):461–70. doi:10.1080/13561820600921915.
9. Edmondson AC. Teaming: how organizations learn, innovate, and compete in the knowledge economy. San Francisco: Jossey-Bass; 2012.
10. Valentine M, Edmondson AC. Team scaffolds: how mesolevel structures enable role-based coordination in temporary groups. Organ Sci. 2015;26(2):405–22.
11. Tuckman B, Jensen MAC. Stages of small-group development revisited. Group Organ Manage. 1977;2(4):419–27.
12. Pentland A. Building great teams. Harv Bus Rev. 2012;90(4):60–70.
13. Hart P, Irving L. Janis' victims of groupthink. Political Psychol. 1991;12(2):247–78.
14. Ungerleider JD, Ungerleider RM. Seven practices of highly resonant teams. In: Da Cruz ME, Ivy D, Jaggers J, editors. Pediatric and congenital cardiology, cardiac surgery and intensive care. London: Springer London; 2014. p. 3423–50. doi:10.1007/978-1-4471-4619-3_78.
15. Edmondson AC. Teamwork on the Fly. Harv Bus Rev. 2012;90(4):72–80.
16. Edmondson AC. The kinds of teams health care needs. Harv Bus Rev. 2015. p. 2–5.
17. Berwick DM. A primer on leading the improvement of systems. BMJ. 1996;312(7031):619–22. doi:10.1136/bmj.312.7031.619.
18. Langley G, Moen R, Nolan K, et al. The improvement guide: a practical approach to enhancing organizational performance. 2nd ed. San Francisco: Jossey-Bass; 2009.
19. Lewis Software testing and continuous quality improvement, vol. 3. Boca Raton: Auerbach Publications; 2009.
20. Kon A. The shared decision-making continuum. J Am Med Assoc. 2010;304(8):903–4.
21. Institute of Medicine. Crossing the quality chasm: a new health system for the 21th century. Inst Med. 2001:1–8. doi:10.17226/10027.
22. Internet Citation: The SHARE approach: a model for shared decision making - fact sheet. Content last reviewed September 2016. Rockville: Agency for Healthcare Research and Quality. http://www.ahrq.gov/professionals/education/curriculum-tools/shareddecisionmaking/tools/sharefactsheet/index.html.

23. Batalden M, Batalden P, Margolis P, Seid M, Armstrong G, Opipari-Arrigan L, Hartung H. Coproduction of healthcare service. BMJ Qual Saf. 2016;25(7):509–17.
24. Kaplan M. Co-production: a new lens on patient-centered care. April 1 2016. Institute for Healthcare Improvement. http://www.ihi.org/communities/blogs/_layouts/ihi/community/blog/itemview.aspx.
25. Clauss SB, Anderson JB, Lannon C, Lihn S, Beekman RH, Kugler JD, Martin GR. Quality improvement through collaboration: the National Pediatric Quality Improvement Collaborative Initiative. Curr Opin Pediatr. 2015;27(5):555–62.
26. Lihn SL, Kugler JD, Peterson LE, Lannon CM, Pickels D, Beekman RH. Transparency in a pediatric quality improvement collaborative: a passionate journey by NPC-QIC clinicians and parents. Congenit Heart Dis. 2015;10(6):572–80.
27. Brown DW, Mangeot C, Anderson JB, Peterson LE, King EC, Lihn SL, Neish SR, Fleishman C, Phelps C, Hanke S, Beekman RH, Lannon CM. Digoxin use is associated with reduced interstage mortality in patients with no history of arrhythmia after stage 1 palliation for single ventricle heart disease. J Am Heart Assoc. 2016;5(1)

Chapter 5
QI Methods and Improvement Science

Lori Rutman and Selena Hariharan

Definition of Improvement

On its own, improvement is a difficult term to define. Improvement is most clearly understood when it is defined by characteristics with a positive connotation like faster, easier, more efficient, safer, or less expensive. All of these characteristics have one thing in common—they require change from a current state, the baseline. Thus, improvement is the outcome achieved when a system has undergone some fundamental change for the better. In an ideal state, the effects of the improvement are sustained and have a lasting impact on the system.

Not all changes will lead to improvement. Improvement is driven by the application of knowledge about the current state, the desired state, and the context of the system you are working in. There are a variety of methods by which the quality of patient care can be improved, such as Lean and Six Sigma [1, 2]. The Institute for Healthcare Improvement (IHI) supports a method based on the Model for Improvement. The Model for Improvement, described in Chap. 2, is a framework for applying the following five principles of improvement.

Five guiding principles of improvement [3]:

1. Knowing why you need to improve
2. Having a feedback mechanism to tell you if the improvement is happening
3. Developing an effective change that will result in improvement

L. Rutman (✉)
Division of Pediatric Emergency Medicine, Seattle Children's Hospital,
4800 Sand Point Way NE, Seattle, WA 98105, USA
e-mail: Lori.Rutman@seattlechildrens.org

S. Hariharan
Division of Pediatric Emergency Medicine, Cincinnati Children's Hospital Medical Center,
3333 Burnet Avenue, Cincinnati, OH 45229, USA
e-mail: Selena.hariharan@cchmc.org

© Springer International Publishing AG 2017
C.E. Dandoy et al. (eds.), *Patient Safety and Quality in Pediatric Hematology/Oncology and Stem Cell Transplantation*, DOI 10.1007/978-3-319-53790-0_5

4. Testing a change before attempting to implement broadly
5. Knowing when and how to make the change permanent (implement the change)

We will explore each of these principles in more detail through this chapter using the following example:

> As the quality leader in your oncology division, you would like to improve time to antibiotics (TTA) for oncology patients who present to the emergency department (ED) with fever and concern for infection. You recognize the national benchmark for TTA is 60 minutes or less, and after reviewing your hospital's data over the past year, you find the average TTA in your ED is currently twice that, 120 minutes. In fact, only 25% of immunosuppressed patients with fever receive antibiotics within 60 minutes. Further, in the past 6 months the hospital patient safety team has identified an increase in ICU transfers for oncology patients related to need for initiation of vasoactive medications. The team believes one reason for the clinical deterioration of these patients is delay of initial antibiotics. When the individual patient charts are reviewed, the team finds a number of problems, ranging from port access issues to protocol deviations and communication failures.

The first principle of improvement, knowing why you need to improve, is sometimes referred to as the aim or purpose of the improvement project. The improvement aim of the oncology team above was clear; they first needed to make changes to the processes surrounding TTA to deal with the time delays.

Selection of a Global and Project Aim

Improvement projects should begin by addressing the first question of the Model for Improvement, "What are we trying to accomplish?" This requires development of an aim statement. To be effective, an aim statement should be developed in collaboration with leadership and frontline staff in response to an observed problem [4]. A clearly written aim statement is critical for a successful improvement project and serves several purposes. For example, a clearly written aim statement provides leadership with an understanding of the purpose of your project and therefore promotes leadership buy-in and support. Further, an aim statement will help clarify who should be part of the improvement team. It also reduces variation from the project's original purpose; when stakeholders begin to push different agendas, an aim statement serves as an effective reminder of the project's intended scope. Finally, an aim statement defines the magnitude of the expected improvement and sets an expected timeline for achieving results.

The aim statement may be divided into a global aim, which describes the long-term goals of the process under evaluation, and a project, or specific aim, which is narrow in scope and related to the current team's work. The specific aim for a project, often referred to as a SMART aim, should be specific, measurable, actionable, relevant, and time bound [3]. To do this, the specific aim statement should clearly state the process/system which will be the subject of the work, the desired outcome, the timeline during which the team will accomplish the work, and the magnitude of change that is expected.

With this information, you write down the following global and specific aim statements for the TTA improvement project:

Global aim: Improve outcomes by providing timely and effective care to immunosuppressed patients with fever.

Specific aim: Increase and maintain the percentage of febrile immunosuppressed (F&I) oncology patients who receive their antibiotics in the ED within 60 minutes from 25% to 90% over the next 12 months.

Analysis of the Existing Process

Prior to attempting any improvement project, a thorough analysis of the existing process should be undertaken. All stakeholders, which may include but are not limited to physicians, nurses, patient services, ancillary staff, administrators, patients and their families, consultants, and external supports, should be included [5]. Representatives from this group then create a comprehensive operational map of the flow of the process from the first to the last step. If the process map is created properly, potential areas of operational failure, both those that currently exist, and potential future areas of weakness can be identified more easily. These can be described in a healthcare failure mode and effect analysis (HFMEA). First used in engineering, the failure modes and effects analysis (FMEA) uses a proactive approach to identify vulnerabilities in a system or product to prevent failures [6]. The HFMEA expands the engineering approach to a more comprehensive, systematic approach that can be applied to healthcare operations to improve processes and hopefully prevent safety failures [6]. This is particularly relevant in healthcare where the product is the process itself [7].

You assemble a quality improvement (QI) team that includes key stakeholders in oncology and emergency medicine (physicians, nurse practitioners, nurses, clerical staff, clinic managers) as well as a few interested oncology patients and families. You review the aim statements with the team and develop an HFMEA for the process (Fig. 5.1). The QI team then pictographically represents potential failures as a Pareto chart which shows a cumulative histogram of failures from the direct observation period. (Fig. 5.2)

The next step is to create a process map. To start, key stakeholders meet and discuss the process from start to finish. They then observe the process "in action." When the group meets again, depending on the improvement theory the team has chosen to implement, they create a map of the process. Process maps help clarify complex processes by showing decisions, events, wait times, and delays in care. The process map helps draw a picture of how a process works and serves as a base that can be used as the team transforms the currently existing process.

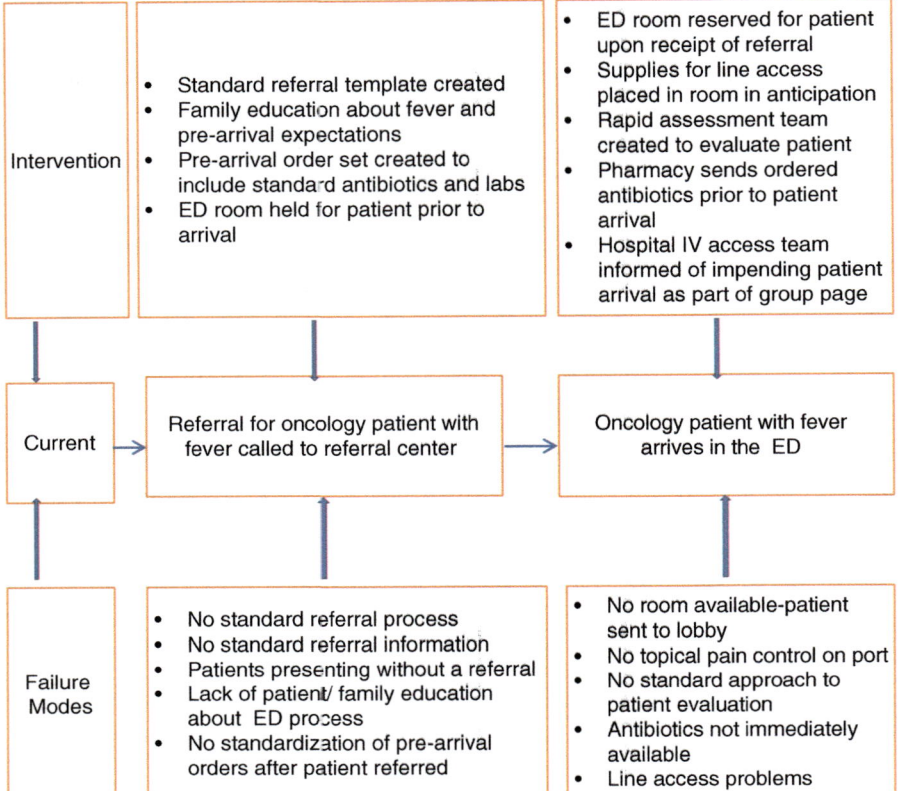

Fig. 5.1 Healthcare failure modes and effects analysis (HFMEA) for time to antibiotics for oncology patients who present to the emergency department with fever

Steps to Create a Process Map

It is important to have representatives of all the roles involved in the process that participate in the creation of the process map. Start with a high-level process map which will contain the various steps that are imperative to the process (Fig. 5.3). After the high-level process map is finished, a detailed process map should be completed. The detailed process map includes decisions as well as all subprocesses (Fig. 5.4). After completing the process maps, the team should validate them with other individuals.

At that time, potential interventions are reviewed and a first series of trials are planned based on improvement theory. Theories are grand (global and general), big (concepts that can be applied across projects), and small (pragmatic and applicable

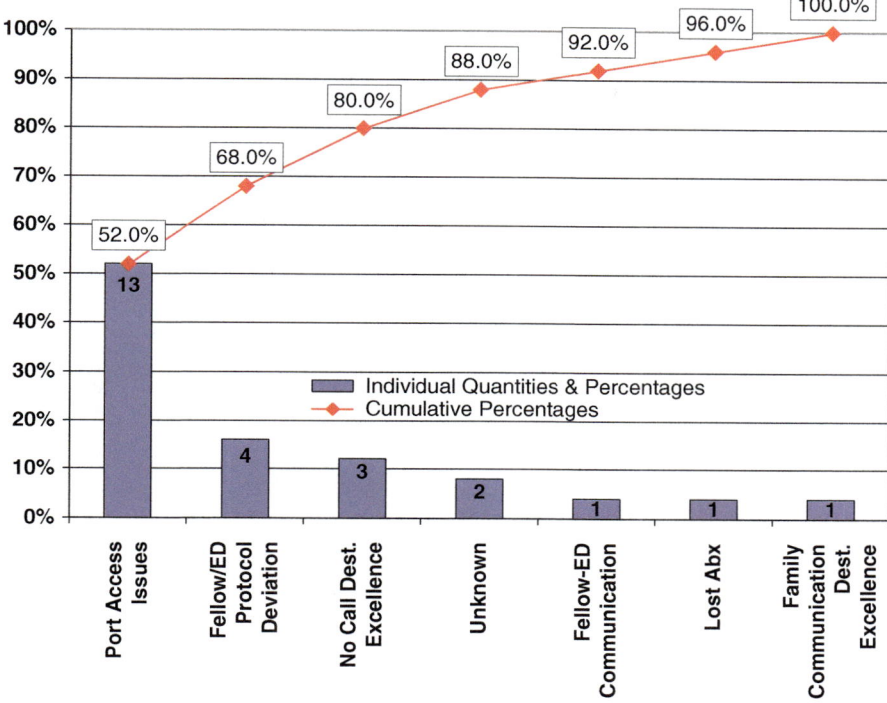

Fig. 5.2 Pareto chart: Oncology patients who did not receive antibiotics within 60 min of arrival in the ED

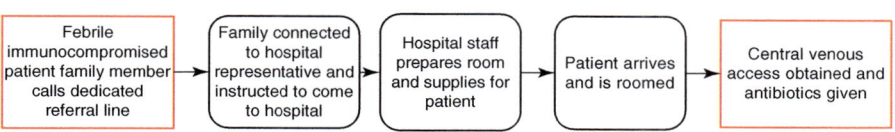

Fig. 5.3 High-level process map

to a specific improvement) [8]. After the failures are identified and the Pareto chart created, the team can identify barriers to improvement, develop key drivers, and plan the first improvement intervention. On the other hand, if the project is focusing on Lean methodology and eliminating waste, the observation period will identify process steps that are valuable to the patient (value added) and those that may be necessary but are non-value added [9].

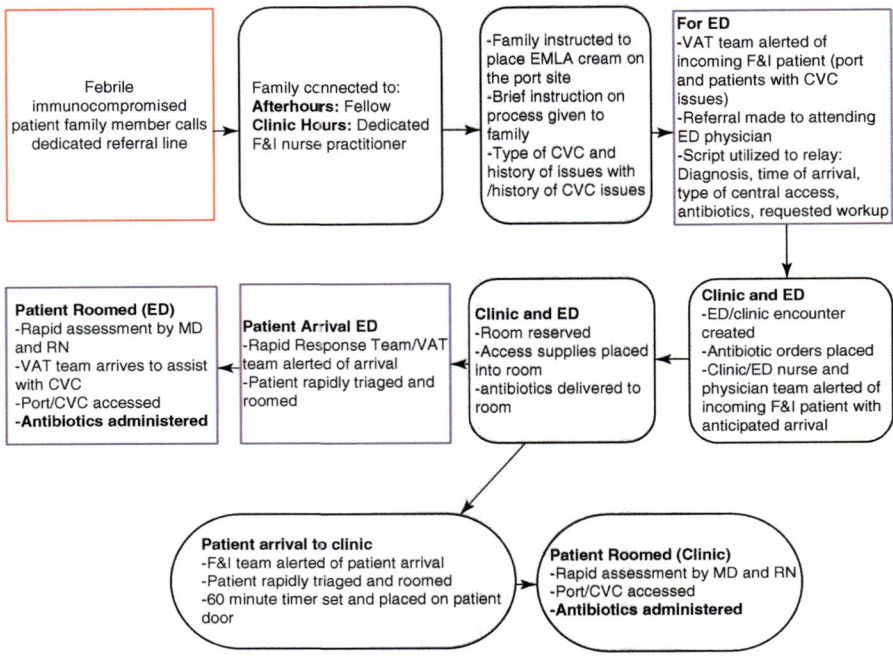

Fig. 5.4 Detailed process map

Identification of Barriers

Inevitably, the people involved in an improvement team are enthusiastic, optimistic, and invested in the success of the new process. Unfortunately, this can cause them to overlook potential barriers to success. During the analysis of the existing process, it is essential that the members of the group honestly evaluate potential pitfalls that may be associated with changing the process in an attempt to improve. This starts by looking at the existing culture and infrastructure theoretically then directly observing the providers. Once the barriers are identified, they further inform the key drivers, described below:

After further consideration and honest discussions, the QI team identified the following potential barriers to improving TTA:

1. A culture that was resistant to standardizing patient care
2. Staff entropy
3. Comfort with silos of care and a lack of collegiality between services
4. Family expectations that did not align with standards of care
5. Acceptance of failure as a part of business as usual

Honesty is essential when identifying impediments to process improvement. It is human nature to believe that fault lies elsewhere—another person, another service, and another team within the hospital—but for any process to succeed, the silos must be razed and staff engaged. Obstacles are best removed when the staff as a whole perceives themselves to be part of the team as opposed to drafted soldiers being forced into labor; indeed, in those situations, the staff simply becomes another hurdle to overcome in the path of improvement.

Barriers can also be divided into organizational and personal. Though quality improvement is a growing field, some organizations simply do not have the infrastructure or the financial resources to undertake a large-scale quality improvement project [10]. Some organizations are ineffective at communicating the underlying vision of the quality improvement; hence, leadership does not attain support for the process at the grassroots level. Even if employees are ready to undertake quality improvement, sometimes leadership does not understand how to empower frontline providers, so these individuals are not ready to accept the responsibility for the process [11]. Individually, barriers include resistance to standardizing care (i.e., disdain for "cookbook medicine"), personal biases about patients, the organization and leadership, and limitations in skill [11].

Identification of Key Drivers

A driver diagram is a tool for building a testable hypothesis. It illustrates the structures, processes, and norms that may need to change in order for the system to operate at a new, improved level. Similar to conceptual models, a well-designed driver diagram clarifies the theory behind an improvement project and informs the strategy for achieving the aim (outcome). Driver diagrams also provide a framework for measurement, inform evaluation, and allow for comparison of projects across different organizations and researchers.

When creating a driver diagram, the aim statement (desired outcome) is traditionally located on the far left; everything to the right of the aim statement depicts a theory about what must change and how it must change to achieve the desired outcome. The items to the right of the aim statement are known as key drivers. Generally speaking, key drivers are the elements present in a system that must be considered as leverage points when developing a plan for change. Key drivers may be further broken down into primary and secondary drivers.

Primary drivers are high-level elements in the system that must change to accomplish the outcome of interest. These include the structures (physical space, equipment, technology), processes (workflow, protocols), and operating norms (culture, organizational psychology) that define the system in its current state [12]. Depending on the scope of the improvement project, secondary drivers may also be relevant. Secondary drivers are more specific, actionable items within the system that can be acted upon when introducing change.

Ideally, a driver diagram should be constructed by working closely with subject matter experts who work directly with the system of interest; they will know the

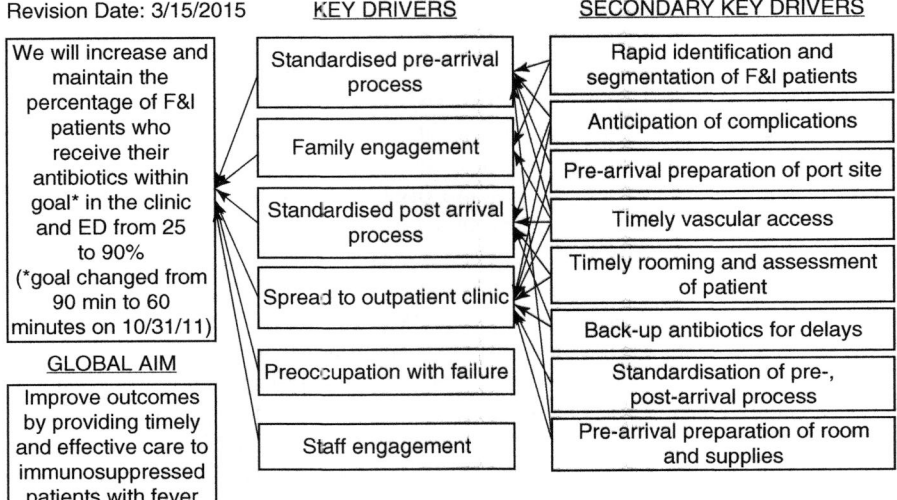

Revision Date: 3/15/2015   KEY DRIVERS   SECONDARY KEY DRIVERS

Fig. 5.5 Driver diagram: Improving time to antibiotics in febrile oncology patients

system best and will likely be able to provide a high-yield list of key drivers. The following steps may then be followed to create a driver diagram:

1. Write out the global aim and SMART aim statements for your improvement project.
2. List all key leverage points or "drivers" in your system that will require change to achieve your aim.
3. Logically group drivers and identify high-level primary drivers (structure/process/culture) and more specific, actionable elements (secondary drivers).
4. Draw connecting arrows to show causal relationships.

The QI team identified key drivers related to structures (spread to the outpatient clinic), processes (standardized pre-arrival and post-arrival processes), and operating norms (family and staff engagement, preoccupation with failure). Further, the team was able to identify secondary drivers such as pre-arrival preparation of port sites, timely rooming and assessment of patients, and availability of back up antibiotics for delays. These drivers were organized into a driver diagram for your improvement project. (Fig. 5.5)

Root Cause Analysis and Understanding of Failures

Root cause analysis (RCA) is a structured method used to analyze failures and serious events and is utilized as an error analysis tool in healthcare. RCA helps identify underlying problems that increase the likelihood of errors utilizing a systems approach to identify both active errors (errors occurring at the point of interface between humans and a complex system) and latent errors (the hidden problems within healthcare systems that contribute to adverse events).

Plan-Do-Study-Act

In order to effectively create solutions in quality improvement, study the effects and determine if the process change versus any of a number of potential confounders created the improvement; a quality improvement team must use a systematic approach. The most commonly adopted in quality improvement is a variation of the "Deming Wheel" or the "Plan-Do-Study-Act" (PDSA) approach [11]. In the PDSA model, during the **P**lan, a hypothesis is generated; while "**D**oing," data is collected; the data is **S**tudied; this data creates the foundation for future **A**ctions [14]. These are also called "PDSA ramps" as each phase builds on the previous to become more comprehensive. As each PDSA cycle is looking to show a specific and causal improvement, often only one or two subjects are included in the initial test ramp to establish a baseline; as additional cycles are undertaken, more subjects can be included [4, 14]. Additionally, in the interest of time and resources, while in the initial phase with small groups of subjects, multiple PDSA cycles can be run in parallel then aggregated to create the next PDSA ramp using the data collected. It is important, however, to note each of these interventions on a run chart so those analyzing or attempting to recreate the process can do so accurately [4]. Once all ramps are complete, interventions that fall into similar categories can be grouped for ease of data reporting, but the discrete data should be maintained for integrity, so anyone who wants to recreate the process can do so.

Looking at each step individually:

Plan

During the planning phase, several questions must be asked. Done properly, the answers obtained from the first PDSA cycle will generate questions for the next PDSA, so asking relevant and answerable questions for the first ramp is integral to the success of the project. These include [4]:

– The objective
– Key drivers to be tested
– How to measure the impact (for this PDSA may not be the final project measure)
– Predictions

> One of the key drivers your team identified in trying to improve TTA was to standardize the pre-arrival process. This involved multiple steps, so a PDSA was created for one of the steps, the pre-arrival referral, which was a secondary driver of the key driver of interest, standardization of the pre-arrival process. The objective was to evaluate if creating a standard referral page and template in the electronic medical record would improve standardization of information available to providers. The process owners hypothesized that physicians in the ED who input patient referrals would be more compliant with referral standardization after creation of an accessible template than before. Referrals for oncology patients with fever who presented to the emergency department were analyzed before and after the intervention to determine if the intervention was successful [13].

Do

Doing the test involves the following [4]:

– Do the test.
– Collect data and feedback.
– Make note of unexpected outcomes so these can be incorporated in planning for the next cycle.

The referral template was introduced to providers at a staff meeting. Additionally, the process owners spoke to individual providers and were in the ED during the initial phases of the PDSA ramp. The template included a pre-populated check list that automatically pulled data like diagnosis, last clinic weight, and allergies about the patient from the existing medical record. The physician would then only have to answer a few questions including antibiotic of choice, time of arrival and type of access. During the initial phase, there were several free text questions asked. Process owners measured compliance with use of the template. They also spoke with all the stakeholders in the referral process to reveal any barriers to success [13].

Study

Studying the test requires analyzing both the test itself and the data collected [4]:

– Was the test done as planned?
– Was the test feasible and reasonable in the existing system?
– Was the hypothesis upheld or disproven?

The QI team assessed whether the referral template was used during the proposed testing period and surveyed providers about the ease of use, effect on work flow, and content. They then analyzed whether the providers working during the test period in fact used the available template and whether this referral increased standardization of information available to providers [13].

Act

Learnings from the test are used to either adapt the test process and create the next PDSA ramp, to adopt the new process if it was successful, or to abandon the process altogether if the test was unsuccessful and the data showed the hypothesis was unfounded [4]. Abandoning an idea should not be considered a failure but rather an example of the PDSA process working as wasting time on unsuccessful ramps in a desire to prove an unfounded hypothesis is a waste of resources and energy that could be spent on creating a new PDSA cycle.

The initial test on the oncology referral template demonstrated that providers were in fact willing to use a standard process for referral for a select population; however, they found the template itself difficult to find in the electronic medical record and the information within the template too extensive. As a result, subsequent PDSA ramps focused initially on making the template easier to access in the medical record then on improving the content. The current iteration is the result of several improvement cycles with small volumes of patients [13].

Ultimately, while there are many ways to trial new quality improvement ideas, the PDSA format allows for small trials with a few subjects at a time and mirrors traditional research methodology that most providers are familiar with. It also encourages a stepwise approach and rapid abandonment of an unsuccessful process, hopefully saving time and resources. As a result, even small practices can trial the PDSA format.

Testing (Adapt or Abandon)

After testing a potential improvement, the team must decide whether to adopt, adapt, or abandon the new process. While the testing team often has a personal investment in showing that the new process was successful, it is important to avoid personal bias when deciding whether to implement the improvement on a widespread basis or not.

Most hospital systems have processes already in place that are amenable to small, initial tests of change and PDSAs that focus on the improvement team's SMART aim. By using existing systems and personnel, the team has a better chance to convince staff and administration that the PDSA is worthwhile and will not unnecessarily strain the existing infrastructure. If the small test is successful, ensuing PDSAs can be more ambitious. All tests are temporary, and by making preliminary endeavors small and manageable, the team can learn what works best in the existing hospital system and with the current staff. Hopefully, this will also increase buy-in for future testing.

If the test does not show any improvement or if the risk/benefit ratio is not favorable, the team should not be hesitant to abandon an improvement trial. Admitting failure and moving onto another test of change demonstrates an understanding of the underlying PDSA process and shows both peers and administration that the team is open-minded and willing to continually consider the consequences of all actions.

Implementation (Adopt)

If the improvement team is fortunate enough to find that the test of change created a positive change in the tested environment, the members of the team can choose to adopt the new process. To adopt a new process, the team should first discuss the process with the providers who will be responsible for implementing the change in the clinical environment to ensure acceptance. Once this is done, widespread education can begin. Once the newly adopted process is an established part of the clinical routine, it can be used as a starting point for the next PDSA.

Pitfalls of PDSA Cycles

While the PDSA cycle is not a traditional hypothesis-driven method for research, sloppy methodology can still result in inaccurate improvement testing and, as a result, an unpleasant or even dangerous clinical environment. As a result, it is important to follow rigorous methods when doing improvement testing. First, prior to starting the PDSA cycle, the team should have a clear aim and prediction in mind about the test cycle. The members should write down the aim and the method of the PDSA and review these with the team both before and after testing. While it is acceptable for a PDSA cycle to be small and involve only a few subjects, it should not be so small that the data collected is unreliable or biased, especially if the results are skewed in favor of the results the team desires. Finally, the test should be run a few different times in a few different but appropriate clinical environments to ensure that the outcome is accurate prior to implementation.

> When your testing group implemented the fever, immune compromise order set and tested for the first time, there was an ice storm. As a result, the emergency department had record low volumes and only one oncology patient presented during the week of testing He received his antibiotics in 20 minutes. The team was ecstatic and ready to change the system entirely. Two weeks later, after school had restarted, the clinic had a flood so all oncology patients were referred to the ED and ED census was at a record high, 10 oncology patients were seen in the ED and 3 did not receive antibiotics within sixty minutes.

PDSA Ramp

Small tests are rarely stand alone; therefore, you should start to prepare the next test based upon your predictions. Often a change idea will go through multiple PDSA cycles as data is collected (this is called a PDSA ramp); large-scale tests of changes may require multiple concurrent PDSA ramps before implementation.

Large-scale implementation is viewed in quality improvement as a series or "ramp" of PDSAs, each one larger or under different conditions. When you have evidence that an idea is reliable in one area, further tests and ramps can be spread to the new environment.

Sustainability

Once a QI process has been tested and modified through a robust PDSA ramp, and successfully implemented, it is imperative that infrastructure is in place to sustain improvement. There are several key components of sustainability, described below.

Supportive Management Structure

In order to support sustainability, the division's leadership must consider the process a high priority, devoting regular attention, creating accountability systems for improvement, and recognizing successes.

Structures to "Foolproof" Change

To further support sustainability, the organization should build structures that make it difficult—if not impossible—for providers of care to revert to old ways of doing things. For example, clear documentation of the process in the form of guidelines, job aids, and training materials may reduce variability and prevent drift from the improved state. In addition, tools such as checklists, prepackaged "kits" or carts of materials needed for the intervention, and technology to support sustained implementation of the intervention may be developed and employed.

Robust, Transparent Feedback Systems

As much of the organization as possible should be aware of performance on key indicators, reviewing information generated by a measurement system, comparing it to clear standards set by management, and taking part in improvements devised in response.

Formal Capacity-Building Programs

Once an organization has been successful in developing, implementing, and sustaining improvements, it is important to develop formal capacity-building programs. Such programs promote growth of the improvement efforts and also ensure that future generations of providers maintain and sustain the work that has already been implemented.

Finally, while less tangible than the components of sustainability described above, perhaps one of the most important factors resulting in sustainability is the culture of the division or organization. In an ideal state, the culture should be one that supports change and is willing to work to sustain improvements. This culture of improvement is most easily attained when key stakeholders have been engaged from the start and there is a shared sense of the systems to be improved.

Conclusion

Improvement is driven by the application of knowledge about the current state, the desired state, and the context of the system you are working in. Setting clear aims and using tools such as process maps and driver diagrams early in your improvement work will establish a foundation and rationale for your efforts and will inform the selection of changes you test. Testing changes through multiple Plan-Do-Study-Act cycles will enable further refinement prior to formal implementation and spread. Finally, developing infrastructure and culture to sustain improvements over time is of key importance.

References

1. D'Andreamatteo A, Ianni I, Lega F, Sargiacomo M. Lean in healthcare: a comprehensive review. Health Policy. 2015;119(15):1197–209.
2. DelliFraine JL, Wang Z, McCaughey D, Langabeer II JR, Erwin CO. The use of six sigma in health care management: are we using it to its full potential? Qual Manag Health Care. 2014;23(4):240–53.
3. Langley GJMR, Nolan KM, Nolan TW, Norman CL, Provost LP. The improvement guide: a practical approach to enhancing organizational performance. 2nd ed. San Francisco: Jossey-Bass; 2009.
4. Kurowski EM, Schondelmeyer AC, Brown C, Dandoy CE, Hanke SJ, Cooley HLT. A practical guide to conducting quality improvement in the health care setting. Curr Treat Options Pediatr. 2015;1(4):380–92.
5. Curtis JR, Cook DJ, Wall RJ, Angus DC, Bion J, Kacmarek R, et al. Intensive care unit quality improvement: a "how-to" guide for the interdisciplinary team. Crit Care Med. 2006;34(1):211–8.
6. DeRosier J, Stalhandske E, Bagian JP, Nudell T. Using health care failure mode and effect analysis™: the VA National Center for patient safety's prospective risk analysis system. Jt Comm J Qual Improv. 2002;28(5):248–67.
7. Guo L, Hariharan S. Patients are not cars and staff is not robots: impact of differences between manufacturing and clinical operations on process improvement. Knowledge Process Manage. 2012;19(2):53–68.
8. Davidoff F, Dixon-Woods M, Leviton L, Michie S. Demystifying theory and its use in improvement. BMJ Qual Saf. 2015:1–11. doi:10.1136/bmjqs-2014-003627.
9. Toussaint JS, Berry LL. The promise of lean in health care. Mayo Clin Proc. 2013;88(1):74–82.
10. Guo, L, Hariharan SL. Is process improvement the ultimate solution? Physician Leadership Journal. 2016;3(5):26–30.
11. Walley P, Gowland B. Completing the circle: from PD to PDSA. Int J Health Care Qual Assur. 2004;17(6):349–58.
12. Bennett B, Provost L. What's your theory? Driver diagram serves as a tool for building and testing theories for improvement. Qual Prog 2015;38–43.
13. Dandoy CE, Hariharan SL, Weiss B, Demmel K, Timm N, Chiarenzelli J, et al. Sustained reductions in time to antibiotic delivery in febrile immunocompromised children: results of a quality improvement collaborative. BMJ Qual Saf. 2015:1–10. doi:10.1136/bmjqs-2015-004451.
14. Speroff T, O'Conner GT. Study designs for PDSA quality improvement research. Qual Manage Healthcare. 2004;13(1):17–32.

Chapter 6
Measuring for Improvement

Rachel Thienprayoon, Kathy Demmel, and Lloyd P. Provost

Successful measurement is a cornerstone of successful improvement. How do you know if the changes you are making are leading to improvement? To answer this fundamental question, some type of feedback loop is required. Measurement is usually the best way to provide that feedback.

In healthcare organizations, measurements are often used for reporting aggregate results using summary statistics to government authorities, payors, and other parties that evaluate the data against specific standards or guidelines. This "measurement for judgment" can be understandably daunting to staff and become a central focus for measurement efforts in an organization. So measurement for improvement has to compete with this existing demand for data. Here are some guidelines in developing measures for improvement teams [1]:

- A few key measures that clarify the aim of the improvement effort and make it tangible should be regularly reported throughout the project (5–8 measures reported daily, weekly, or monthly, depending on the length of time for the project).
- Be careful about overdoing process measures. A balance of outcome, process, and balancing measures is important (see following discussion).

R. Thienprayoon (✉)
Division of Palliative Care, Department of Anesthesia, Cincinnati Children's Hospital Medical Center, University of Cincinnati College of Medicine, Cincinnati, OH, USA
e-mail: Rachel.Thienprayoon@cchmc.org

K. Demmel
Cancer and Blood Diseases Institute, Cincinnati Children's Hospital Medical Center, Cincinnati, OH, USA
e-mail: Kathy.demmel@cchmc.org

L.P. Provost
Associates in Process Improvement, 2000 Red Hawk Road, Wimberley, TX 78676, USA
e-mail: provost.lloyd@gmail.com

© Springer International Publishing AG 2017   81
C.E. Dandoy et al. (eds.), *Patient Safety and Quality in Pediatric Hematology/ Oncology and Stem Cell Transplantation*, DOI 10.1007/978-3-319-53790-0_6

- Plot data visually on the key measures over time.
- Make use of existing databases and data already collected for developing measures.
- Whenever feasible, integrate data collection for measurement into the daily work routine.

Developing Measures for Improvement

Objectives for Improvement Measures

In improvement work, measurement and feedback are used in multiple ways:

- Identify problems and establish baseline performance.
- Provide insights into opportunities and problems in the current system to focus changes.
- Using specific measures for learning about changes during PDSA test cycles.
- Using key measures to assess progress toward the project's aim.
- Using balancing measures to assess whether the system as a whole is being improved.

Patient feedback is an important source of data for identifying potential areas for improvement. This feedback can come from complaint systems, chart notes, formal surveys, or focus groups. Another mechanism for evaluating current performance is through continuous monitoring of organization measures. For example, if performance gaps are detected in the unit's infection rate, leadership can initiate improvement projects with the aim of reducing the infection rate.

Throughout an improvement project, a balanced set of outcome, process, and balancing measures is monitored and used to assess project toward the projects aim.

The primary use of measurement in improvement projects is to inform and guide the development, testing, and implementation of changes. PDSA cycles are designed to answer specific questions about changes that the improvement team is testing. The "plan" step of the PDSA cycle involves specifying these questions and developing a data collection plan that will answer them. The measures used in these tests are specific process measures related to the change(s) being evaluated in the cycle.

Outcome, Process, and Balancing Measures

As discussed above the family of measures for an improvement project should include three types of measures:

Outcome measures are directly connected to the aim of the improvement effort. They answer the question: "How is the system performing or what are the results?" Often outcome measures are based on clinical data or the voice of the customer or patient.

Table 6.1 Example of a family of measures, taken from a project regarding cardiac monitoring alarms [2]

Type of measure	Example
Process measure	Percent compliance with cardiac monitor care process bundle (defined as the percentile of the number of completed components of the CMCP over the number of opportunities)
Process measure	Percent of patients with age-appropriate alarm settings ordered on admission
Outcome measure	Cardiac monitor alarms per monitor per day
Balancing measure	Number of code blue events that could have been avoided in the absence of the change of cardiac monitor care process

Process measures answer the question: "Are the parts/steps in the system performing as planned?" These measures provide feedback on whether the planned changes are being put in place, for example, the use of an infection reduction bundle or timely administration of antibiotics prior to surgery.

Balancing measures provide feedback on whether the changes are resulting in unintended consequences elsewhere in the system. For example, if changes in the clinical protocol implemented to accomplish the aim of improved health outcomes, some useful balancing measures might be length of stay, patient wait time, or patient satisfaction.

See Table 6.1 for an example of a family of measures for an improvement project with an aim to reduce cardiac monitoring alarms [2].

An appropriate statistic to summarize data from a period should be selected of each measure. Use percentages or rates to adjust for the impact of natural changes to the systems, such as number of patients or visits. The numerator is the key measure (costs, patients waiting, etc.), and the denominator is the unit of production or volume (total visits, total patients). Percentages or rates usually give a more useful picture than simply counting numbers of incidences. For example, if patients with complications increased dramatically, you might draw one conclusion. But if you knew that overall volume had also increased (which would show in the percent of patients with complications), you'd mostly likely draw another conclusion. Sometimes it is useful to present numerators when it is important to emphasize each case.

Collection of Data for the Measures

Types of Data

Data come from documenting observations or results of some measurement process. The two basic types of data are quantitative (numeric) and qualitative (non-numeric). Most qualitative data comes from observations, but measurements can be qualitative (e.g., blood type). Examples of qualitative data are "the customer was unable to assemble the product," "the meeting was not on schedule," and "people seemed interested in the exhibit"; the form was not completed.

While quantitative data are usually preferred for learning, there are a number of reasons to use qualitative data:

- Quantitative data can be difficult to obtain or expensive.
- The information of interest is so dramatic that qualitative data are sufficient to meet all needs.
- Observations of people best describe the phenomena of interest.

Rating scales can be used to obtain data on personal experience. These qualitative scales can be converted to quantitative data by establishing a point scale that corresponds to the word scale (e.g., 1–5). These scales along with common measurements such as time and cost will allow those improving quality in service or administrative applications to use quantitative data as readily as their manufacturing counterparts.

Traditionally from the science of improvement, there are three types of data: *classification, count,* and *continuous.* Classification and count data are often grouped together as attribute data to distinguish them from continuous data. Continuous data are often referred to as variables data. For classification data, attributes are recorded in one of two categories. Examples of these classes are conforming units/nonconforming units, go/no-go, either/or, pass/fail, or good/bad. Count data focuses on attributes that occur that are unusual or undesirable: number of mistakes, number of accidents, or number of no-shows. Often we are counting to obtain the volume or amount of a particular entity, for example, a hospital census, the number of visits to a clinic, or the volume of lab tests completed. These counts are treated as continuous data because of their intent.

Sources of Data

Data are documented observations or the results of performing a measurement process. The concept of data refers to strings or patterns of characters (e.g., computer bits) that describe some aspect of the world. The availability of data offers opportunities to obtain information and knowledge through inquiry, analysis, or summarization of these strings or characters. Data can be obtained by perception (e.g., observation) or by performing a measurement process. Table 6.2 shows sources of data each of the measures from the example above regarding decreasing cardiac monitor alarms [2].

Observations come from perceptions: sight, taste, smell, hearing, and touch. Observations are a valuable source of data, but there are some weaknesses with relying only on observations when learning or testing changes for improvement:

1. Recent observations tend to be more heavily weighted in our minds than observations from the more distant past.

Table 6.2 Sources of data for each of the measures in Table 6.1 [2]

Example	Source of data
Percent compliance with cardiac monitor care process bundle (defined as the percentile of the number of completed components of the CMCP over the number of opportunities)	Monitor log
Percent of patients with age-appropriate alarm settings ordered on admission	Patient electronic medical record
Cardiac monitor alarms per monitor per day	Monitor log
Number of code blue events that could have been avoided in the absence of the change of cardiac monitor care process	Intensive care unit data

2. New observations depend on previous observations. If we are used to a temperature of 30 degrees, a temperature of 60 degrees feels warm. But if we are used to a temperature of 95 degrees, 60 degrees feels cool.

3. Our minds automatically filter perceptions. Sometimes we observe what we want or expect to observe.

Because of the first three issues, improvement teams learn better from data based on measurements than on observations. Measuring a patient's temperature may help us learn more and faster than the patient's perception of whether or not they have a fever.

This doesn't mean that data from observation isn't useful; sometimes it's very important to learning and improvement. Recording data from patient's perceptions of their pain level, for instance, could be a valuable aid to learning about and improving patient pain levels. And many times, no measurement process is available. Combining observation and measurement data is a useful approach to obtaining data for improvement, for example, measurement on cycle time for admitting patients combined with patient and staff observations related to their experience of the process.

Operational Definitions

If we are going to obtain data useful for improving a healthcare process, we need that data to help us learn when changes we make are an improvement. Earlier in this chapter, we addressed the importance of ensuring that measures are useful for improvement. Many measures start as accountability measures, and, while useful for judgment, they are of limited usefulness for improvement. If the data are collected differently by different people, or differently each time we collect the data, it makes it hard to know if changes in the data are due to the changes we hope are an improvement or from inconsistencies in our data collection. In order to learn from our data, we need an agreement as to how the data will be collected in order to maintain data collection consistency.

Operational Definition: Codes Outside the ICU
Measurement: Codes Outside the ICU

1. Description and Rationale

This measure answers the question: Are we recognizing and acting upon the patient conditions that indicate a potential or imminent code, and moving such patients to an ICU?

This measure is the number of code alerts requiring chest compressions or assisted ventilation that occur outside the Critical Care Areas per 1000 hospital patient days. Hospital Patient days exclude PICU, CICU, RCNIC and College Hill patients.

2. Population Definition (Inclusions/Exclusions)

All Inpatients (including Short Stays)

3. Data Source(s)

CCHMC Division of Critical Care Medicine

4. Sampling and Data Collection Plan

All patients admitted to the hospital as inpatients or short stay patients are included.

5. Calculation

Numerator: Number of code alerts requiring chest compressions or assisted ventilation that occur outside the Critical Care Areas

Denominator: Number of hospital patient days. Hospital Patient days will exclude PICU, CICU, RCNIC and College Hill patients.

This is reported as a rate per 1000 patient days ((numerator/denominator)*1000)

6. Analysis Plan and Frequency of Reporting

Data is collected and reported quarterly. A run chart is available.

7. Reporting Venues

Results are reported on the CCHMC Hospital Scorecard under "Health Care Delivery"

Results are reported on the Inpatient CSI Dashboard

Quarterly run chart is posted on Centerlink under Patient Safety (link entitled, "CPR Aggregate Data")

An operational definition is the term used for such an agreement. An operational definition is a definition that gives communicable meaning to a concept (such as error, waiting time, and appropriate care) by specifying how the concept is applied within a particular set of circumstances. An important component of an operational definition is the statement of the measurement process used. We use operational definitions in collecting healthcare data. The example above shows an operational definition for code blue events outside of the intensive care unit (ICU) at Cincinnati Children's Hospital Medical Center.

To develop an operational definition, we need to come to agreement on two things:

1. A method of measurement or test
2. A set of criteria for judgment

Measurements could be for physical characteristics, like pulmonary capacity, and make use of a measurement device. The operational definition then needs to bring clarity to which device(s) will be used, how they will be used, how the users will know the devices' precision (calibration and statistical stability), and to what degree of discretion the data will be collected (i.e., whole number or one or more decimal place).

A set of criteria for judgment may be necessary in some situations. What constitutes an error, a fall, or a delay? Sometimes we need to take a measurement and convert it to an attribute that was either possessed or not possessed when we obtained the measurement. For example, to operationally define "late," we measure time in an agreed-upon fashion. We still need some criteria to judge at what point "late" is declared. What are the agreed-upon criteria for deciding something is "late" or "appropriate"? Agreed-upon criteria for judging such concepts are crucial if we are going to learn whether or not our change was an improvement.

Often an operational definition is converted into a checklist or form that delineates what is meant by "appropriate" or "complete" and helps multiple data collectors to remain consistent in their use of the operational definition. Table 6.3 is an example of a checklist for patients who undergo code events outside of the intensive care unit or critical care areas. In this example, if the answer is "yes" to the first question and any other question in the checklist, the event qualifies as a code event outside of critical care areas.

In some cases, consider sampling when developing the data collection plan to get "just enough data" to see if changes are leading to improvement. In general, a bigger sample creates more stable and reliable results. However, it may not show the effect of interventions or changes over time, which is most important when pursuing

Table 6.3 Operational definition example: a checklist for patients who undergo code events outside of the intensive care unit

Criterion	Yes or no
Patient is not located in a critical care area	
Patient received chest compressions	
Patient was not previously receiving positive pressure ventilation and received bag-mask ventilation	
Patient received code-dose epinephrine[a]	
Patient received defibrillation	

[a]May not fully qualify as code event, but triggers data manager to review the chart for further details

improvement. Large sampling efforts command a large investment in resources. Yet often a year's efforts have the same results as that of 3 months, but at four times the cost. In addition, the feedback cycle is longer, making change a much slower process. Graph and display your measures often enough to give your team feedback in a timely manner, both to keep momentum going and to stop changes that are having adverse effects. Monthly graphs are recommended, as weekly graphs may be too variable to detect patterns and trends. Time should be set aside to allow staff to review the results and develop improvement strategies.

Also, build the data collection into the daily work of staff, instead of making it a separate project that is "done to them" rather than "with them." This not only aids timely, relevant collection of data but also reduces stress by making measurement something that's "easy" to do. Create data collection forms that include only the information you need and are easy to complete. When integrating measurement into a staff member's role, be sure to build in a contingency plan for ongoing collection should that person become unavailable.

Learning from the Measures

All measures will exhibit some level of variation from period to period. Rather than view this as a problem, the science of improvement emphasizes learning from variation in data. Effective visual presentations of data, instead of tabular displays, provide the most opportunity for learning to take place. There are five basic graphical tools to study variation in data. All of these tools rely on a visual display to gain insights from variation in data:

- Run chart. Study variation in data over time; understand the impact of changes.
- Frequency plot. Understand location, spread, shape, and patterns of data.
- Pareto chart. Focus on areas of improvement with greatest impact.
- Scatterplot. Analyze the associations or relationship between two variables.
- Shewhart chart. Distinguish between special and common causes of variation.

When presenting improvement measures on graphs, always annotate graphs so that the reader can see the effect of the changes that you are testing. Since improvement happens over time, some type of time series chart (run chart or Shewhart) should always be used to analyze and report the measures from improvement projects. Multiple charts may be appropriate for the same project, depending on the audience and the goal of the project.

Run Charts

A run chart is a graphical display of data plotted in some type of order. The run chart is also called a trend chart or a time series chart. Figure 6.1 shows a simple example

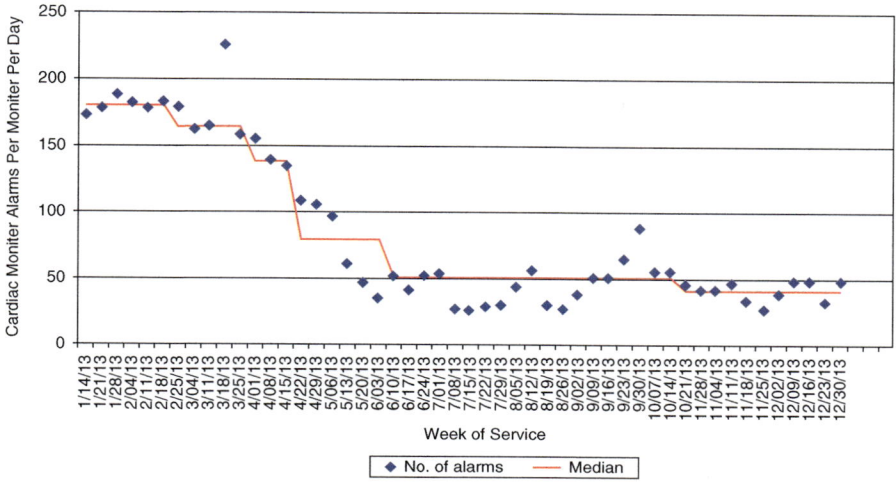

Fig. 6.1 Run chart example from a project studying cardiac monitor alarm frequency by day

of a typical run chart for the number of alarms per patient day. A run chart was a useful tool with which to display their data in time order to see changes in the number of alarms.

A run chart is easy to construct and simple to interpret. The simplicity makes it one of the most important methods for communicating and understanding variation. The tool encourages users to listen to the story the data are trying to tell. Important uses of the run chart in improvement activities include:

- Display data to make process performance visible.
- Determine if our change resulted in improvement.
- Determine if we are holding the gain made by our improvement.
- The run chart allows us to learn a great deal about the performance of our process with minimal mathematical complexity. Displaying data on a run chart can also be the first step in developing a Shewhart control chart. This chapter describes the construction, interpretation, and use of run charts.

The primary use of run charts in improvement work is to answer the second question in the model for improvement: "How will we know that a change is an improvement?" There are both practical and statistical answers to this question. A change in the data might be practically important, but not provide any probability-based "signal" of change. Or a change might be a nonrandom signal, but not of practical importance. Or a change in the data could be both practically important and also exhibit a signal of nonrandomness.

One important caution is to be aware of the impact of unequal denominators when viewing data on a run chart, if the basis for the data points varies by more than 25% from period to period.

Frequency Plot

A frequency plot is designed to present information about the location, spread, and shape of a particular measure. A frequency plot is constructed by putting the scale of the measure of interest on the horizontal axis and then number of occurrences of each value (or groups of values) on the vertical axis. The number at each value can be represented by bars, stacked symbols, or lines. When bars are used, the graph is often called a histogram. When "dots" are used to display the number of each unique value in the data set, the graph is called a dot plot. A stem-and-leaf plot is a type of frequency plot where whole numbers are used to define the horizontal axis and the decimal value (1, 2, 3, etc.) is plotted as the symbol on the chart. See Fig. 6.2 for an example of a frequency plot for number of alarms by patient day.

The frequency plot is most useful after examining a run chart or Shewhart chart for stability. For a stable measure, the frequency plot can be used to summarize the capability of the process performance for the measure. The frequency plot is useful for finding patterns in the data like rounding errors, missing values, truncation, and favorite values of the measure. Useful information about measures with an unusually shaped distribution can also be seen from a frequency plot.

To construct a frequency plot for data on a continuous scale, the range of data for the measure of interest is divided into 5–20 cells, defined by intervals encompassing the total range of the measure. The more data that is available, the more cells can be used. For discrete data (like patient satisfaction data using a 1–5 scale), the cells can be defined by the possible values of the discrete measure.

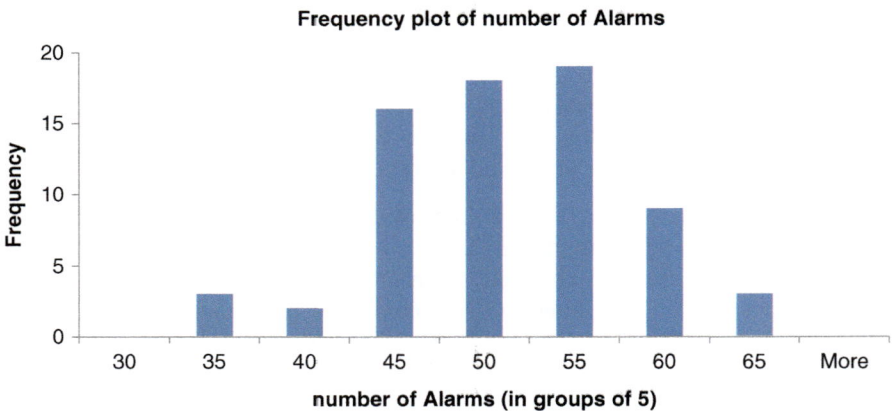

Fig. 6.2 Frequency plot example: number of alarms per patient day

Pareto Chart

A Pareto chart for attribute data is the equivalent of the frequency plot for a continuous measure. It is most useful to help focus improvement efforts and is a manifestation of the 80/20 rule (80% of problems are due to 20% of the reasons). Problems, errors, defects, adverse drug events, patient complaints, etc. can often be organized into categories or classifications. Typical categories for the horizontal scale are DRG, location, operating room, procedure, physician, failure mode, etc. Since there is no natural scale for the order of the categories, they are ordered from the most frequently occurring to least occurring on the horizontal axis of the chart. The chart was named by Juran with the name coming from the work of an economist named Pareto.

A useful Pareto chart will have 30 or more incidents. Charts with just a few data points can be misleading. When just a few observations are available, present the categories in a table. Data for a Pareto chart are collected by recording some type of category to further describe the occurrence of interest. On the horizontal axis, put the categories ordered from most frequent to fewest. Then graph a bar to identify the number of occurrences in each category. Following the 80/20 rule (or Pareto principle), the categories on the left side of the graph are called the "vital few," while the rest are considered the "useful many."

Figure 6.3 shows an example of a Pareto chart from a quality improvement initiative regarding safe opioid prescribing by a palliative care team. Providers

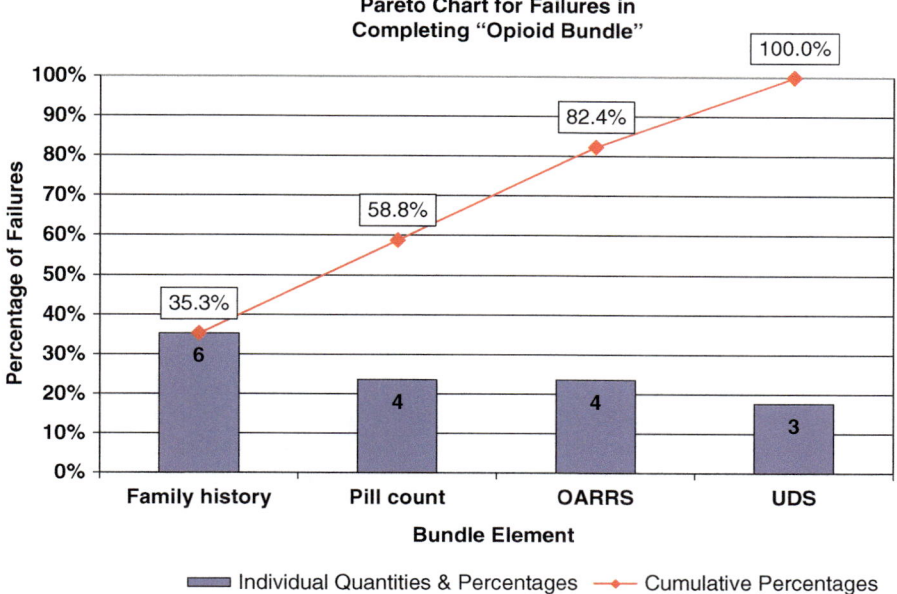

Fig. 6.3 Pareto chart example: reasons for failures in completing the "opioid bundle"

were required to review, obtain, or complete four elements of a "bundle" (a family history questionnaire, a pill count, an OARRS [Ohio Automated Rx Reporting System] report, and urine drug screen or UDS) for each patient to whom opioids were prescribed, in order to apply a risk-stratification scheme for likelihood of opioid misuse to each patient. At the beginning of the project, several patient charts were examined to determine which elements the team had failed to complete.

Scatterplot

The scatterplot is a tool for learning about associations or relationships between two continuous variables. If a cause and effect relationship exists between the variables, the scatterplot will show this relationship. The patterns on the charts indicate if two variables are associated.

To develop a scatterplot, select the two measures of interest and record pairs of measures (same patient, same time period, same clinic, etc.). Plot the pairs on a scale such that the range of variation takes up the full range of data. The axes should be of approximately equal length for each variable (square graph). The correlation statistic (r) can be calculated as a statistical measure of the association between the two variables, and a regression analysis can be done to quantify the relationship between two variables after examining the scatterplot. Stratification can be accomplished with a scatterplot by plotting different symbols to represent a third stratification variable.

As with the frequency plot and Pareto chart, the scatterplot may be a useful tool with which to contrast and learn about the difference between a common cause and special cause timeframe evident on a Shewhart chart. By creating a pair of scatter charts, one using data from the common cause timeframe and another using data from the special cause timeframe, we can contrast the two timeframes enhance our understanding of the variation in the process.

Shewhart Control Chart

The Shewhart chart is a statistical tool used to distinguish between variation in a measure due to common causes and variation due to special causes (Ref Shewhart). The common name used by Shewhart and other authors to describe the chart is a "control chart." But this name is misleading since the most common uses of these charts in improvement activities are to learn about variation and to evaluate the impact of changes. Also the word "control" has other meanings often associated with specifications or targets. A more descriptive name might be "learning charts" or "system performance charts."

A fundamental concept for the study and improvement of processes, due to Walter Shewhart [5], is that variation in a measure of quality has its origins in one of two types of causes:

Common causes—those causes that are inherent in the system (process or product) over time, affect everyone working in the system, and affect all outcomes of the system

Special causes—those causes that are not part of the system (process or product) all the time or do not affect everyone but arise because of specific circumstances

(Note: Shewhart initially used the term assignable rather than special and chance rather than common to describe these two types of causes. Deming popularized the common and special cause nomenclature [3].)

A system that has only common causes affecting the outcomes is called a *stable system*, or one that is in a state of statistical control. A stable process implies that the variation is *predictable* within statistically established limits. A system whose outcomes are affected by both common causes and special causes is called an *unstable system*. An unstable system does not necessarily mean one with large variation. It means that the magnitude of the variation from one time period to the next is unpredictable.

This distinction between common and special causes of variation is fundamental to developing effective improvement strategies. When one is made aware that there are special causes affecting a process or outcome measure, it is feasible and usually economical to identify, learn from, and take action based on the special cause. Often this action is to remove the special cause and make it difficult for it to occur again. Other times, the special cause produces a favorable situation, so the appropriate action is to make it a permanent part of the healthcare process.

As special causes are identified and removed, the process becomes stable. Deming gives several benefits of a stable process [3].

Figure 6.4 shows a typical Shewhart chart. Shewhart charts created with equal subgroups size (each subgroup or "dot" contains the same number of data values) will have straight upper and lower limits. More common in healthcare applications are Shewhart charts made with unequal subgroup sizes. These will have varying limits as in Fig. 6.2. These varying limits are adjusted to be appropriate for each subgroup size.

The method of Shewhart charts includes:

- Selection of a measure and a statistic to be plotted
- A method of data collection: observation, measurement, and sampling procedures
- A strategy for determining subgroups of measurements (including subgroup size and frequency)
- Selection of the appropriate Shewhart chart
- Criteria for identifying a signal of a special cause

Shewhart charts include a center line and an upper and lower limit. Shewhart called the limits of the chart "three-sigma" limits and gave a general formula to calculate the limits for any statistic to be charted. Let S be the statistic to be charted, then

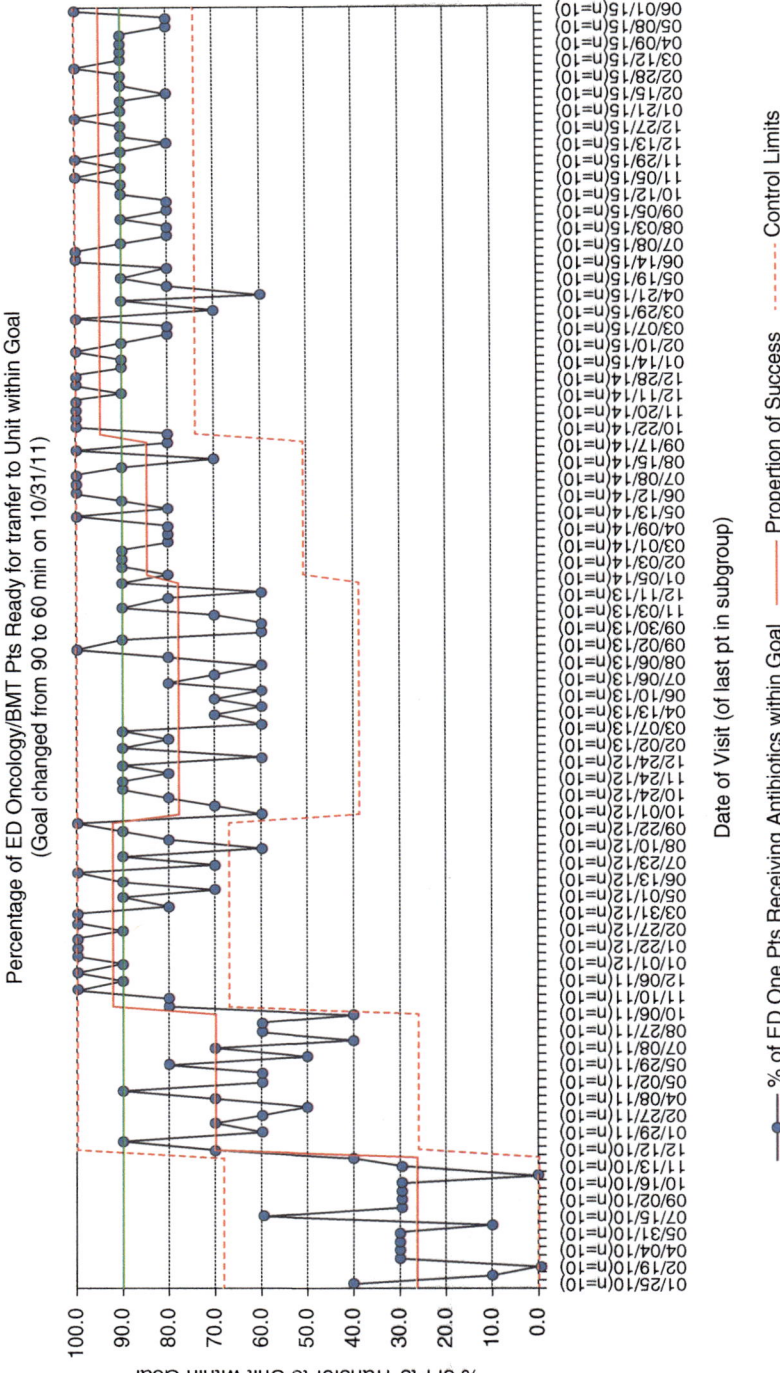

Fig. 6.4 Example of Shewhart chart for varying subgroup size

$$\text{the centerline} : CL = \mu_s$$
$$\text{the upper limit} : UL = \mu_s + 3 \times \sigma_s$$
$$\text{the lower limit} : LL = \mu_s - 3 \times \sigma_s$$

where μ_s is the expected value of the statistic and σ_s is the standard deviation (or standard error) of the statistic. Shewhart emphasized that statistical theory can furnish the expected value and standard deviation of the statistic, but empirical evidence justifies the width of the limits (the use of "3" in the limit calculation).

A Shewhart chart provides a basis for taking action to improve a process. A process is considered to be stable when there is a "random distribution" of the plotted points within the control limits. For a stable process, action should be directed at identifying the important causes of variation common to all of the points. If the distribution (or pattern) of points is not random, the process is considered to be unstable, and action should be taken to learn about the special causes of variation.

There is general agreement among users of control charts that a single point outside the control limits is an indication of a special cause of variation. However, there have been many suggestions for systems of rules to identify special causes which appear as nonrandom patterns within the control limits. Figure 6.5 contains five rules which are recommended for general use with Shewhart charts. These rules are consistent in the sense that the chance of occurrence of rules #2 through #5 in a stable process is close to the chance of rule #1 occurring in a stable process [1].

The concept of subgrouping is one of the most important components of the control chart method. Shewhart said the following about subgrouping [5]:

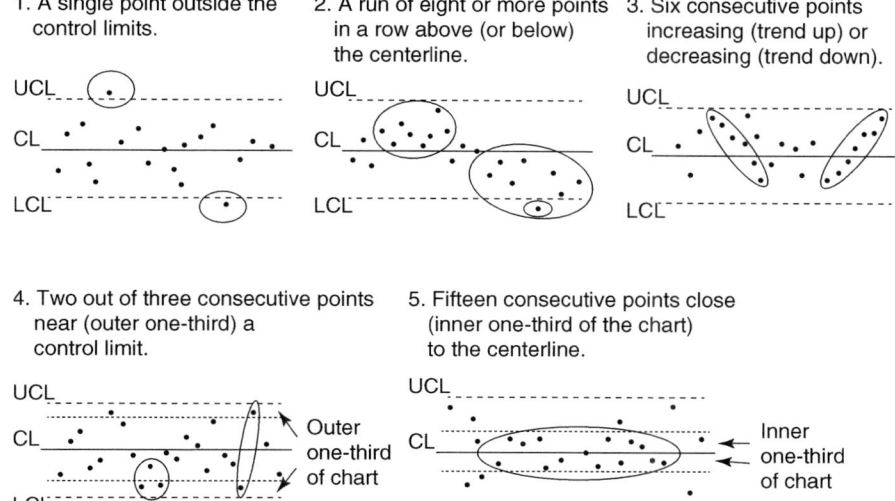

Fig. 6.5 Rules for detecting signals of special cause on Shewhart charts

Obviously, the ultimate object is not only to detect trouble but also to find it, and such discovery naturally involves classification. The engineer who is successful in dividing his data into rational subgroups based upon rational hypotheses is therefore inherently better off in the long run than the one who is not thus successful.

Shewhart's concept was to organize data from the process in a way that is likely to give the greatest chance for the data in each subgroup to be alike and greatest chance for data in other subgroups to be different. The aim of rational subgrouping is to include only common causes of variation within a subgroup, with all special causes of variation occurring between subgroups.

The most common method to obtain rational subgroups is to hold time "constant" within a subgroup. Only data taken at the same time (or for some selected time period) are included in a subgroup. Data from different time periods will be in other subgroups. This use of time as the basis of subgrouping allows the detection of causes of variation that come and go with time.

There are five types of basic Shewhart charts which depend on the type of data used to create the measure and the method of forming subgroups. Figure 6.6 shows how each of these charts connects with the type of data [1].

The following Fig. 6.7 shows example of a U chart. Further information on the use of Shewhart charts in healthcare is available in references [3–5].

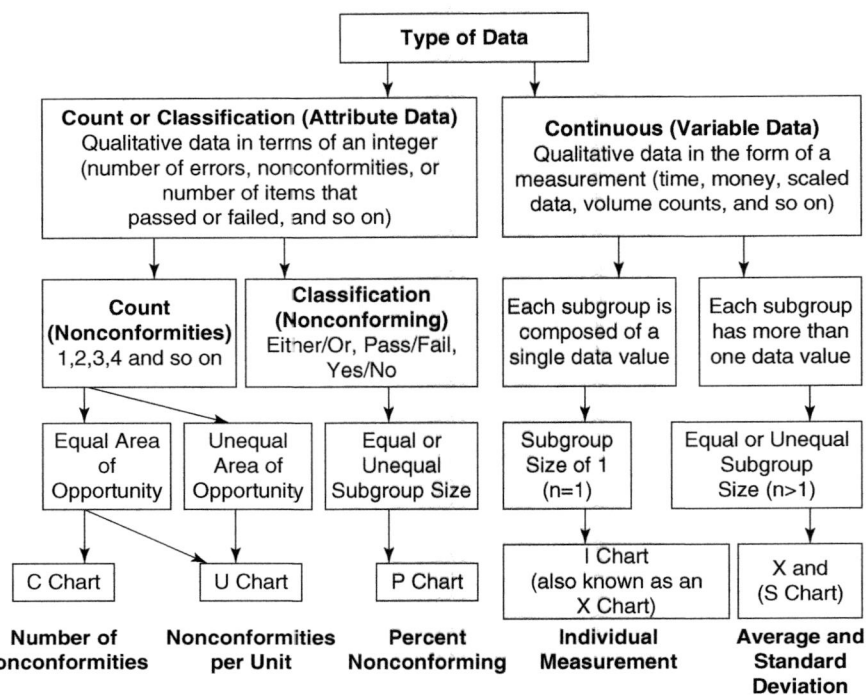

Fig. 6.6 Selection of type of Shewhart chart [1]

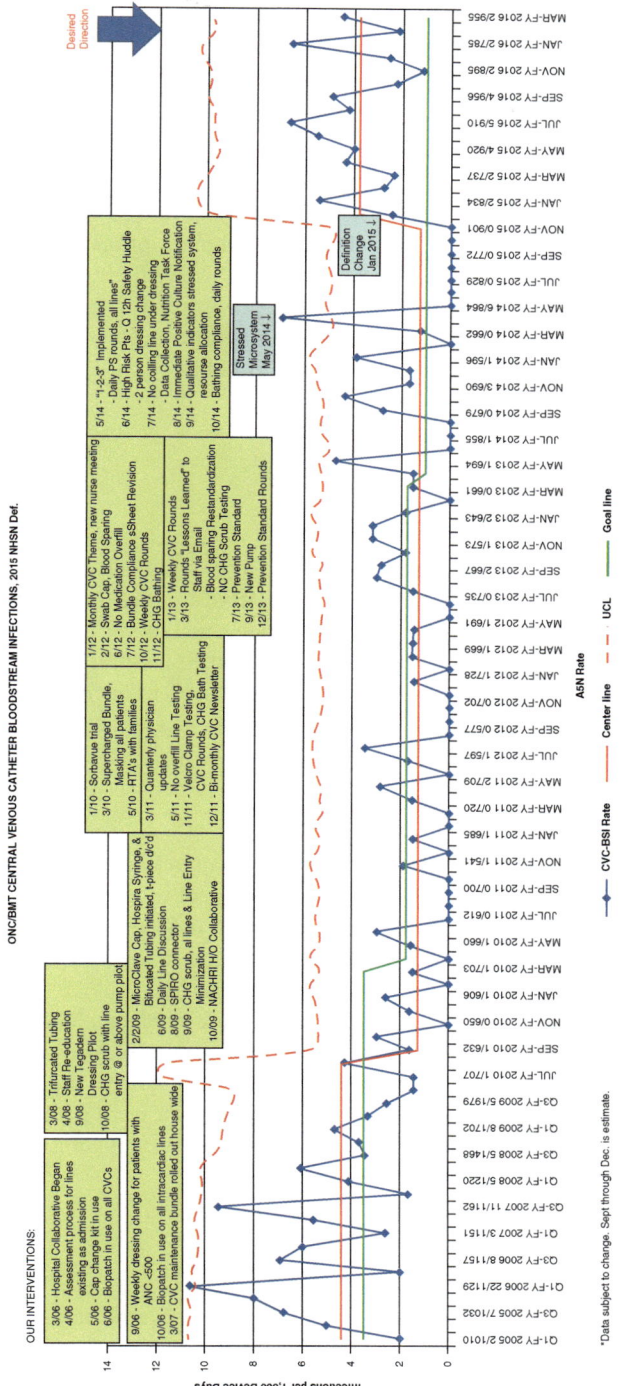

Fig. 6.7 U chart example: central venous catheter bloodstream infections in oncology and bone marrow transplant patients

Putting It All Together: A Case-Based Example

Dr. Amy Fowler is a pediatric oncologist in Austin, Texas. During her fellowship in pediatric hematology-oncology, she noticed that, frequently, physicians and nurse practitioners in that group did not follow the COG protocol guidelines for titrating 6-MP and methotrexate in patients with pre-B acute lymphoblastic leukemia in maintenance therapy. A chart review revealed that guidelines were followed only 39% of the time. She decided to build an improvement project with the goal of improving adherence to these guidelines [6]. The SMART aim was: "In children with pre-B ALL who are in maintenance therapy, we will improve provider adherence to guidelines for oral chemotherapy dose adjustments from 39% to >75% and to improve patients' average absolute neutrophil count (ANC) from 2,180 to less than 1,900 from January 1, 2011 to June 30, 2011."

Step 1

Select balanced set of measures related to the improvement aim.

For this project, Dr. Fowler chose percentage of provider adherence by month as the primary process measure. To monitor the impact of increased adherence to guidelines upon the patient's CBC, the average absolute neutrophil count (ANC) of all patients in maintenance by month was a second outcome measure. Due to concern that increased adherence to guidelines could cause increased frequency of neutropenia, episodes of neutropenia per patient per month were chosen as a balancing measure.

Step 2

Operationally define each measure (including data collection and sampling).

Provider adherence was defined as the percentage of time a dose escalation was made when indicated by the guidelines, by month. A trained set of providers evaluated each outpatient encounter during the study period to determine if the decision made was consistent with the dose delivery guidelines [6].

ANC was defined as the value reported on the complete blood count (CBC) drawn in clinic on the day of the patient's visit; this was tracked as an average for all clinic patients by month. ANC was obtained from the electronic medical record.

Neutropenia was defined as ANC <500, and these data were tracked as episodes of neutropenia per patient per month. Evidence of neutropenic episodes was obtained from the electronic medical record.

Step 3

Collect historic baseline data and then continue regular basis throughout the project.

Dr. Fowler undertook a chart review of patients in maintenance therapy, which revealed that provider adherence to guidelines before the project was 38%. Mean average ANC prior to the project was 2180/μL, and median was 2117/μL. Baseline frequency of neutropenic episodes was 0.15 episodes per patient per month.

Steps 4 and 5

Report data on SPC charts (at least monthly), and use SPC charts of measures to assess the impact of changes and to determine when the aim is accomplished.

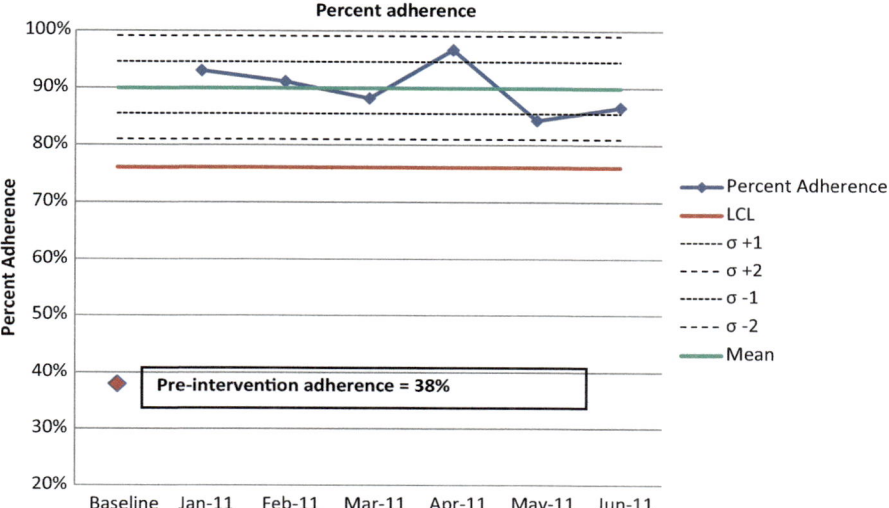

Fig. 6.8 P chart of mean and median percent adherence to maintenance guidelines by month

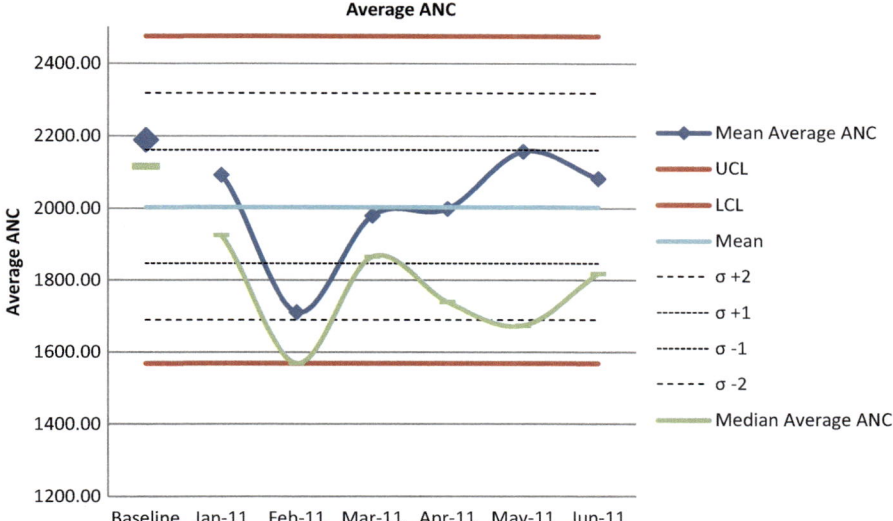

Fig. 6.9 X-bar chart of average ANC by month

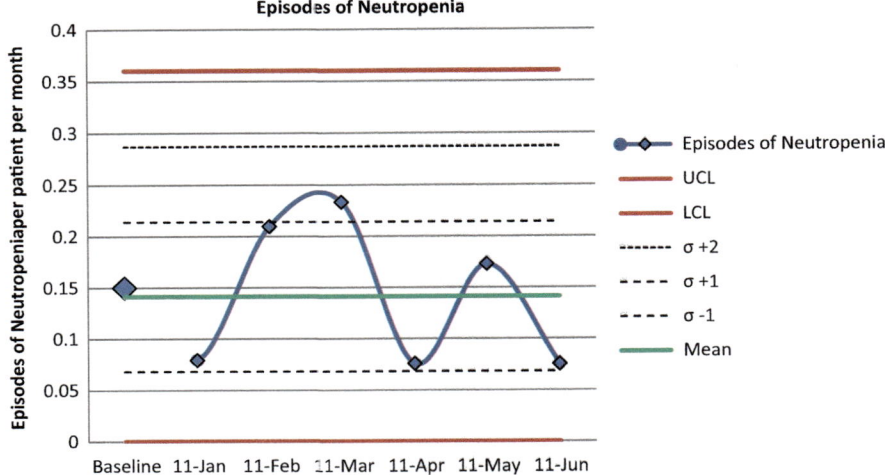

Fig. 6.10 U chart of episodes of neutropenia per patient per month

Dr. Fowler created three SPC charts to plot her data. For percent adherence to guidelines per month, Dr. Fowler chose a P chart (Fig. 6.8): her data was attribute data, each month offered differing subgroup sizes, and she was counting a percentage that did not conform to guidelines. For average ANC per month, she created an X-bar chart (Fig. 6.9) as she followed the mean and median of the average value. For episodes of neutropenia, she created a U chart (Fig. 6.10), as she was counting "Is the patient neutropenic?" (yes/no) and tracking this value per patient per month. These charts indicated that percent adherence to guidelines improved to 90% by June 2011 (Fig. 6.8), mean average ANC improved to 2080/µL, and median ANC improved to 1819/µL (Fig. 6.9), and there was no change (increase) in frequency of neutropenic episodes (Fig. 6.10).

References

1. Provost LP, Murray SK. The health care data guide: learning from data for improvement. 1st ed. San Francisco: Jossey-Bass; 2011.
2. Dandoy CE, Davies SM, Flesch L, et al. A team-based approach to reducing cardiac monitor alarms. Pediatrics. 2014;134:e1686–94.
3. Deming WE. Out of the crisis. Cambridge: Massachusetts Institute of Technology, Center for Advanced Engineering Study; 1986.
4. Randolph G, Esporas M, Provost L, Massie S, Bundy DG. Model for improvement - part two: measurement and feedback for quality improvement efforts. Pediatr Clin N Am. 2009;56:779–98.
5. Shewhart WA. Economic control of quality of manufactured product. New York: D. Van Nostrand Company, Inc.; 1931.
6. Fowler A, Leonard D, Slone T. Tellinghuisen C, Kennedy A, Griffith P, Winick N. Provider adherence to oral chemotherapy dose adjustment guidelines in the treatment of childhood acute lymphoblastic leukemia (ALL). Platform Session 4018. Abstracts of the 2014 American Society of Pediatric Hematology-Oncology Annual Meeting. Chicago: Pediatric Blood and Cancer; 2014. P. S1–S104.

Chapter 7
Sustainability and Spread

Mona D. Shah, Jacqueline R. Ward, and Angelo P. Giardino

All systems and organizations are faced with the challenge of implementing new practices at one time or another, yet many of the innovations that are initially successful fail to become part of the habits and routines of the host organizations and communities. Why do some take root and flourish while others languish? ([1], p. 2)

Introduction

By any standard of success, implementation and dissemination of quality improvement and/or patient safety innovations are essential elements in enhancing patient care. Prior and subsequent chapters of this book document the critical components for a robust quality program, detailing technical aspects of effective initiatives. However, the sustainability and spread of quality improvement and/or patient safety innovations are often elusive, presenting continuous challenges to clinicians and healthcare leaders, as noted by Wiltsey-Stirman et al. [1] above. In fact, depending on the study, 33–70% of all innovations are reportedly not sustained, as measured by a number of different organizational design methods [2]. One group from the United Kingdom (UK) refers to this elusive goal of measurable sustained change as the "evaporation of improvements,"

M.D. Shah, MD, MS (✉)
Associate Clinical Director, Texas Children's Cancer and Hematology Centers, Texas Children's Hospital, Baylor College of Medicine, Houston, TX, USA
e-mail: mdshah@texaschildrens.org

J.R. Ward, MSN, RN, NE-BC
Vice President of Nursing, Texas Children's Hospital, Houston, TX, USA
e-mail: jaward@texaschildrens.org

A.P. Giardino, MD, PhD
SVP/Chief Quality Officer, Texas Children's Hospital, Professor & Section Head, Academic General Pediatrics, Baylor College of Medicine, Houston, TX, USA
e-mail: apgiardi@texaschildrens.org

© Springer International Publishing AG 2017
C.E. Dandoy et al. (eds.), *Patient Safety and Quality in Pediatric Hematology/Oncology and Stem Cell Transplantation*, DOI 10.1007/978-3-319-53790-0_7

alluding to the seemingly mysterious inability of many institutions to maintain the enhanced improvement on the team or throughout the organization ([3], p. 22).

The immediate question becomes: "How can this be?" Clearly, sustainability and spread of healthcare quality improvement and/or patient safety innovations must be difficult to achieve. Harkening back to Paul Batalden, who is often quoted as saying, "every system is perfectly designed to get the results it gets," we must conclude that sustainability and spread are not inherently built into a system or its design ([4]; p. 1). This is not exclusively a limitation of the healthcare delivery industries, but as the literature demonstrates, other industries also encounter this sustainability and spread challenge [1, 5].

In the pursuit of excellence, discouragement is not a viable option. Detailed assessments and targeted process improvements directed at addressing the systems' vulnerabilities are essential. Careful evaluation of the currently available literature on sustainability and spread is a necessary first step, followed by process improvement, and finally, adoption of best practices to address any barriers to the implementation of quality and/or patient safety innovations.

To understand the factors that influence and facilitate sustainability and spread of effective innovations in the healthcare setting, this chapter will focus on:

(1) emerging definitions for sustainability and spread;
(2) models for understanding sustainability and spread (within the health care context);
(3) case examples from a hematology/oncology clinical program, illustrating elements of the aforementioned frameworks; and finally,
(4) considering the value of addressing the pre-conditions and characteristics essential to the eventual success of sustainability and spread upfront, during the quality improvement process.

Review of Literature: Definitions and Models/Frameworks

Definitions

A number of reviews have been performed summarizing and synthesizing the findings of various empiric studies that examine the sustainability and spread of innovation, both in and outside of the healthcare industry [5–9]. Most of these reviews comment on the differing definitions of sustainability; and to a lesser extent, spread. The Institute for Healthcare Improvement (IHI) uses straightforward language to define sustainability, as locking in progress, while continually building upon that foundation. Fleiszer et al. [2] constructed an inventory of definitions of sustainability (reproduced in Table 7.1), supplementing the straightforward language in the IHI definition, but with adaptations to various settings. The IHI, in a similar manner, defines spread as actively disseminating best practice and knowledge about every intervention, and then implementing each intervention in every available care setting [10].

According to Greenhalgh et al. [8], spread, diffusion, and dissemination are similar terms that are often used interchangeably, when, in fact, they have subtle but important distinctions between them. Spread (e.g., within an organization) involves the exchange of knowledge and experience via clear communication and education on specific work practices, maximizing process improvements, and the development

Table 7.1 Definitions of sustainability

Source and domain/setting	Definition	Characterized as		
		benefits	persistence/ continuation	development
Merriam-Webster [20] (English dictionary)	• "able to be used without being completely used up or destroyed" • "able to last or continue for a long time"		X	
Rogers (2003) [21] (sociology; diffusion of innovations)	• "the degree to which an innovation continues to be used after initial efforts to secure adoption is completed" (p. 429) • "the degree to which a programme of change is continued after the initial resources provided by a change agency are ended" (p. 376)		X	
Bowman et al. (2008) [22] (health care)	• "the continued use of core elements of an intervention and persistent gains in performance as a result of those interventions" (p. 11)	X	X	
Scheirer [5] Scheirer and Dearing (2011) [23] (public health; health care)	• "the programme components developed and implemented in earlier stages are (or are not) maintained after the initial fundings or other impetus is removed" (p. 322) • "the continued use of programme components and activities (beyond their initial funding period) for the continued achievement of desirable programme and population outcomes" (p.2060)	X	X	
Stetler et al. [24] (nursing)	• "changes (practice and outcomes) … that continue over time as related to specific projects" (p.19)	X	X	
Davies and Edwards (2013) [25] (health care)	• "the continued implementation of innovations over time and depends on the ability of workers, organizations and healthcare delivery systems to adapt to change" (p. 237)		X	?
Mancini and Marek (2004) [26] (health promotion)	• "the capacity of programmes to continuously respond to community issues" (p. 339)	X	?	X

(continued)

Table 7.1 (continued)

Source and domain/setting	Definition	Characterized as		
		benefits	persistence/ continuation	development
Gruen et al. (2008) [27] (public/ community health; health care)	• "complex systems that encompass programmes, health problems targeted by programmes and programmes' drivers or key stakeholders, all which interact dynamically in any given context" (p. 1579) • "capability of being maintained at a certain rate or level" (p. 1580)	?	X	?
Buchanan et al. [7], Buchanan et al. [3] (management; health care)	• "the process through which new working methods, performance goals and improvement trajectories are maintained for a period appropriate to a given context" (p. 189; p. xxii)	X	X	X
Johnson et al. (2004) [28] (health promotion)	• "the process of ensuring an adaptive prevention system and a sustainable innovation that can be integrated into ongoing operations to benefit diverse stakeholders" (p.137)	X	X	X
Bevan et al. (2002) [29] (health care)	• "when new ways of working and Improved outcomes become the norm … the process and outcome [are] changed … the thinking and attitudes behind them are fundamentally altered … the systems surrounding them are transformed in support… it has [withstood] challenge and variation … evolved alongside other changes in the context and perhaps has actually to improve over time" (p. 12)	X	X	X

Fleiszer et al. [2]. Used with permission

of interventions. In contrast, diffusion refers to the unplanned, informal, and decentralized process of spread. Dissemination is the spread of innovation that is planned, formal, and centralized, but occurs through vertical hierarchies. Greenhalgh et al. [11] summarize these definitions of spread (as seen in Table 7.2). Two additional terms are equally notable: (1) assimilation, which describes more complex adoption processes, including formal decision making, an evaluation phase (or phases), and

Table 7.2 Definitions of spread

Source	Definition	Comments
Damanpour and Gopalakrishnan (1998) [30]	"… an organization's means to adapt to the environment, or to pre-empt a change in the environment, in order to increase or sustain its effectiveness or competitiveness. Managers may emphasize the rate or speed of adoption, or both, to close an actual or perceived performance gap"	Adoption of innovations
Rogers ([13], p. 5)	Diffusion is the process by which an innovation is communicated through certain channels over time among the members of a social system	Diffusion refers to spread of abstract ideas and concepts, technical information, and actual practices within a social system, from a source to an adopter, typically via influence or communication
Wejnert (2002, [31] p. 297)	"… identifying the factors that influence the spread of innovations across groups, communities, societies, and countries … an area of inquiry referred to formally, as diffusion"	
Mowatt and colleagues (1998, [32] p. 669)	Dissemination is actively spreading a message to defined target groups.	
The Modernisation Agency (NHS Modernisation Agency, 2003 [33])	Spread is the extent to which learning and change principles have been adopted in other parts of the organization that could benefit from them. This includes not only those parts of the organization that are the same as the original improvement site but also spread to other parts of the service that have similar processes or face similar issues. Spread means that the learning which takes place in any part of an organization is actively shared and acted upon by all parts of the organization. Improvement knowledge generated anywhere in the healthcare system becomes common knowledge and practice across the healthcare system.	Berwick prefers the term "re-invention" to spread

Adapted from Greenhalgh et al. [11]

planned sustained efforts at implementation; and (2) implementation, which encompasses the active and planned efforts to mainstream an innovation within an organization [12].

Inherent to any discussion of sustainability and spread is the concept of innovation. Ideally, it is an innovation which improves care that we hope is sustained and spread throughout the clinical setting. It should be noted that not all innovations are improvements. Rogers [13] defines an innovation as, "an idea, practice, or object that is perceived as new by an individual or other unit of adoption." Four core characteristics of innovation, as identified by Osbourne [14], are particularly relevant to the healthcare setting:

1. Innovation represents newness (but not necessarily improvements).
2. It is not the same thing as invention (the latter is concerned with the discovery of new ideas or approaches whereas innovation is concerned with their application).
3. It is both a process AND an outcome.
4. It involves discontinuous change (as opposed to incremental development of practice).

Fraser et al. [15] and Osbourne [14] also classify innovations into four categories with application to the healthcare setting, namely:

1. Developmental innovations (existing services to a particular user group are improved or enhanced);
2. Expansionary innovations (existing services are offered to new user groups);
3. Evolutionary innovations (new services are provided to existing users); and
4. Total innovations (new services to new users).

Understanding the nuances between each of these categories is essential to the improvement leader, whose knowledge of the innovation to be "hardwired," and then spread to other colleagues or units throughout the healthcare organization is ideally conducted from a position of expertise. Having one's conceptual frameworks clearly in mind and recognizing the multi-variate factors at play in a complex, unpredictable environment can help facilitate change, even anticipate barriers or resistance should they arise. Finally, Buchanan, Fitzgerald, and Ketley [3] from the UK expand upon this discussion, by taking a more ecological or systems-based approach, describing different levels at which change may occur, which can be simplified for the purposes of our discussion as, change and adoption of innovation occurring at the (1) individual, (2) unit, and (3) across organizational levels.

Models/Frameworks

With the definitions provided above, Fleiszer et al. [2] frame sustainability as a multi-dimensional, multi-factorial concept that may ideally be viewed as having three characteristics and four pre-conditions; all drawn from their comprehensive concept analysis (Fig. 7.1). These three characteristics include: (1) benefit, (2) routinization/institutionalization, and (3) development. Briefly, the benefit characteristic of sustainability relates to the idea that only effective and valuable innovations should be sustained. There are two perspectives when considering the benefit characteristic, namely (1) objective (quantifiable results that formally confirm the achievement of an outcome), and (2) subjective (perceived value that is more informal in nature that confirms the positive results to involved stakeholders).

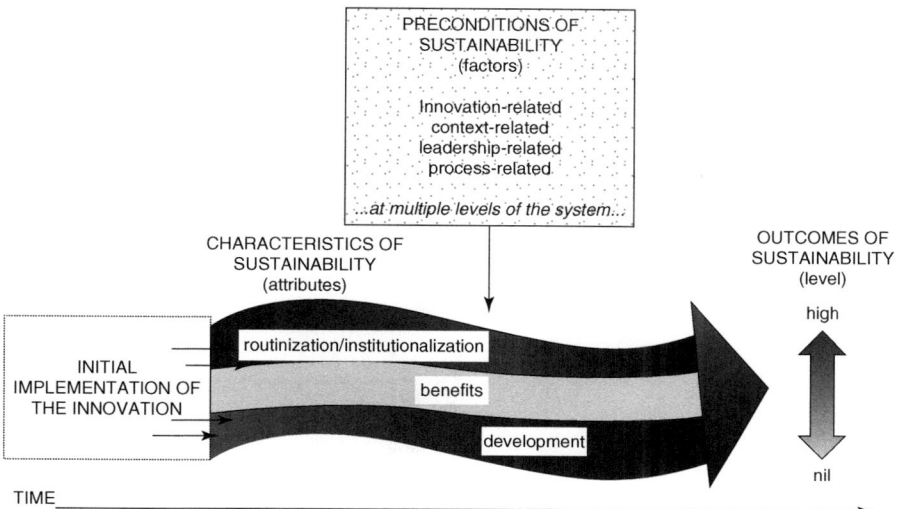

Fig. 7.1 Concept analysis for the sustainability of healthcare innovations. Fleiszer et al. [2]. Used with permission

The routinization/institutionalization characteristic of sustainability refers to the adoption of practices that indicate that the innovation has moved from "new" to "accepted," and its structures and processes are now woven into the fabric of a specified setting. In the clinical setting, this embedding process would be referred to as being accepted as a "standard of care" or as a "best practice."

Development, as a characteristic of sustainability, describes the sense of ownership by key stakeholders, who: (1) invest in the ongoing study and enhancement of the initial innovation, but (2) address the need to apply the innovation in continually evolving environments. This requires constant renewal, re-invention, and resilience. The ability to adjust and refine an innovation allows stakeholders to recognize that the ideas and improvements are ultimately their own. The recognition that development can occur reinforces the sense of ownership and desire to invest and re-invest in maintaining (or sustaining) the change process.

In addition to characteristics essential to sustaining an innovation, Fleiszer et al. [2] articulate several pre-conditions that influence sustainability. These four pre-conditions include: (1) innovation, (2) context, (3) leadership, and (4) processes. Briefly, the innovation pre-condition relates to aspects of the innovation itself. This can best be summarized as, the "fit" with the mission, and its relevance towards addressing the need (or solving the problem). The pre-condition related to context addresses both internal and external aspects of a given setting. Internal context involves organizational culture and project management capacity to keep an innovation on track. External context relates to policy, regulations, legislation, and financial pressures (i.e., funding or market-place associated). The leadership pre-condition addresses the prowess of the improvement champions and management

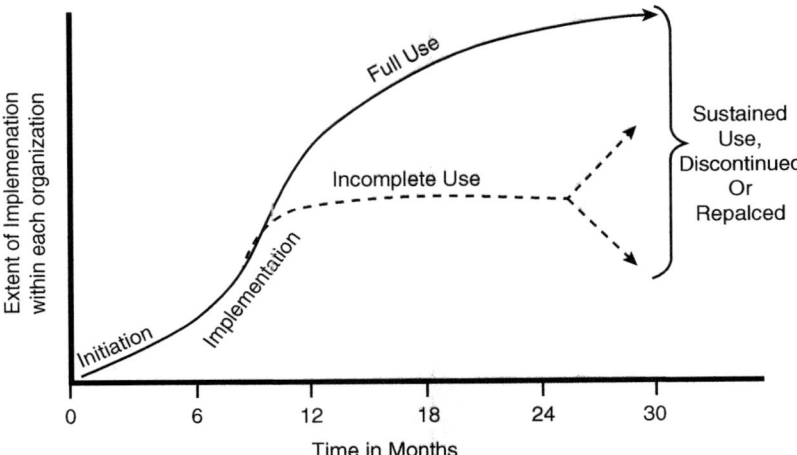

Fig. 7.2 Implementation of an innovation and possibility of sustained use. Scheirer [5]. Used with permission

team to generate support and inspire engagement. Finally, the process pre-condition resembles quality improvement paradigms, such as performance monitoring and the ability to plan, trial, and implement.

Scherier [5] conducted a review of the empirical literature around program sustainability, and graphically represents the chronology of sustaining an innovation in Fig. 7.2. He suggests that the change process begins with the introduction of the innovation into the setting (initiation), and then progresses through implementation, and finally, adoption within the setting. Over time, the innovation is either fully or partially implemented, as determined by an evaluation of the effort. The innovation is then seen to either be sustained, abandoned, or replaced.

Both Scheirer [5] and Fleiszer et al. [2] agree that sustainability hinges on: (1) perceived benefits by stakeholders involved in the innovation, (2) the existence of effective processes to implement and ultimately routinize (institutionalize) the change going from new to expected practice, and (3) the existence of some level of flexibility, such that unique contextual aspects can be recognized and accommodated. Both authors also recognize the need for leadership in the form of a "champion" for a given innovation, as well as the need for the innovation to fit within the mission of the key stakeholders.

In addition, Scheirer [5] specifically draws attention to the observation that innovations may be either fully or partially implemented over time. A number of factors affect the extent to which an innovation is fully implemented. She specifically advocates for the use of established evaluation methods and tools (e.g., logic models, key driver diagrams), to assist in defining the components that are essential in achieving the desired outcome. Linking her work on sustainability to the field of implementation science, Scheirer [5] addresses the concept of spread (or specifically, dissemination) as an important dimension after an innovation is sustained in its original setting.

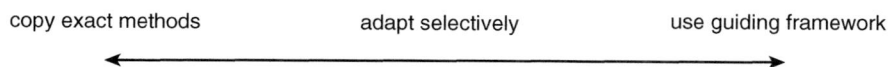

Fig. 7.3 The spread continuum. Buchanan et al. [3]. Used with permission

Type of spread	Definition	Reinvention issues
Scatter	One simple behaviour or practice is disseminated to and adopted by many	*Not much:* ideas are simple and obviously better
Switch	Transferring good practice from one sector to another context	*Significant:* ideas from outside require a new language
Share	Copying practices in one division to others in the organization	*Moderate:* practice hard to share due to internal competition
Stretch	Expanding good practice across internal divisional boundaries	*Significant:* crossing boundaries increases complexity of process

Fig. 7.4 Type of spread. Buchanan et al. [7]. Used with permission

Spread, essentially the adoption of an innovation beyond its original implementation site, may occur in a variety of ways. Buchanan et al. [3] offer the idea of spread as occurring across a continuum (Fig. 7.3): moving from copying the innovation exactly as it was previously implemented to the other extreme, where the original innovation serves only as a guiding framework for action in the new setting.

Figure 7.4 provides a categorization of the types of spread: scatter, switch, share, and stretch. By referencing the development characteristic of the sustainability framework from Fleiszer et al. [2], the resilience of an innovation (embodied by its ability to be adapted into varying contexts), including the ease of incorporating modifications and enhancements from engaged stakeholders, is a critical element to spread. The ownership of an innovation is only enhanced if more participants perceive that they have a role in "shaping" the innovation to apply to their individualized environments and specific clinical contexts.

Case Scenarios

To illustrate the aforementioned models, we shall discuss two case examples that represent current and ongoing quality improvement efforts. Case 1 describes an initiative designed around reducing central line associated blood stream infections (CLABSIs). Case 2 describes an initiative designed around managing pediatric oncology patients with febrile neutropenia (FN). Each of these case scenarios is chronicled using the vocabulary common among those well versed in quality improvement. In each case, we shall highlight the previously discussed frameworks, including the characteristics and pre-conditions of sustainability, as well as the continuum of spread.

Innovations that are successfully sustained and spread are, by definition, valued quality and patient safety improvements. Central to both Case 1 and Case 2 are innovation fundamentals commonly found in health care: (1) key driver diagrams that visually describe the core elements of the innovation that must be addressed [5]; (2) measurement and data displays to ground the improvement effort in transparent data sharing; and (3) cascading responsibility diagrams that communicate the role and responsibility of each participant in the effort, thereby reinforcing the participants' sense of ownership of the change process [2].

Case 1: Central Line Associated Blood Stream Infections

Texas Children's Hospital, a quaternary pediatric hospital with 687 licensed beds, cares for the highest acuity patients in the community, providing a wide range of subspecialty services, including pediatric hematology-oncology. The Texas Children's Hospital Pediatric Hematology-Oncology inpatient service includes a 36-bed inpatient unit, with an average daily census of 35 patients, with 100% of these patients being either primary pediatric hematology or oncology patients; and 80% of those patients requiring some form of intravenous central line. Additionally, the inpatient service includes a 15-bed pediatric bone marrow transplant unit, with an average daily census of 14 patients, with 100% of these patients being primary bone marrow transplant patients, who also require some form of intravenous central line access. Due to the complexity of care, long-term treatment regimens, and the need for frequent intravenous access, the pediatric hematology-oncology patient population has the highest demand for central line access. This patient population generally maintains this type of access for a prolonged (years) period of time. Due to the nature of being severely immunocompromised, they are at greater risk for an untoward outcome secondary to central line associated blood stream infections (CLABSIs). Consequently, using central venous access in this patient population directly impacts morbidity and mortality [16].

There is a plethora of recent literature highlighting CLABSI prevention and key strategies to mitigate impact. Due to the increased risk to this particular patient population, an intense focus to reduce the incidence of CLABSIs was endorsed. Texas Children's Hospital participates in the nationally recognized Solutions for Patient Safety (SPS) initiative. Through this collaborative, the foundation of improving performance was identified. Initially, in 2013, the pediatric hematology-oncology unit had 15 recorded CLABSIs over 9310 line days, equating to a rate of 1.6 CLABSIs/1000 line days. In 2014, 15 CLABSIs were recorded over 9489 line days, equating to a rate of 1.6 CLABSIs/1000 line days. Finally, in 2015, the same unit had 25 CLABSIs recorded over 9841 lines days, resulting in a rate of 2.5 CLABSIs/1000 line days (Fig. 7.5).

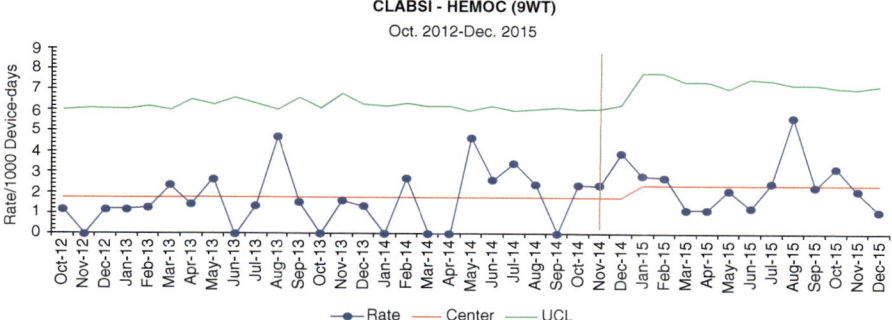

Fig. 7.5 Case 1: Central line associated blood stream infections (CLABSIs)

With these performance metrics, there was an urgent need from a patient out-comes perspective, to institute a structured framework and to develop new processes to mitigate this increasing CLABSI rate. Using our characteristics for sustainability perspective, at the outset of the case, prior to describing the quality improvement effort that eventually unfolded:

(1) the *benefit* of an innovation around CLABSIs reduction was clear (reduce risk of mortality and morbidity);
(2) the need for a standardized process, that could be *routinized,* was supported both by the literature around successful efforts at other comparable institutions and by the focus on bundle compliance within the national patient safety collaborative of which the unit was a member; and
(3) the *development* characteristic would be embraced, since ownership of any practice change was essential to tenets of quality improvement.

Furthermore, the pre-conditions for a sustainable program were also present in this case, namely:

(1) innovation—appropriate "fit with mission";
(2) context, both internal and external (unit wanted to reduce CLABSIs from a patient safety perspective, and wanted to comply with expectations as a member of the patient safety collaborative and other external data reporting initiatives— i.e., the hospital rankings that include CLABSIs rates such as US News & World Report);
(3) leadership—management and inspiration necessary for effective interdisciplin-ary health care delivery; and
(4) processes—well-functioning quality improvement and patient safety capacity.

The primary goal of this initiative was to utilize key quality improvement prin-ciples to implement evidence-based practices across the hospital system to address this concern. The first step involved developing an interdisciplinary structure to manage the work of the initiative. This team had the responsibility of addressing the current gaps in performance and making recommendations for improvement. Additionally, an executive steering committee was formed to provide governance, oversight, and support for the initiative. This executive team removed barriers, provided direction, and served as a report-out function for the interdisciplinary team.

The interdisciplinary structure involved the redesign of the organization's SPS Hospital Acquired Conditions (HAC) team. The team was redesigned to include key clinicians from all high risk areas, including pediatric hematology-oncology. Each high risk area had representation from a triad—a nurse leader, a physician champion, and a clinical nurse specialist. Additionally, separate from the broader HAC team, the pediatric hematology-oncology triad developed a service-line specific structure to address key findings that were unique to their service.

The first step in understanding the desired outcomes of a quality project is to identify and clearly state the aim. The interdisciplinary team worked diligently on the key driver diagram (Fig. 7.6) which outlined the pathway to improved outcomes. The key driver diagram outlined the key drivers, vital interventions, and measures of success that would support achieving the identified aim. Each decision made by the team was cross-referenced with the key driver diagram to validate alignment.

The structure comprised of four distinct teams, each with a key focus—Catheter, Catheter Maintenance, Hygiene, and Policy and Procedure. Each of these teams worked in parallel to implement Plan-Do-Study-Act (PDSA) cycles founded in the SPS framework of quality improvement. The most impact was seen in the Catheter Maintenance team, as these key drivers were critical.

Through countless hours of collaboration between nurse and physician experts, the Catheter Maintenance team focused on the following key strategies:

- Standardizing the bundle compliance definition to ensure minimization of variability from front line staff when conducted audits.
- Standardizing catheter maintenance practice across the system.
- Educating the system on the definition of CLABSIs to assess the knowledge gap.
- Establishing an accountability rounding process (see Appendix 1: Cascading of Accountability) for all levels of leadership and staff including physician leadership and front line physician roles.
- Creating the top ten essential practices to reduce CLABSIs as referenced by the literature in The Society for Healthcare Epidemiology of America [17].
- Developing a CLABSI prevention champion model for front line staff engagement and involvement for sustainability.

The key driver diagram supported the aforementioned key areas of focus. These essential practices included, but were not limited to: standardizing the nursing practice, technique, and maintenance criteria for managing all central lines. This team created, developed, and implemented a system-wide education curriculum for all 2400 nurses at the institution. This training included both didactic lectures and direct observation of key practices, in which every nurse had to return demonstrate compliance, while receiving active coaching and positive support. In parallel to the line maintenance initiative, this team (in partnership with Infection Control) also implemented a house-wide hand hygiene campaign.

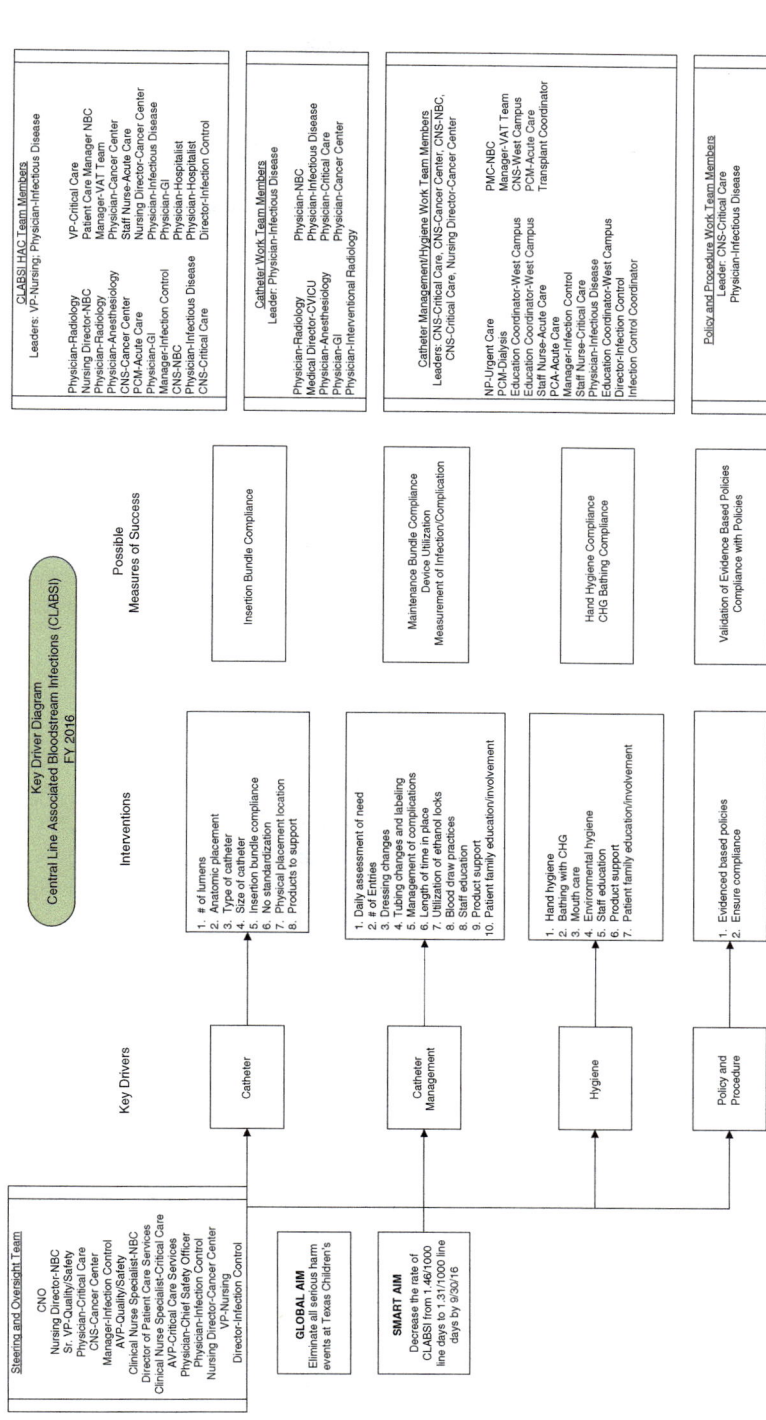

Fig. 7.6 Case 1: CLABSIs key driver diagram

Through key strategies, variability in practice has been minimized. At the outset, focusing heavily on the design of this work prepared the team for high impact execution.

Continued focus on dissemination of best practices across all areas of the organization is critical for continued success and impacting positive patient care outcomes. Sustaining a culture of being a high reliable system of care by ensuring staff are engaged and are provided formidable ongoing feedback will remain of top priority. In order to achieve sustainability, organizations must incorporate processes at the individual, organizational, and system level that adhere to uniformity within practice.

The key concepts of sustainability and spread are pivotal in process improvement. Once a process/performance improvement initiative, such as CLABSI prevention, has been identified as successful among the original participants, then the team can move on to considering how to sustain the innovation considering the characteristics for sustainability as well as the presence of the pre-conditions described above. The spread of best practice (to ensure similar work practices are occurring throughout the organization) occurs through sharing of knowledge and expertise among various teams within the larger healthcare organization. Consistency, in the enhanced practice, is valued as a reliability factor throughout the individual units as well as across the entire organization.

Case 2: Febrile Neutropenia

In addition to CLABSIs, febrile neutropenia (FN, also known as neutropenic fever) is also one of the most serious adverse events in children with malignancies, who receive chemotherapy for treatment or patients with bone marrow failure syndromes. Infections in neutropenic patients can progress rapidly, leading to life-threatening complications. Prompt initiation of empiric antibiotic therapy is critical for patients with FN in order to avoid progression to sepsis, regardless of whether bacteremia is detected [18].

Neutropenia is defined as an absolute neutrophil count (ANC) of less than 500/μL, or less than 1000/μL with an anticipated decline to less than 500/μL within the next 48-h period. Neutropenic fever is a single oral temperature of 38.3°C (101°F) or a temperature of greater than 38.0°C (100.4°F) sustained for more than 1 h in a patient with neutropenia [18].

FN is considered a medical emergency, as infections can rapidly progress without broad spectrum antibiotic treatment initiated within 1 h of fever [12]. The spectrum of bacterial pathogens isolated from FN patients has shifted from gram-negative organisms (noted in the 1970s) to gram-positive species (since mid-1980s), related to the use of antibacterial prophylaxis and indwelling catheters [18].

Numerous studies have sought to stratify patients at presentation into those at high- versus low-risk for complications of severe infection. Categorizing these neutropenic patients according to presenting signs and symptoms, underlying cancer, type of therapy, and medical comorbidities has become essential to determining the appropriate treatment algorithm. Risk stratification is a recommended starting point for managing patients with fever and neutropenia. What has not changed is the indication for immediate empirical antibiotic therapy. It is universally accepted that all patients who present with fever and neutropenia should be treated swiftly and broadly with antibiotics to treat both gram-positive and gram-negative pathogens [18].

Although several guidelines for the management of FN have been developed, none were initially focused on children. To address this critical gap, a panel of pediatric experts was convened to develop an evidence-based guideline for the empiric management of pediatric FN. The International Pediatric Fever and Neutropenia Guideline Panel included representatives from oncology, infectious disease, nursing, and pharmacy, as well as a patient advocate, from ten different countries [19].

Yet, how do we imbed the structure and process of these recommendations into the habitual practices of individuals, divisions, and hospital systems, all within the context of competing medical care, financial, and resource priorities? Despite two universally accepted international guidelines [18, 19] and the clinical experience/knowledge of bedside providers regarding the necessity of timely antibiotic administration, hospital practices continue to be variable. Just as many of our colleagues do, our hospital system has institutional, evidence-based practice guidelines based on industry standards and recommendations. These guidelines are carefully reviewed and approved by internal content experts, and disseminated into practice via various educational and clinical operational mechanisms (see Appendix 2).

The guidelines were implemented and determined to represent an improvement over previous practices. Subsequently, we considered how best to sustain this enhanced practice. From the sustainability perspective, we again consider the characteristics of sustainability described previously. From this vantage point, at the outset of the case:

(1) the *benefit* of an innovation around identification and early response to FN is clear (reduce risk of mortality and morbidity);
(2) the need for a standardized process that could be *routinized* like the previous CLABSI case was supported by the literature and readily available practice standards; and
(3) the *development* characteristic focused on clarity around accountability as well as its value at promoting ownership of the practice change.

Additionally, as in the CLABSI example, the pre-conditions for a sustained program were again present in that: (1) innovation—the "fit with mission"; (2) context, both internal and external; (3) leadership (same institutional support and structure); and (4) processes, including a well-functioning quality improvement and patient safety capacity.

The first step in addressing these challenges was to clearly identify and state the specific aim. The interdisciplinary team worked on the key driver diagram to create a pathway to improved outcomes. The key driver diagram was critical to delineating the key drivers, clear interventions, and ultimately metrics to measure success (Fig. 7.7).

Febrile Neutropenia – Key Drivers Diagram

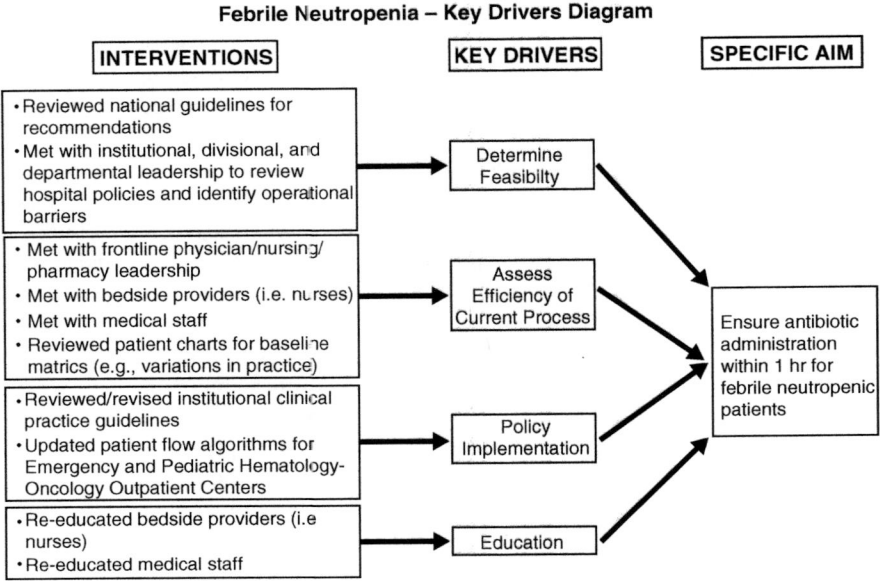

Fig. 7.7 Case 2: FN key driver diagram

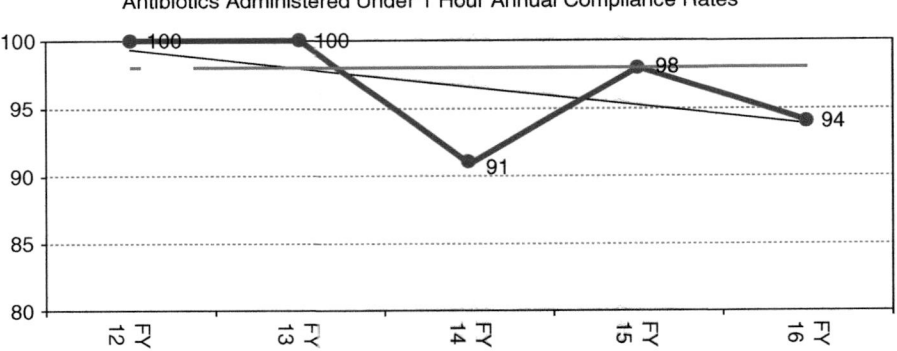

Fig. 7.8 Febrile neutropenia (FN, also known as neutropenic fever) compliance rates

The structure comprised of four key drivers—determining feasibility, assessing the efficiency of the original process, implementing the newly revised/reviewed policy, and re-educating the pertinent stakeholders on the changes to the existing process. A multidisciplinary team of physician and nursing partners worked on each of these drivers in a sequence of PDSA cycles. By implementing these key strategies, we anticipated that variability in practice would be minimized (Fig. 7.8).

We developed working relationships with our Emergency Department partners, to appropriately collect data, but also partnering with them in educating their providers, nursing, and pharmacy to prioritize our population of patients (sometimes in advance of other patients awaiting seen), and were educated our inpatient and outpatient staff. We consequently saw a significantly bump in FY15 back to 98% compliance. However, with an influx of hundreds of new nursing and provider trainees, we experienced another decline to 94% this past fiscal year. This illustrates the need for persistent attention to the quality initiative over time in order to ensure full implementation as well as sustained practice change.

Discussion/Conclusion

At the most basic level, sustainability refers to when a valuable quality innovation that improves care moves from being seen as "new" to becoming part of the standard of delivering care. Spread, in equally simple terms, is when that improvement moves from the original developers to other areas, and eventually to every available care setting, within a health care organization or system [10]. Case 1 and Case 2 (CLABSI and FN, respectively) each have elements of well-designed, realistic quality improvement efforts, with stops and starts, successes, and challenges. From a sustainability and spread perspective, each case occurs at the individual and unit level has varying levels of implementation, and shares characteristics associated with sustainability as well as the pre-conditions previously described.

The sustained innovation is fundamentally connected to the value or benefit perceived by the clinicians on the original team, becomes a standard of care that is measured and reported by the clinical care team and is owned by the various team members who embrace the change as a part of their own patient care. Additionally, the sustained innovation fits with the mission of the clinical care team, occurs in a clinical context that is responding to both internal and external factors, is led by effective leaders, and trialed, modified, and operationalized by a team well versed in quality improvement processes and techniques. Sustaining innovation is not easy as the literature demonstrates but those that have the highest chances for success tend to share the characteristics and pre-conditions described. Sustained improvements should be spread or disseminated in a planned formal manner to other teams and throughout the organization. Of course, depending on the clinical context the spread occurs along a continuum from making an exact replica of the innovation elsewhere to seeing the innovation as a general framework or guiding principle that can be embraced, modified, and applied to a variety of clinical settings.

We started this chapter recognizing that the "evaporation of improvement" seems omnipresent and of great concern in the health care quality improvement arena. No magic bullet has been identified that ensures automatic sustainability and spread. We recognize that a good first step is a well-functioning, quality improvement-oriented team. Ideally, this team is sensitive to the characteristics and pre-conditions associated with sustained improvement as well as understanding the concepts associated with improvements that spread beyond the initial stakeholders. It seems reasonable to diminish the evaporation of improvement by having quality improvement efforts condense around concepts and frameworks that speak to sustainability and spread both in and outside of health care.

Appendix 1: Case 1: Central Line Associated Blood Stream Infection (CLABSI)

CLABSI – Cascading of Responsibility

What role do I play in CLABSI prevention?					
SVP	**VP/AVP**	**Director**	**Frontline Leadership**	**Bedside Provider**	**Patient Family**
• Eliminate CLABSIs	• Eliminate CLABSIs	• Eliminate CLABSIs	• Eliminate CLABSIs	• Eliminate CLABSIs	• Eliminate CLABSI's
• Support the removal of operational barriers experienced by the clinical team to prevent CLABSIs.	• Promote a culture of safety, accountability and teamwork • Ensure collaboration across all inter-professional teams in support of CLABSI prevention is achieved	• Ensure standardization of practice within clinical area • Conduct monitoring and surveillance for compliance • Report key quality metrics and compliance on a monthly basis.	• Monitor and investigate practice and policy variations. • Provide education and training to ensure all staff are deemed competent.	• Strict adherence to bundle elements and infection control standards • Partner with frontline leadership in identifying barriers for compliance • Provide patient and family education	• Partner more closely with patients and families regarding CLABSI prevention • Empower patients to verbalize any concerns regarding central line care to direct caregiver or leadership team member

CLABSI – Cascading of Responsibilities – Medical Staff

What role do I play in CLABSI prevention?				
SVP/In Chief	**Quality Officer/Safety Officer**	**Service Chief/Medical Director**	**Decentralized Quality Physician or designee**	**Bedside provider**
• Eliminate CLABSIs	• Eliminate CLABSIs	• Eliminate CLABSIs	• Eliminate CLABSIs	• Eliminate CLABSIs
• Support the removal of operational barriers experienced by the clinical team to prevent CLABSIs.	• Promote a culture of safety, accountability and teamwork • Support process to enhance best practices for central line care and team collaboration • Remove barries as necessary	• Ensure standardization of approach and enhance accountability for adherence to guidelines	• Monitor lines for cleanliness, necessity and usage. Instruct and remediate as necessary	• Uniform adherence to bundles infection control standards • Provide patient and family education

What actions do I perform in CLABSI prevention?						
SVP	**VP/AVP**	**Director**	**Frontline Leadership**	**Bedside Provider**	**Medical staff**	**Patient Family**
• *ACTIONS*	• *ACTIONS*	• *ACTIONS*	• *ACTIONS*	• *ACTIONS*	• *ACTIONS*	• *ACTIONS*
• *1. "Executive Rounding" monthly throughout high risk clinical areas*	• *1. "Executive Rounding" weekly throughout high risk clinical areas* • *2. Recognize clinical areas for good performance*	• *1. Round weekly with physician partner.* • *2. Review performance metrics for "Pratice Must Haves" on a weekly basis.* • *3. Report key quality metrics and compliance on a monthly basis in CLABSI streering mtg*	• *1. Round daily to monitor and investigate practice and policy variations on 100% of lines.* • *2. Track bundle complieance on a weekly basis and report to Director* • *3. Implement training plan for new staff, travelers, float and existing staff*	• *1. Implement maintenance bundle for every central line.* • *2. Follow all infection control standards for hand hygiene, fingernail policy, and isolation* • *3. Educate each family on CLABSI prevention and document education*	• *1. Rounding weekly with nursing leadership* • *2. Strict adherence to bundle elements and infection control standards* • *3. Monitor lines for necessity and usage* • *4. Partner in identifying barriers*	• *1. Serve as a central line care consultants by communicating practice opportunities to leader during rounds*

Appendix 2: Febrile Neutropenia (FN, Neutropenic Fever)

Neutropenic Fever – Cascading of Responsibility

What role do I play ensuring antibiotic administration <1 hour after fever?

SVP	VP/AVP	Director	Frontline Leadership	Bedside Provider	Patient/Family
• Timely antibiotic administration	• Timely antibiotic administration	• Timely antibiotic administration	• Timely antibiotic administration	• Timely antibiotic administration	• Timely antibiotic administration
• Support the removal of operational barriers experienced by the clinical team to ensure antibiotics are administered <1 hour after fever	• Promote a culture of safety, accountability and teamwork • Ensure collaboration across all inter-professional teams such that timely antibiotic administration is achieved	• Ensure standardization of practice within clinical areas • Conduct monitoring and surveillance for compliance • Report key quality metrics and compliance on a quarterly basis	• Monitor and investigate practice and policy variations • Provide education and training to ensure all staff are deemed competent	• Strict adherence to evidence based Clinical Practice Guidelines • Partner with frontline leadership in identifying barriers for compliance (Hematology-Oncology-Transplant, Emergency Center) • Provide patient and family education	• Partner more closely with patients/families regarding timely antibiotic administration • Empower patients to verbalize any concerns regarding medical care directly to direct caregiver or leadership team member

Neutropenic Fever – Cascading of Responsibilities – Medical Staff

What role do I play in ensuring antibiotic administration <1 hour after fever?

SVP/In Chief	Quality Officer/Safety Officer	Service Chief/Medical Director	Decentralized Quality Physician or designee	Bedside provider
• Timely antibiotic administration	• Timely antibiotic administration	• Timely antibiotic administration	• Timely antibiotic administration	• Timely antibiotic administration
• Support the removal of operational barriers experienced by the clinical team to ensure antibiotics are administered <1 hour after fever	• Promote a culture of safety, accountability, and teamwork • Support process to enhance collaboration across all inter-professional teams such that timely antibiotic administation is achieved • Remove barries as necessary	• Ensure standardization of approach and enhance accountability for adherence to guidelines	• Monitor and investigate practice and policy variations • Conduct monitoring and surveillance for compliance	• Uniform adherence to evidence based Clinical Practice Guidelines • Provide patient and family education

What actions do I perform in ensuring antibiotic administration <1 hour after fever?

SVP	VP/AVP	Director	Frontline Leadership	Bedside Provider	Medical staff	Patient Family
ACTIONS	*ACTIONS*	*ACTIONS*	*ACTIONS*	*ACTIONS*	*ACTIONS*	*ACTIONS*
1. Recognize clinical areas for good performance	1. Recognize clinical areas for good performance	1. Report key quality metrics and compliance on a quarterly basis in Texas Children's Cancer and Hematology Centers Quality Transformation Crore meeting	1. Investigate practice and policy variations of 100% of admissions. 2. Track compliance on a quarterly basis and report to Director 3. Implement training plan for new staff, travelers, float and existing staff	1. Strict adherence to evidence based clinical practice guidelines 2. Educate each family on evidance based clinical practice guidelines and document education	1. Consistent communication with nursing and pharmacy partners 2. Strict adherence to evidance based clinical practice guidelines 3. Partner in identifying barriers	1. Serve as madical care consultants by communicating practice opportunities to medical staff during rounds

References

1. Wiltsey-Stirman S, Kimberly J, Cook N, Calloway A, Castro F, Charns M. The sustainability of new programs and innovations: a review of the empirical literature and recommendations for future research. Implement Sci. 2012;7:17–35.
2. Fleiszer AR, Semenic SE, Ritchie JA, Richer M, Denis JL. The sustainability of healthcare innovations: a concept analysis. J Adv Nurs. 2015;71(7):1484–98.
3. Buchanan DA, Fitzgerald L, Ketley D, editors. The sustainability and spread of organizational change. Abingdon, Oxon: Routledge; 2007.
4. Carr, S. Editor's notebook: a quotation with a life of its own. Patient safety & quality healthcare editor's notebook. http://www.psqh.com/analysis/editor-s-notebook-a-quotation-with-a-life-of-its-own/. Accessed 1 July 2008.
5. Scheirer MA. Is sustainability possible? A review and commentary on empirical studies of program sustainability. Am J Eval. 2005;26:320–47.
6. Berwick DM. Disseminating innovations in health care. J Am Med Soc. 2003;289(15):1969–75.
7. Buchanan D, Fitzgerald L, Ketley D, Gollop R, Jones JL, et al. No going back: a review of the literature on sustaining organizational change. Int J Manag Rev. 2005;7(3):189–205.
8. Greenhalgh T, Robert G, MacFarlane F, Bate P, Kyriakidou O. Diffusion of innovations in service organizations: systematic review and recommendations. Milbank Q. 2004a;82(4):581–629.
9. Racine DP. Reliable effectiveness: a theory on sustaining and replicating worthwhile innovations. Adm Policy Ment Health Ment Health Ser Res. 2006;33:356–87.
10. 5 Million Lives Campaign. Getting started kit: rapid response teams. Cambridge, MA: Institute for Healthcare Improvement; 2008. IHI.org.
11. Greenhalgh, T., Robert, G., Bate, P., Kyriakidou, O., Macfarlane, F., & Peacock, R. (2004b). How to spread good ideas: a systematic review of the literature on diffusion, dissemination and sustainability of innovations in health service delivery and organisation. National Institute for Health Research (NIHR). http://www.nets.nihr.ac.uk/__data/assets/pdf_file/0017/64340/FR-08-1201-038.pdf.
12. Slaghuis S, Strating M, Bal R, Nieboer A. A measurement instrument for spread of quality improvement in healthcare. Int J Qual Health Care. 2013;25(2):125–31. doi:10.1093/intqhc/mzt016.
13. Rogers EM. Diffusion of innovations. New York: Free Press; 1995.
14. Osbourne SP. Naming the beast defining and classifying service innovations in social policy. Hum Relat. 1998;30:1133–54.
15. Fraser SW, Burch K, Knightly M, Osborne M, Wilson T. Using collaborative improvement in a single organisation; improving anticoagulant care. Int J Healthcare Qual Assur. 2002;15:152–8.
16. Wilson MZ, Rafferty CR, Deeter D, Comito MA, Hollenbeak CS. Attributable costs of central line-associated bloodstream infections in a pediatric hematology/oncology population. Am J Infect Control. 2014;42:1157–60.
17. Marschall, J., Mermel, L., Fakih, M., Hadaway, L., Kallen, A., et al. (2014). Strategies to prevent central line-associated bloodstream infections in acute care hospitals. Infect Control Hosp Epidemiol, 35, 753–771. (On behalf of The Society for Healthcare Epidemiology of America).
18. Freifeld AG, Bow EJ, Sepkowitz KA, et al. Clinical practice guideline for the use of antimicrobial agents in neutropenic patients with cancer: 2010 update by the infectious diseases society of America. Clin Infect Dis. 2011;52(4):e56–93.
19. Lehrnbecher T, Phillips R, Alexander S, et al. Guideline for the management of fever and neutropenia in children with cancer and/or undergoing hematopoietic stem-cell transplantation. J Clin Oncol. 2012;30(35):4427–38.
20. Merriam-Webster. Sustainability. Springfield: Merriam-Webster Online Dictionary; 2013.
21. Rogers EM. Diffusion of innovations. New York: Free Press; 2003.
22. Bowman CC, Sobo EJ, Asch SM, Gifford AL. Measuring persistence of implementation: QUERI series. Implement Sci. 2008;3:3–21.

23. Scheirer MA, Dearing JW. An agenda for research on the sustainability of public health programs. Am J Public Health. 2011;101(11):2059–67.
24. Stetler CB, Ritchie JA, Rycroft-Malone J, Charns MP. Leadership for evidence-based practice: strategic and functional behaviors for institutionalizing EBP. Worldviews Evid Based Nurs. 2014;11(4):219–26.
25. Davies B, Edwards N. Sustaining knowledge use. In: Straus SE, Tetroe J, Graham ID, editors. Knowledge translation in health care: moving from evidence to practice. West Sussex: Wiley-Blackwell; 2013. p. 165–73.
26. Mancini JA, Marek LI. Sustaining community-based programs for families: conceptualization and measurement. Fam Relat. 2004;53(4):339–47.
27. Gruen RL, Elliott JH, Nolan ML, Lawton PD, Parkhill A, McLaren CJ, Lavis JN. Sustainability science: an integrated approach for health-programme planning. Lancet. 2008;372(9649):1579–89.
28. Johnson K, Hays C, Center H, Daley C. Building capacity and sustainable prevention innovations: a sustainability planning model. Eval Program Plann. 2004;27(2):135–49.
29. Bevan H, Christian D, Cottrell K, Easton J, Fraser S, Green L, Green R, Godfrey-Harris L, Hargadon J, Kennedy R, Ketley D, Kulkarni M, McBride M, Maher L, Mudd D, O'Neil S, Penny J, Plsek P, Riley N, Rogers H. Improvement leaders' guide to sustainability and spread. Ipswich: N. H. S Modernization-Agency; 2002.
30. Damanpour F, Gopalakrishnan S. Theories of organizational structure and innovation adoption: the role of environmental change. J Eng Technol Manag. 1998;15:1–24.
31. Wejnert B. Integrating models of diffusion of innovations: a conceptual framework. Annu Rev Sociol. 2002;28:297–326.
32. Mowatt G, Thomson MA, Grimshaw J, Grant A. Implementing early warning messages on emerging health technologies. Int J Technol Assess Health Care. 1998;14:663–70.
33. NHS Modernisation Agency. The improvement leader's guide to spread and sustainability. London: Department of Health; 2003.

Chapter 8
Principles of Patient Safety in Pediatric Hem/Onc/HSCT

Patrick Guffey and Daniel Hyman

Introduction

> First do no harm…. I will follow that system which, according to my ability and judgment, I consider for the benefit of my patients, and abstain from whatever is deleterious and mischievous—The Hippocratic Oath

Patients want three things from their healthcare experience: "Don't hurt me, heal me, and be nice to me"—in that order [1]. Until recently, the focus of healthcare has been on developing novel cures and advances in how to treat a disease. In the past 15 years, there has been a dramatic expansion of efforts focused on improving systems of care and understanding the science of quality and patient safety. The 1999 Institute of Medicine's seminal report "To Err is Human: Building a Safer Healthcare System" publicized the analysis that approximately 100,000 deaths annually are due to preventable medical errors, at a cost of between $17 and 29 billion [2]. This report was a significant catalyst in engaging a broad group of stakeholders in identifying and addressing the reasons why medical errors occur and how they can be prevented.

Patient safety is also intrinsic to health system efforts to increase the value of the care provided to patients and families. As healthcare costs continue to rise and increasingly stress the economy (17.5% of US gross domestic product in 2014) [3], there has been an increasing focus on improving the *value* of care. Value is defined as the patient outcomes achieved per dollar expended [3]. Patient safety impacts

P. Guffey (✉)
Associate Chief Medical Information Officer, Division of Pediatric Anesthesiology, Department of Anesthesiology, Children's Hospital Colorado, University of Colorado School of Medicine, Aurora, CO, USA
e-mail: patrick.guffey@childrenscolorado.org

D. Hyman
Chief Medical and Patient Safety Officer, Department of Pediatrics, Children's Hospital Colorado, University of Colorado School of Medicine, Aurora, CO, USA
e-mail: daniel.hyman@childrenscolorado.org

© Springer International Publishing AG 2017
C.E. Dandoy et al. (eds.), *Patient Safety and Quality in Pediatric Hematology/Oncology and Stem Cell Transplantation*, DOI 10.1007/978-3-319-53790-0_8

value both in that adverse occurrences both worsen outcomes and increase costs. Consider the example of central line-associated blood stream infections, often (but not always) preventable with consistent adherence to infection prevention practices. There are estimated 250,000 cases of CLABSI per year in the USA at a cost in excess of $25,000 per episode and a mortality of approximately 15% [4]. A hematopoietic stem cell transplant (HSCT) may be seriously affected by one provider forgetting to "scrub the hub" prior to injecting a medication. Preventing 10% of these infections would save millions of dollars and prevent a significant number of deaths. Increasing patient safety is an incredibly effective method to add value to the care patients receive.

Structure of Safety Oversight

The governance of a hospital's quality and safety program begins with the organization's board of directors, which often has a distinct committee whose focus is in the area of quality and patient safety. The hospital's medical board and management team share in this governance the responsibility, but case law and regulatory requirements over the past several decades have established that the board itself is explicitly accountable for the quality and safety of patient care in its hospital. Clinicians and program leaders should have the opportunity to periodically interact with the hospital's board (or its quality/safety committee) to review key performance indicators and identify issues needing strategic management.

The hospital board of directors, medical board, hospital management team, and clinical program leaders together establish, develop, nurture, and maintain the culture of safety in their organization. There is a dynamic tension between individual actions and organizational structures, policies, and processes that seek to limit autonomy and promote consistency and reliable safety practices [5]. Therefore, the institution's quality and safety system must influence individual and team performance in order to impact patient outcomes and reduce rates of preventable harm. We propose that the most effective structure is one that begins with the board and then extends throughout the organization to the bedside and the healthcare team providing care to patients and families.

Individual clinical programs achieve program-specific outcomes in quality, safety, service, and efficiency in the context of their organizational approach to these efforts but can actively and positively impact program performance with focused attention on improvement. Avedis Donabedian focused on the importance of structures and processes in achieving improved outcomes in his early descriptions of quality improvement in healthcare settings [6, 7]. Units or programs (clinical microsystems) benefit from establishing multidisciplinary committees of providers, nurses, and allied health staff that care for patients. The first step in an effective safety program is unit-level quality and patient safety committees. The purpose of these groups is to monitor and effect change at the local level. Key leaders and stakeholders should meet at a reasonable interval, review data on patient harm (and its root cause) and preventative process measures, and identify and implement solutions to increase safety. Including patients and families on improvement teams and safety governance committees is increasingly a standard in Children's Hospitals. These team members ensure that program leaders keep the patient and family's needs central to these discussions.

The program's quality and safety committee can also provide the necessary peer review of adverse occurrences for the hospital's medical staff credentialing and ongoing practice evaluation. A system for reporting adverse events as well as near misses is a critical element of a safety program and is discussed below. Events that are reported can be referred to the department's quality improvement and safety committee for determination as to whether the care provided was appropriate or if there are improvements in the system or the provider's methods that may result in safer care.

While much of patient safety improvement is local, the interdisciplinary quality committees require a support system to be maximally effective. Additionally, there are a significant number of patient safety initiatives that are most effective if driven from the organizational level. A quality and patient safety (QPS) department, led by a chief quality (or quality and patient safety) officer (CQO), is one structure that can enable having both the data and support the local groups require while also ensuring accountability for the overall patient safety strategy and culture of the organization.

Many hospitals encounter the same challenges in improving patient safety. A number of national collaboratives have been effective in accelerating both individual and collective hospital improvements and providing the ability to compare results and share the various methodologies used to achieve them. The Children's Hospitals' Solutions for Patient Safety Network is one example of a collaborative that has seen dramatic results, including significant reductions in various hospital-acquired conditions and other serious safety events [8]. Another example is the Children's Hospital Hematology/Oncology central line-associated blood stream infection (CLABSI) collaborative. Through the National Association of Children's Hospitals and Related Institutions (NACHRI), this group developed a quality improvement collaborative to study the impact of consistent care bundles on the incidence of CLABSI. The member institutions saw a 20% decrease in infections over a 12-month period [9]. The initial CLABSI rate of 2.85 CLABSIs per 1000 line days decreased by 28% to 2.04 CLABSIs per 1000 line days. This group has also published the incidence of CLABSI in different kinds of central lines [10].

Safety Reporting Systems

We cannot fix what we do not know about preventing adverse events requires an understanding of current practice and then strategies to influence that practice so as to produce the desired result. This typically requires learning from previous adverse events or "near misses" and then adjusting the system to prevent adverse events from occurring again

The first step in preventing adverse events is detection and reporting of individual occurrences and near misses. Aggregating this information at both the individual hospital level and through specialty societies permits continuous learning and improvement. Generally, the healthcare team members involved in an event, or alternatively the patient or family, are the first to recognize an error or adverse event. Other sources of information about adverse events include "trigger tools," data mining from electronic health records, the sharing of safety stories in group meetings, and, much later, through notification of legal action.

A patient safety incident is defined by the World Health Organization as *an event or circumstance, which could have resulted, or did result, in unnecessary harm to a patient* [11]. A *near miss* is defined as *an incident that did not reach the patient* but reasonably could have resulted in harm [11, 12]. Most medical errors are multifactorial, and it often takes a series of individual errors that align to cause significant patient harm.

Voluntary Incident Reporting Systems

The single greatest impediment to error prevention in the medical industry is that we punish people for making mistakes—Lucian Leape, MD

Voluntary incident reporting is widely used to report near misses as well as cases of harm. Voluntary reporting to a central repository can take many forms, ranging from highly complex electronic systems to a paper form. The most important part is that the system is reliably used to report cases of harm or near misses.

An organization's safety culture is a key factor in the likelihood of incidents being voluntarily reported into incident reporting systems. A culture that recognizes and rewards reporting is much more likely to become aware of latent system risks so they can be addressed than one which punishes people for making errors, especially in the context of a system that does not prevent those errors. Several studies have suggested that only a small fraction of adverse occurrences and near misses are captured in voluntary incident reporting systems [13–15]. For instance, Cullen found that reporting of adverse drug events was highly unreliable and variable across a 1300-bed tertiary hospital [16]. Another problem associated with voluntary reporting is that healthcare providers report events at different rates. Milch found through an analysis of 92,547 reports across 26 hospitals that physicians were the least likely to report a case of harm to a patient [17].

Despite these problems, it is possible to increase the use of reporting systems and access this data. Systems that are well-designed, easy to use, and customized to the specialty can result in higher rates of use [14, 18, 19]. For example, when a reporting system was customized to the needs of anesthesiologists at two major academic medical centers, reporting increased by two orders of magnitude compared to the baseline hospital system [18]. Tables 8.1 and 8.2 illustrate some of the reasons why reporting systems are not used adequately and the methods to increase reporting [19].

Table 8.1 Disincentives for reporting adverse events [13–15, 19–21]	Disincentives for reporting adverse events
	Poor education about what constitutes an event
	Concern over legal or credentialing consequences
	Personal shame
	Fear of implicating others
	Time-consuming processes
	Systems that are difficult to access
	Lack of anonymity
	Potentially discoverable information
	Slow infrastructure
	Arduous, poorly designed interfaces
	Lack of feedback and follow-up, no perceived value to the department

Table 8.2 Features of a successful incident reporting system [21]	Factors that incentivize reporting
	Secure and non-discoverable data
	Quick entry time (less than 1 min) and ease of use
	Accessibility of the system
	The capture of both near misses and incidents of patient harm
	An option of anonymity for entering reports
	Data searchable by the department QI committee
	Summary reports to department and hospital
	A culture of learning, not blame, in response to reports

Quality Metrics

Quality metrics can be grouped into volume, structure, outcomes, or process measures [7]. All of these have quality and safety implications, and it is important to understand each in the context of an overall safety program.

- Volume, in and of itself, may be a driver of safer care. The basic concept is that if an organization has a higher volume, that quality will be higher than a comparable institution with a lower volume of the disease or procedure in question. This ratio has been demonstrated in numerous cases, but is not universal [22].
- Structural metrics are defined as the presence or absence of a service, designation, or other designation. An example is the trauma classification of a hospital, for example, Level 1 status. While there may be an association between this and the safety and quality of the trauma program, there is typically not robust evidence that these markers are directly tied to safer outcomes.
- Outcomes are probably the most sought-after metric by the public as an overall marker of safe, effective care. However, defining outcomes is exceptionally difficult. There are many confounding variables, such that a simple comparison between facilities may not yield accurate results. Many outcome measures are derived from administrative data sets, which are typically derived from coding

and billing data. This is fraught with opportunities for bias. This variability in what in many cases is a manual process then confounds any meaningful attempt at risk adjustment. Patient characteristics are variables that have to be controlled in order to generate meaningful outcome measures. However, no standard approach is available for risk or severity adjustment, and typically these adjustments are based on the aforementioned administrative data sets, further compounding any inherent biases. There are examples where the data is analyzed in such a controlled manner as to draw meaningful conclusions, such as the outcomes for children with congenital heart defects. In 2015, the Society of Thoracic Surgeons (STS) released its assessment of outcomes at hospitals that perform pediatric congenital heart surgery. However, even with robust data collection, analysis, and risk adjust techniques, the results are limited—the centers are represented by a star classification of 1–3 and basic adjusted mortality information only [23].

• Process measures assess whether the defined process or standard of care was provided to the patient. These measures are typically abstracted from the medical record rather than from administrative coding data. Provided the compliance with the process is linked to improved outcomes, these measures can add value. For example, a "bundle" exists for central line placement, and following the steps in the process has been linked with a lower CLABSI rate. An example of a process measure is if the clinician was compliant with the bundle. However, it is not an uncommon occurrence for a process measure and an outcome to be discordant. This can be due to confounding variables, or that the process steps are not linked with the outcome.

Trigger tools are an example of a quality metric and an innovative method for measuring the frequency of adverse events. This method consists of performing time-limited screening of charts to find the presence of "triggers" that indicate the possibility of their having been an adverse event. Examples would include the prescribing of reversal agents (e.g., naloxone, diphenhydramine) that may be indicative of an adverse drug event, unplanned return to the operating room that might indicate a surgical complication, etc. In addition to manual chart review approaches to finding and measuring triggers, there are examples now of using automated data mining from electronic medical records to do this. Detailed information on how to use trigger tools to measure harm frequency is beyond the scope of this chapter but available to the interested reader [24, 25].

Adverse Event Management

Management of an adverse event occurs in three phases: mitigation, management, and follow-up, including both disclosure and analysis/improvement efforts.

Mitigation is the management of an ongoing adverse event to prevent or minimize resulting harm to the patient. The specific response depends upon the nature of the situation. For example, if a patient is demonstrating signs of an adverse reaction to a transfusion, the transfusion is discontinued and treatment given for fever or other signs and symptoms. In some cases, the mitigation may be urgent, for example, after an overdose of a medication in which a patient is demonstrating potentially life-threatening reactions (e.g., respiratory depression after opiates). It is often possible to start mitigating an adverse event when warning signs of a potential or an impending adverse event first appear. An adverse event that does not reach the patient because of early mitigation is defined as a *near miss*.

A good plan can help the provider to anticipate an adverse event and also enables him or her to determine that there has been a deviation from the plan that requires further action. This in turn allows the contingency plan to be activated. As a result, an impending adverse event can be recognized more quickly, and a pre-formulated contingency plan invoked to mitigate further development of the incident. This may not prevent the adverse event from occurring but may help to mitigate the severity of the outcome.

Consider, for example, unanticipated anaphylaxis to intramuscular PEG-asparaginase. During the pre-chemotherapy briefing, the nurse states that the patient had previously received PEG-asparaginase and did not have a reaction to it. Although the patient does not have a known allergy, anaphylaxis medication should be preordered and at the bedside in case an allergic reaction occurs. If the patient develops a small local reaction including respiratory distress, diphenhydramine should be administered. If the patient develops a systemic allergic reaction, diphenhydramine, corticosteroids, and epinephrine should be administered rapidly. In addition, a rapid response alert should be sent to the appropriate intensive care staff. Finally, if the patient develops respiratory failure despite treatment, the airway management protocol should be initiated. The precise triggers should be set for an individual patient, while the concept is that of escalating the care and management.

In summary, mitigation usually involves three steps: attempting to prevent the event from getting any worse, attempting to improve the situation, and making a diagnosis so that further management can be targeted to a specific cause.

Management follows mitigation and starts with diagnostic assessments and/or therapies directed at managing the presumed diagnosis or complication. The word *presumed* is used because the mode of presentation of the event might lead to an incorrect working diagnosis. This is not a reflection upon the skill or decision-making of the responder, merely, that it is often not possible to make the correct diagnosis until the event has evolved. During the initial management, therefore, one must accept that initial pathways might not be ideal. Until a definitive diagnosis is made (and possibly even afterward), the responder should be aware of alternative possibilities and be prepared to change the working diagnosis.

Imagine for a moment an adolescent patient with lymphoma who has been admitted for fever and neutropenia and is stable on antibiotics. Twenty-four hours into his hospitalization, the nursing staff identify that the patient is wheezing. Albuterol is prescribed for a presumed exacerbation of underlying asthma. If, shortly thereafter, the patient develops urticaria and hypotension, the diagnosis of anaphylaxis would be readily considered. It may initially present with bronchospasm and then be treated according to a specific management protocol, but other causes of bronchospasm should be considered and excluded while this treatment is commenced. In a different situation, the correct diagnosis might be either bronchospasm or anaphylaxis, but this example highlights the importance of keeping an open mind during the management of an adverse event. On occasion a diagnosis is not apparent, or initial efforts at management are insufficient. If a "call for extra help" has not already been made, this is the stage where consultation is appropriate. An example is the initiation of an RRT (rapid response team). Each hospital, clinic, and infusion area should have a mechanism for summoning additional resources, and in many hospitals, patients and family members are informed about their ability to request an emergency response team if they feel their concerns are not being addressed.

Follow-up after adverse occurrences consists of the management of the residual clinical conditions, disclosure, learning from outcomes, improvements in patient safety, as well as risk management and medicolegal considerations. Another follow-up to consider is reporting to an event registry because this may trigger analysis and studies that lead to prevention of the initial event. The reporting may be through an incident report, M&M process, or other means—but a sign of a strong safety culture is that cases of harm or near misses are always reported and evaluated for improvement.

Disclosure After Adverse Events

After an adverse event occurs, consideration should be given to disclosing the event to the patient and family. Multiple studies have shown that physicians and patients believe that when a medical error occurs, it should be disclosed in a timely fashion [26, 27]. Further, in many circumstances, there are benefits to the provider by disclosing the adverse event. According to Robbennolt, a physician, attorney, and expert in medical error, "Patients were less likely to indicate they would seek legal advice when the physician assumed responsibility for the error, apologized, and outlined steps that would be taken to prevent recurrence" [28]. In 2001 the University of Michigan formed an institutionally supported program of full disclosure, investigations, a timely apology, implementation of solutions to prevent the error, and, when appropriate, financial compensation in response to medical errors. This program showed a statistically significant decrease in claims, compensation, and legal costs [29]. Even given agreement on the responsibility to disclose, and potential benefits, multiple studies illustrate that disclosure is not assured [30–32]. Providers are less likely to disclose when the error did not have a tangible effect on the patient's outcome [26, 33]. Barriers to disclosure are legal and financial factors, the physician's reputation, an expectation of perfection by patients and physicians, emotional distress, and a medical culture that focuses on personal responsibility rather than the effect of system-based errors [33]. Implementing an educational program at the department and/or hospital level can reduce these barriers.

A recommended approach to disclosure is summarized below:

1. Contact the hospital's risk management department for support if the practitioner is uncertain of the best practices surrounding event disclosure.
2. State the facts of what happened and that a medical error occurred.
3. Offer an apology.
4. Review the clinical implications of the medical error.
5. Assure the patient the reasons for the error will be investigated and that the patient and family will be informed of the results and how the institution will prevent the error from recurring.
6. Consider waiving charges or offering compensation when appropriate.

Event Review

The goal of event review is to identify the proximate and/or root causes of errors that contribute to adverse events. These errors may be individual human mistakes, but often they are due to underlying systems issues (latent errors) that could lead to future harm. Identifying and addressing the latent errors in the system is a far more effective strategy than simply trying to retrain or write new policies to prevent future human errors.

Root Cause Analysis

A variety of tools have been used to analyze and manage hazards and incidents in healthcare, including various forms of root cause analysis (RCA) or apparent cause analysis (ACA). The Joint Commission requires an RCA to be performed for all adverse events that reach the patient and cause severe temporary harm requiring intervention, permanent harm, or death (*sentinel events*) [34]. Root cause analysis typically includes individual interviews of all team members involved in any serious safety event by two neutral facilitators, trained in interviewing and sensitive to principles of just culture. Facts and perspectives gathered through these discussions are then summarized by the interviewers and presented to a group of peers and/or supervisors of the staff involved in the event. The purpose of this "root cause analysis team" is to identify the proximate and root causes of the occurrence and recommend countermeasures that, if implemented, can prevent a future recurrence. These RCA teams are generally supported by an executive level sponsor who is accountable for the results of the review and the implementation of the action plans. Results of RCAs should be reviewed with appropriate governance committees overseeing organizational safety, and they should ensure timely and effective implementation of action plans.

The relationship between hazards, barriers, and incidents, which may be identified in an event review, is typically complex and difficult to represent in a concise manner. Moreover, root cause analysis can be very time-consuming and is not an appropriate method for analyzing the majority of events and near misses that are reported to a voluntary registry. A number of cognitive aids have been developed to show the causes of an incident including the use of causal trees [34]. Ideally the results of an event review should be depicted in a diagram, so that the accident trajectory can be understood. Diagrams for depicting the accident trajectory include the Swiss cheese model [35], causal trees [34], and more recently bowtie diagrams [36].

Just Culture Algorithm

> The question that drives safety work in a just culture is not who is responsible for failure, rather, it asks what is responsible for things going wrong. What is the set of engineered and organized circumstances that is responsible for putting people in a position where they end up doing things that go wrong? –Sidney Dekker

Another critical part of event review is a determination if the caregivers involved adhered to the standards of care and if not, why? Humans make mistakes, frequently, and human error is unavoidable. A "just culture" is one in which all participants are evaluated in a fair, equitable, and balanced fashion. Tragic examples of dedicated healthcare team members who have been involved in errors that caused serious harm or death of patients who are then "second victims" and are fired, incarcerated, or experience psychological trauma and even harm themselves are the reasons why it is imperative that health system leaders approach adverse occurrences in a just and fair way. There are many similar algorithms for evaluating occurrences using these principles [37]. One such example in use at the authors' hospital and medical school is included here (Fig. 8.1).

While rare cases of intentional harm and periodic situations due to provider impairment must be identified for appropriate discipline or evaluation/support, most cases of harm occur due to some interaction between latent system factors and human error that may be either innocent or due to reckless or risk-taking behaviors. A response to the situation that is based upon this evaluation is much more likely to promote a safety culture in which individuals are treated fairly and that the systems they work in can be continuously improved.

Sidebar: The Just Culture Algorithm in Practice

A 9-year-old girl, recently diagnosed with acute lymphocytic leukemia, is readmitted with fever following completion of induction chemotherapy. After several days of improvement, she begins to complain of increasingly severe diarrhea and abdominal pain. Overnight, her heart rate begins to increase from 120 to 140 to 170 beats per minute. An on-site resident is in communication with a fellow and a fluid bolus is given and labs obtained. In the morning, the patient's abdomen is

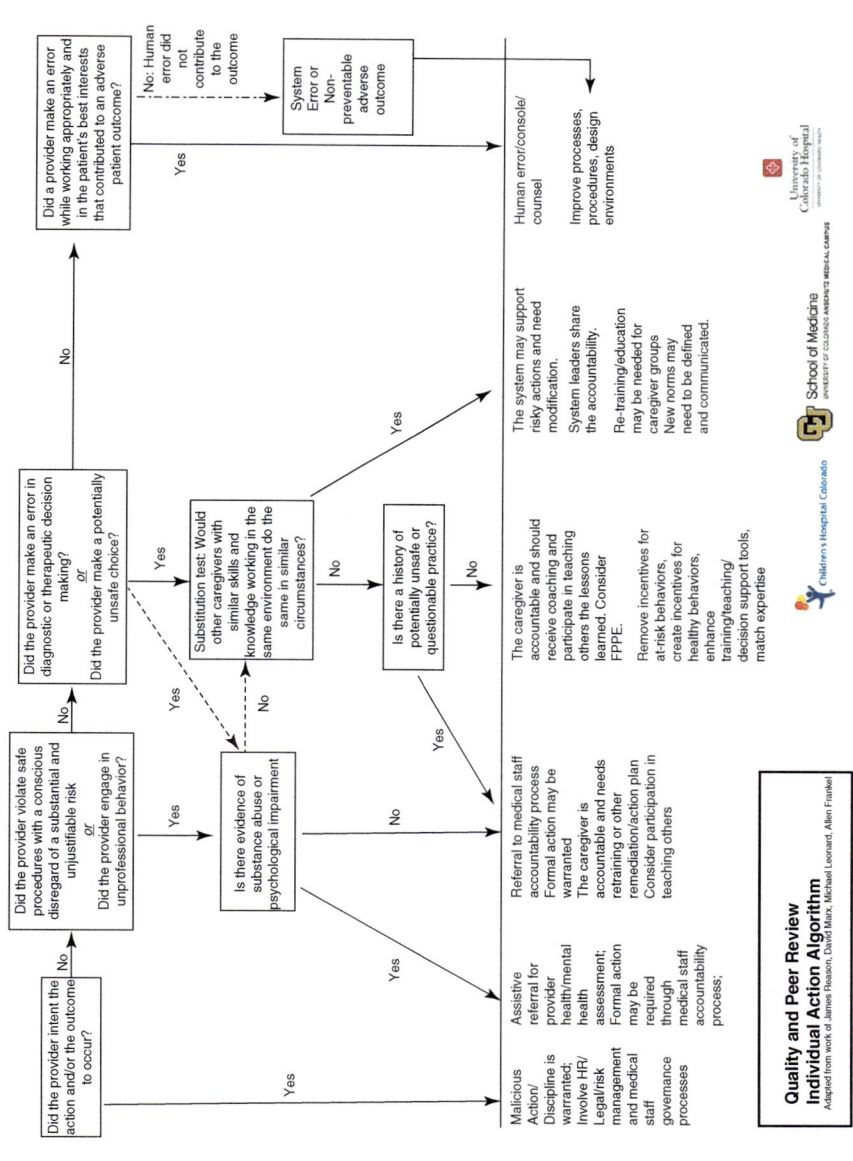

Fig. 8.1 Example individual action algorithm

noted to be distended and tender, and she is emergently taken to the operating room. Unfortunately, she is found to have severe bowel ischemia as a result of typhlitis and not enough viable bowel to survive. Support is withdrawn later that day, and she dies.

The root cause analysis proceeds to identify a number of gaps in the care provided to this patient. Focusing though on a review of provider decision-making, the assessment might be something like:

1. Is there any concern about the intention to cause harm? (Almost always will be no.)
2. Did the provider act unprofessionally or consciously disregard safe practice? Is there evidence of impairment? (This is also generally not the case, but explicit consideration is worthwhile, particularly if someone has been in repeat cases requiring focused review.)
3. Did the provider make an error in diagnostic or therapeutic decision-making? This is often answered positively as it would be in this case. The failure to recognize compensated shock led to a delay in recognition of the need for escalation of care. As described, in this case issues related to training and supervision are also relevant and must be considered. The algorithm would lead a cause analysis team to assess whether the provider was involved in other similar cases and to take action accordingly.

One of the uncomfortable aspects of case review is that the difference between cases with significant adverse events and those that are near misses is often determined less by the causal error than by other factors. Reviewing cases that have no harm or are near misses using the just culture algorithm is equally important to a fair and ethical review process.

FMEA

When reviewing medical errors, one sometimes wonders whether there is a proactive approach to preventing adverse events. A failure modes and effects analysis (FMEA) can be used to identify many if not all of the potential risks in a process and how to mitigate them. FMEAs have been used widely across industry and have been applied successfully in healthcare. In fact, the Joint Commission requires FMEA as a systemic, proactive method to improve safety and reliability. A description of the process can be found at www.fmeainfocentre.com. The FMEA process consists of four steps:

- Identifying all of the steps in a process
- Identifying failure modes for each step in the process (what could go wrong)
- Identifying failure causes (how could it go wrong)
- Identifying failure effects (what would happen)

Once this is complete, a risk score is assigned that takes into account the probability and severity of a failure. One method for ascertaining this information is the "Five Whys" which is an exercise identifying the root cause of a problem. In the case of an FMEA, this tool can be used to trace back to the step in the process that has the potential to lead to a system failure.

Once the FMEA is complete, it can be used to improve care and lower the risk of a failure. For each failure mode that is deemed to have an unacceptable risk score, an intervention can be undertaken. Typically, each intervention will require development, testing, and implementation of system changes designed to reduce the risk. A critical final step is post implementation monitoring and refinement to address unintended consequences of the change as well as further opportunities. The Institute of Healthcare Improvement offers a host of FMEA tools on its website, http://www.ihi.org.

Technology and Patient Safety

The Intersection of Quality and Informatics Is High Reliability

Highly reliable organizations (HROs) are ones that achieve extraordinary levels of safety and reliability under complex conditions expected to cause life-threatening failures. As described by Weick and Sutcliffe, there are five tenets of HROs worth reviewing and striving for a safety culture that embodies these principles [38]:

- Preoccupation with Failure—HROs do not ignore failure. Instead, they detect it and relentlessly pursue it in order to analyze what caused it.
- Reluctance to Simplify—By definition, an HRO is complex and they embrace this complexity in the analysis of events.
- Sensitivity to Operations—Employees and their leadership in HROs are constantly aware of how the system (processes and operations) affects the organization and maintain constant vigilance to recognize evolving risks and then take steps to mitigate them.
- Commitment to Resilience—HROs anticipate failure, are prepared for it to occur, and respond with swift problem-solving and responses that halt the issue.
- Deference to Expertise—Leaders in HROs listen to the individuals with the most knowledge of the issue regardless of hierarchy.

Examples of highly reliable industries include commercial aviation, nuclear power, chemical production, and naval aviation. These industries share another common trait. They rely heavily on informatics to gain information on their processes and respond accordingly. Consider the case of Delta Flight 1889 that was critically disabled by hail. The pilots flew right through a major thunderstorm in what would be considered a human error. The windshield was obliterated such that the pilots had no view out the windows and no visual references to land. This would be expected to cause a severe crash. However, commercial airliners have had the ability to land on autopilot since the early 1980s. The system was engaged, and the plane landed safely, brought itself to a complete stop, and was towed to the gate.

This would not have been possible without a highly advanced application of informatics and is an example of why commercial aviation is a highly reliable industry. In healthcare, clinical informatics is used in many applications to improve patient safety. While this is a relatively new area, informatics will be critical to the healthcare industry achieving high reliability.

Increasing Awareness

Patient safety and quality indicators are of limited use to providers if they are only available in static reports. At a local level, quality and process indicators can be abstracted from the medical record and displayed at the unit level or on dashboards. Clinical decision support (CDS) is an electronic tool that can provide information or suggest treatments at the time the clinician is entering an electronic order. This has been used successfully to increase the rate of influenza vaccination for inpatients prior to their discharge [39]. Another method of increasing awareness is informing the organization of the near misses and harm that occurs. An example report highlighting a deviation from safety practices and how to avoid it in the future is illustrated in Fig. 8.2. At our institution, this innovative program allows all members of the healthcare team access to information to help improve their practice.

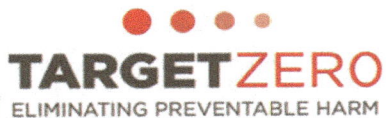

TARGETZERO
ELIMINATING PREVENTABLE HARM

A nurse called an inpatient service specialist (ISS) and asked for an ID band to be printed. The nurse asked if she could give the patient's MRN, but the ISS asked if she could provide the room number instead, which the nurse did. When the ID band arrived, it was for the wrong patient (the room numbers were similar, both ending in "08"). The nurse caught the error, called the ISS back and used the MRN to request a new ID band. Acceptable patient identifiers include MRN, patient name and date of birth. Room number is a locater, not a patient identifier.

TZ Buzz: ARCC & ADE

Sign up here *with your @childrenscolorado.org,*
@childrenscoloradofoundation.org or @ucdenver.edu email address to
receive safety emails, or text TARGETZERO to 2828 to get started.
(Message and data rates may apply).

Privileged and Confidential; Protected by Colorado State Statute 25-3-109.
This document contains information created as part of health care services review and is privileged and confidential and may not be disclosed.

Fig. 8.2 Target zero safety story

Electronic Medical Record

The electronic healthcare record (EHR) has become integral to care delivery, and there are multiple areas where its implementation has been proven to increase patient safety. Computerized physician order entry (CPOE) is one such example. When a CPOE system is installed as part of an enterprise EHR deployment, the physicians and other healthcare providers enter their orders through an electronic interface, in lieu of handwritten orders. This allows for numerous advantages. "CPOE systems help to reduce errors by providing very drug-specific information that can clarify potential confusion due to drug names that sound and look alike" [40]. "Other systems that have positive clinical decision support features further ensure appropriate drug prescription by guiding appropriate choices and providing alerts and recommendations when the drug orders are entered" [41]. CPOE systems can also use preprogrammed clinical decision support (CDS) to assist the physicians in making sound medical decisions. These modules can suggest less expensive and equally efficacious drugs or alert a provider if a study has already been performed. CPOE has been proven to be effective and has resulted in error reductions of 55–83% [42, 43].

Another example of where the EHR has improved patient safety is bar code medication administration (BCMA). When this technology is installed, the nurse scans all medications and the patient's identification prior to administration. BCMA allows the person administering medications, likely a nurse, to scan the drug and the patient to verify the five rights of medication, right patient, right drug, right time, right dose, and right route, and sends an alert if there is a mismatch. [42]. This technology has also been proven to reduce medication errors at a comparable rate as CPOE, 54–87% depending on the implementation [42, 43].

The EHR can be used to assist with patient identification and improvement of process measures. Proper patient identification prior to entering an order with CPOE is a known failure mode. The authors' hospital installed software in their implementation of the Epic EHR to display the patient's photo on a verification screen prior to finalizing an order and saw a dramatic reduction in cases of ordering tests, medications, or other interventions on the wrong patient [44]. The World Health Organization's Surgical Safety Checklist has been proven to reduce the rate of harm for patients undergoing surgical procedures [45]. One difficulty in using the checklist is presenting it at the point of care and integrating it into the surgical workflow. Along with the patient photo described above, the checklist is also filled out with information from the EHR. Figure 8.3 illustrates the checklist used for a lumbar puncture with chemotherapy injection in a procedure room. Process data shows the checklist is used greater than 99% of the time, and the rate of charting on the wrong patient, a common problem with anesthesia information systems, is 1 in 150,000 patients. This is an example of using the EHR to address multiple failure modes (patient identification, right procedure, correct weight and allergies, etc.) in real time. This checklist format could be used in other areas of the healthcare environment, such as a pre-BMT checklist.

Anesthesia Sign In - Performed By Anesthesiologist
Before Induction in Room

Anesthesiologist & Circulator Verify:

1) Patient Identification (Two identifiers - first & last name, MRN)
  Benjamin Jones (DOB: 12/12/2011, Sex: male)
  MRN: 1651144
  Check armband and consent
  Verify with family, if applicable

2) Procedure and Anesthetic
  Lumbar Puncture - Lower - Spine
  Verify on consent
  State anesthetic technique
  Discuss regional block(s) and check for block/surgical site mark(s)
  Blood consent signed, if applicable

3) Weight and Allergies
  Weight: 19 kg
  Allergies: Review of patient's allergies indicates no known allergies.

4) Assessment scores and prevention strategies, as appropriate
  For example:
    ✓ VTE(SCDs)
    ✓ STBUR
    ✓ Braden Q

5) Verify information against whiteboard

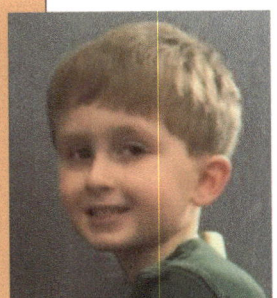

In room time:

Fig. 8.3 Pre-procedure checklist integrated into an EHR

References

1. Press Ganey. Reducing Serious Safety Events. 2016. Accessed at: http://images.health-care.pressganey.com/Web/PressGaneyAssociatesInc/%7B1bbbf571-af42-484d-8664-48726500ff22%7D_PI_Reducing_Serious_Safety_Events.pdf.
2. Institute of Medicine Committee on Quality of Health Care in A. In: Kohn LT, Corrigan JM, Donaldson MS, editors. To err is human: building a safer health system. Washington: National Academies Press (US). Copyright 2000 by the National Academy of Sciences. All rights reserved; 2000.
3. Porter ME. What is value in health care? N Engl J Med. 2010;363(26):2477–81.
4. Reduction in central line-associated bloodstream infections among patients in intensive care units—Pennsylvania, April 2001–March 2005. MMWR Morb Mortal Wkly Rep. 2005;54(40):1013–6.
5. Groves PS, Meisenbach RJ, Scott-Cawiezell J. Keeping patients safe in healthcare organizations: a structuration theory of safety culture. J Adv Nurs. 2011;67(8):1846–55.
6. Donabedian A. Evaluating the quality of medical care. Milbank Mem Fund Q. 1966;44(3):166–206.
7. Donabedian A. Evaluating the quality of medical care. 1966. Milbank Q. 2005;83(4):691–729.
8. Safety SfP. Solutions for patient safety. 2016. http://www.solutionsforpatientsafety.org/.
9. Bundy DG, Gaur AH, Billett AL, He B, Colantuoni EA, Miller MR. Preventing CLABSIs among pediatric hematology/oncology inpatients: national collaborative results. Pediatrics. 2014;134(6):e1678–85.
10. Hord JD, Lawlor J, Werner E, Billett AL, Bundy DG, Winkle C, et al. Central line associated blood stream infections in pediatric hematology/oncology patients with different types of central lines. Pediatr Blood Cancer. 2016;63(9):1603–7.

11. The World Alliance For Patient Safety Drafting G, Sherman H, Castro G, Fletcher M, on behalf of The World Alliance for Patient S, Hatlie M, et al. Towards an international classification for patient safety: the conceptual framework. Int J Qual Health Care. 2009;21(1):2–8.

12. Reason J. Human Error. New York: Cambridge University Press; 1990.

13. Kaldjian LC, Jones EW, Wu BJ, Forman-Hoffman VL, Levi BH, Rosenthal GE. Disclosing medical errors to patients: attitudes and practices of physicians and trainees. J Gen Intern Med. 2007;22(7):988–96.

14. Leape LL. Reporting of adverse events. N Engl J Med. 2002;347(20):1633–8.

15. Taylor JA, Brownstein D, Christakis DA, Blackburn S, Strandjord TP, Klein EJ, et al. Use of incident reports by physicians and nurses to document medical errors in pediatric patients. Pediatrics. 2004;114(3):729–35.

16. Cullen DJ, Bates DW, Small SD, Cooper JB, Nemeskal AR, Leape LL. The incident reporting system does not detect adverse drug events: a problem for quality improvement. Jt Comm J Qual Improv. 1995;21(10):541–8.

17. Milch CE, Salem DN, Pauker SG, Lundquist TG, Kumar S, Chen J. Voluntary electronic reporting of medical errors and adverse events. An analysis of 92,547 reports from 26 acute care hospitals. J Gen Intern Med. 2006;21(2):165–70.

18. Guffey P, Szolnoki J, Caldwell J, Polaner D. Design and implementation of a near-miss reporting system at a large, academic pediatric anesthesia department. Paediatr Anaesth. 2011;21(7):810–4.

19. Guffey PJ, Culwick M, Merry AF. Incident reporting at the local and national level. Int Anesthesiol Clin. 2014;52(1):69–83.

20. Kaldjian LC, Jones EW, Wu BJ, Forman-Hoffman VL, Levi BH, Rosenthal GE. Reporting medical errors to improve patient safety: a survey of physicians in teaching hospitals. Arch Intern Med. 2008;168(1):40–6.

21. Rowin EJ, Lucier D, Pauker SG, Kumar S, Chen J, Salem DN. Does error and adverse event reporting by physicians and nurses differ? Joint Commission Journal on Quality And Patient Safety/Joint Commission Resources. 2008;34(9):537–45.

22. Halm EA, Lee C, Chassin MR. Is volume related to outcome in health care? A systematic review and methodologic critique of the literature. Ann Intern Med. 2002;137(6):511–20.

23. Surgery SoT. STS congenital heart surgery public reporting [Webpage]. 2016. http://www.sts. org/congenital-public-reporting-module-searchSTS.

24. Classen DC, Lloyd RC, Provost L, Griffin FA, Resar R. Development and evaluation of the institute for healthcare improvement global trigger tool. J Patient Saf. 2008;4(3):169–77.

25. Classen DC, Resar R, Griffin F, Federico F, Frankel T, Kimmel N, et al. 'global trigger tool' shows that adverse events in hospitals may be ten times greater than previously measured. Health Aff (Millwood). 2011;30(4):581–9.

26. Hingorani M, Wong T, Vafidis G. Patients' and doctors' attitudes to amount of information given after unintended injury during treatment: cross sectional, questionnaire survey. BMJ. 1999;318(7184):640–1.

27. Witman AB, Park DM, Hardin SB. How do patients want physicians to handle mistakes? A survey of internal medicine patients in an academic setting. Arch Intern Med. 1996;156(22):2565–9.

28. Robbennolt JK. Apologies and medical error. Clin Orthop Relat Res. 2009;467(2):376–82.

29. Kachalia A, Kaufman SR, Boothman R, Anderson S, Welch K, Saint S, et al. Liability claims and costs before and after implementation of a medical error disclosure program. Ann Intern Med. 2010;153(4):213–21.

30. Wu AW, Folkman S, McPhee SJ, Lo B. Do house officers learn from their mistakes? JAMA. 1991;265(16):2089–94.

31. Christensen JF, Levinson W, Dunn PM. The heart of darkness: the impact of perceived mistakes on physicians. J Gen Intern Med. 1992;7(4):424–31.

32. Lamb RM, Studdert DM, Bohmer RM, Berwick DM, Brennan TA. Hospital disclosure practices: results of a national survey. Health Aff (Millwood). 2003;22(2):73–83.

33. Fein S, Hilborne L, Kagawa-Singer M, Spiritus E, Keenan C, Seymann G, et al. Advances in patient safety a conceptual model for disclosure of medical errors. In: Henriksen K, Battles JB, Marks ES, Lewin DI, editors. Advances in patient safety: from research to implementation (volume 2: concepts and methodology). Rockville: Agency for Healthcare Research and Quality; 2005.
34. Williams PM. Techniques for root cause analysis. Proc (Baylor Univ Med Cent). 2001;14(2):154–7.
35. Reason J. Human error: models and management. West J Med. 2000;172(6):393–6.
36. Pitblado R, Weijand P. Barrier diagram (bow tie) quality issues for operating managers. Process Saf Prog. 2014;33(4):355–61.
37. Frankel AS, Leonard MW, Denham CR. Fair and just culture, team behavior, and leadership engagement: the tools to achieve high reliability. Health Serv Res. 2006;41(4 Pt 2):1690–709.
38. Chassin MR, Loeb JM. High-reliability health care: getting there from here. Milbank Q. 2013;91(3):459–90.
39. Gerard MN, Trick WE, Das K, Charles-Damte M, Murphy GA, Benson IM. Use of clinical decision support to increase influenza vaccination: multi-year evolution of the system. J Am Med Inform Assoc. 2008;15(6):776–9.
40. Bobb A, Gleason K, Husch M, Feinglass J, Yarnold PR, Noskin GA. The epidemiology of prescribing errors: the potential impact of computerized prescriber order entry. Arch Intern Med. 2004;164(7):785–92.
41. Minesh P. Computerized physician order entry (CPOE) systems—an introduction. J Pharm Res. 2012;5(10):4962–7.
42. Agrawal A. Medication errors: prevention using information technology systems. Br J Clin Pharmacol. 2009;67(6):681–6.
43. Bates DW, Leape LL, Cullen DJ, Laird N, Petersen LA, Teich JM, et al. Effect of computerized physician order entry and a team intervention on prevention of serious medication errors. JAMA. 1998;280(15):1311–6.
44. Hyman D, Laire M, Redmond D, Kaplan DW. The use of patient pictures and verification screens to reduce computerized provider order entry errors. Pediatrics. 2012;130(1):e211–9.
45. Haynes AB, Weiser TG, Berry WR, Lipsitz SR, Breizat AH, Dellinger EP, et al. A surgical safety checklist to reduce morbidity and mortality in a global population. N Engl J Med. 2009;360(5):491–9.

Chapter 9
Implementation of Evidence-Based Care

Pauline A. Daniels and Jared D. Capouya

Principles of Evidence-Based Care

Heraclitus once said "The only thing that is constant is change." In the ever-changing world of health care, there is a need to not only adapt to these changes but also to continue to provide quality care for patients. In the early twentieth century reform of medical education to integrate public health into medicine, the shift in viewpoint of hospitals as merely shelters for the ill to reputable institutions that serve as the technological and scientific centers of medicine, the birth of modern epidemiology, and the concern for the economic sustainability of health care were just some of the factors contributing to the development of evidence-based medicine [1, 2].

Prior to the evolution of evidence-based medicine, and even today, clinical decisions are often based on personal experience. While personal experience can be beneficial in practice, it is, unfortunately, subject to bias which can negatively impact the clinical decision-making process. Over time it was recognized that basing medical practice on personal experience and widely accepted but unproved theories often resulted in negative patient outcomes. It became increasingly evident that a method which combines clinical experience, the best research evidence, and patient values/preferences to guide clinical practice and develop standardized processes was needed.

In 1996, Sackett, et al. defined evidence-based medicine as "the conscientious, explicit and judicious use of current best evidence in making decisions about the care of individual patients. The practice of evidence-based medicine means

P.A. Daniels
Bone Marrow Transplantation and Immune Deficiency, Cincinnati Children's Hospital Medical Center, Cincinnati, OH, USA
e-mail: Pauline.Daniels@cchmc.org

J.D. Capouya (✉)
Quality, Pediatrics, Mary Bridge Children's Hospital and Health Network, Tacoma, WA, USA
e-mail: Jared.Capouya@multicare.org

© Springer International Publishing AG 2017
C.E. Dandoy et al. (eds.), *Patient Safety and Quality in Pediatric Hematology/Oncology and Stem Cell Transplantation*, DOI 10.1007/978-3-319-53790-0_9

integrating individual clinical experience with the best available external clinical evidence from systematic research" [3]. Muir Gray subsequently expanded upon the definition to highlight the importance of the patient by stating that " … the clinician uses the best scientific evidence available, in consultation with the patient, to decide upon the option which suits the patient best" [4].

The original model for evidence-based medicine was proposed in 1992 in the article *Evidence-Based Medicine Working Group. Evidence-based medicine: a new approach to teaching the practice of medicine* published in the Journal of the American Medical Association (JAMA). Per this model, a patient encounter typically triggers a clinical question. At that point the physician should perform a literature search, select the best articles to evaluate, and subsequently determine the validity of the results. The physician should then decide the best course of action based on information obtained [5].

The evidence-based model encompasses five steps:

1. Ask
2. Acquire
3. Appraise
4. Apply
5. Assess

Step 1: Ask

When presented with a clinical problem, the first step of the evidence-based model is to develop an answerable question. Sackett et al. proposed that a good clinical question should consist of four components: (1) the patient or problem in question; (2) the intervention, test, or exposure of interest; (3) comparison interventions (if relevant); and (3) the outcome, or outcomes, of interest. The PICO format is often employed to construct an answerable clinical question.

PICO is a mnemonic standing for:

P = *Patient/problem*: Who are the relevant patients? What is the health concern?
I = *Intervention*: What diagnostic/therapeutic measures are of interest?
C = *Comparison*: Is there an alternative intervention, or no intervention, to be considered?
  = *Outcome(s)*: What is the intended effect/result to be measured, accomplished, or improved upon?

Some also add two additional components (PICOTT) for evaluation where "TT" stands for:

T = *Type of question*: Is the question about a therapy/treatment? diagnosis? prognosis? or harm/etiology?
T = *Type of study*: The type of question being asked can help identify the best study designs to look for once the practitioner is ready to start his/her literature search.

For example, if the question is regarding the best treatment for a particular diagnosis, randomized controlled trials would provide more relevant information than a case report.

Step 2: Acquire

Once the clinical question has been constructed, the next step is to perform a literature search to obtain information relevant to the clinical question. There are numerous articles and databases that can be utilized to search the literature. Some of these resources are considered evidence-based practice (EBP) resources, such as DynaMed, UpToDate, Essential Evidence, and the Cochrane Database of Systematic Reviews.

Step 3: Appraise

After obtaining relevant articles that can potentially answer the clinical question, the next step is to read the articles and evaluate them for validity and clinical utility. The validity of study can be assessed by looking at the study methodology. Some research designs are more powerful than others. Systematic reviews and meta-analyses of randomized controlled trials are considered to be the strongest body of evidence, while case series/case reports are viewed as the least powerful (Fig. 9.1).

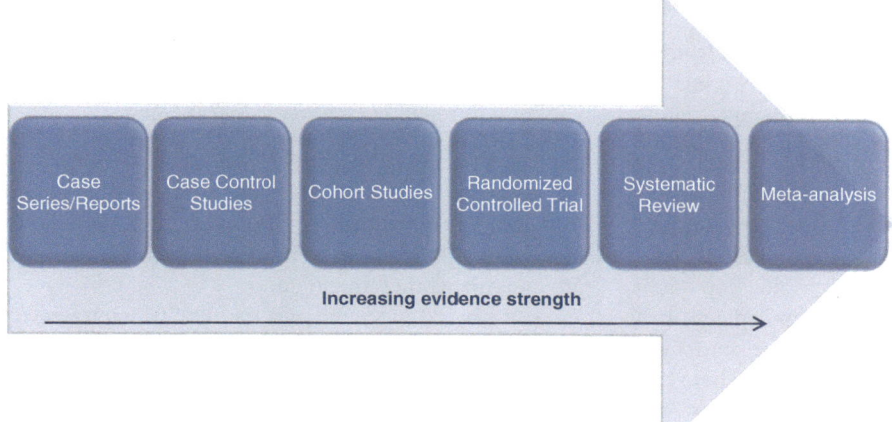

Fig. 9.1 Hierarchy of study methodologies progressing from lowest (*left*) to highest (*right*) strength of evidence

Step 4: Apply

Once an article is deemed as valid, it should then be determined if the evidence can be applied to the patient(s) in question. It is important to remember in this step to discuss potential risks and benefits with the patient and/or parents so that their personal values can also be taken into consideration.

Step 5: Assess

Taking an evidence-based approach to patient care requires evaluating current approaches/processes frequently in order to determine if improvements can be made.

Using Evidenced-Based Models to Guide Practice Change

With the practice of evidence-based medicine also came the need to improve current processes in order to continually provide quality, patient-centered care. While evidence-based medicine focuses on answering a clinical question and making the best clinical decision based on scientific literature, quality improvement focuses more so on addressing recurrent problems within systematic practice.

In the 1980s the Model for Improvement was developed by the Associates in Process Improvement in order to address the needs of people seeking to make improvements in various settings from manufacturing plants and industry to hospitals and schools [6]. The Model for Improvement is based on the W. Edwards Deming's System of Profound Knowledge and focuses on three fundamental questions:

1. What are we trying to accomplish? (Aim)
2. How will we know that a change is an improvement? (Measures)
3. What changes can we make that will result in improvement? (Changes)

The Model for Improvement as first set forth by API has been subsequently adopted by and tailored to meet the needs of various fields, including health care. In 1995, the Institute for Healthcare Improvement (IHI) used the Model for Improvement to develop the Breakthrough Series in order to help health-care organizations develop quality improvements while reducing costs.

A proposed link between evidence-based medicine and the quality improvement model was set forth by Glasziou et al. in 2011 [7]. If after performing the first four steps of the evidence-based model, it appears that the clinical problem is one that is frequently seen and not being optimally addressed with current practices, this would trigger the need for quality improvement measures to then optimize the current clinical practices.

Once a need for improvement is identified, the first step of the QI process should be engaged. In order to identify what is to be accomplished, an aim statement should be established. The aim statement should not only identify the process that needs to be improved but also the desired result and the time frame in which the change will be accomplished. After establishing the aim statement, the current process should be mapped out and potential failures within the system identified. A key driver diagram should subsequently be developed to identify factors that will result in the desired improved outcome. The key driver diagram also includes interventions that will potentially result in the desired change. The next step in the QI process is establishing appropriate measures to track progress. There are three types of measures: outcome measures (how are patients being impacted?), process measures (is the system performing as planned?), and balancing measures (are changes meant to improve one part of the system resulting in new problems?). The third step of the QI process involves use of the Plan-Do-Study-Act (PDSA) cycle to determine the appropriate mechanism to reliably implement evidence-based practices into the health-care delivery system (see Chap. 5).

Implementing Evidence-Based Care

The eighteenth century philosopher, Goethe, commented, "to put your ideas into action is the most difficult thing in the world," and also, "Knowing is not enough, we must apply." Implementing evidence-based medicine into health-care organization practice is a very difficult and highly complex activity. This evolution has been described to take approximately 17 years, from the time evidence is discovered to the time it is implemented [8]. Further once a best practice is identified, it has been found they are only followed around 55% of the time [9]. Past success in implementation does not guarantee future success, as there is generally a complex ever-adapting environment present [10]. There are a few formalized ways in which to introduce evidence into practice in health care, three of which are policy, procedure, and guidelines [11]. Each of these applies a mechanism to standardize and decrease variation within a specific focus area. These terms will be used throughout this section of this chapter and are defined in Table 9.1. When evidence has been organized into a policy, procedure, or guideline, there has to be an accompanying strategy to implement on a micro-, meso-, or macrosystem level within an organization or

Table 9.1 Definitions for policy, procedure, and guideline [13]

Term	Definition
Policy	A concise statement outlining the context, goal, or purpose of a specific procedure. A statement that is the guide to any decision-making in relation to processes or activities that regularly take place or might be expected to occur
Procedure	The desired, intentional action steps taken by specified persons to achieve a certain objective n a defined set of circumstances. Protocol is synonymous with procedure. Often used when describing clinical patient care-related interventions
Guideline	Recommended actions for a specific situation, diagnosis, or patient case. For example, the specific care recommended for a patient being admitted for sickle cell disease pain crisis. These are generally a guide and require clinician judgment

similar structure [12]. There may be many drivers that dictate success or failure. Some of these include the following: an organization's capacity to change, the structure to implement, the associated strategy, institutional culture, guideline context, and external influences [13]. These will be explored in more detail below.

MultiCare Connected Care, an accountable care organization (ACO) associated with MultiCare Health System, in Tacoma, Washington, has identified five key steps in taking knowledge into action (Fig. 9.2). These are: establishing an aim, investigating the current evidence, developing and testing ideas, implementation, and stabilization. This chapter will focus on the last three of these categories.

Guidelines, Policy, and Procedure

Once evidence is formalized into a guideline, probably more so than a policy or procedure, there should be a period of testing and adjusting that follows to ensure the best practice is ultimately implemented. One of the most common methods for doing this is the Plan-Do-Study-Act (PDSA) model that is a part of the Institute for Healthcare Improvement (IHI), model for improvement, as discussed previously in this chapter. This will allow the organization or unit to measure what effects the new changes are having on the system in which the process was intended to work [14]. This will also involve defining the measures from process, outcome, balancing, and possibly structure to define success or mitigate untoward consequences of change. It can also helpful to relate these measures to one or more of the eight domains suggested by the Institute for Medicine around organizational transformation. These are access, coordination, safety, timeliness, effectiveness, efficiency, equity, and patient centered [15].

Brili et al. demonstrated an effective implementation strategy utilizing domains from the perspective of the patient and family: Do not harm me, cure me, treat me with respect, navigate my care, and keep us well, in an effort to connect the work to the target population [16]. One specific example provided, from the domain of treat me with respect, involves having families provide advice at the different levels of hospital operations, including on the quality committee of the board. The relationship between measure type and domain will better allow for a description of value in terms of the process being implemented. The last step in implementation, after measures have been defined and PDSA cycles have occurred, is sustaining the process or in some circumstances adapting as time goes on.

Guideline Implementation

As mentioned previously there are many drivers that will dictate success and failure when implementing a guideline. In the next section, the following six areas will be highlighted: capacity to change, guideline context, institutional culture, the associated strategy, the structure to implement, and external influences [12] (Fig. 9.3).

Detailed Process

MCC

	Prioritize/ Establish Aims	Investigate	Development	Development/ Implementation	Stabilization
Detailed Process	Confirm objectives, KPIs (outcomes) & assumptions	Gather baseline data & map current state process through direct observation & available data.	Implement test of proposed Pathway & measure outcomes.	Set timeline for Pathway and order set rollout across sites.	Define and mitigate risks
	Confirm scope and timing	Research current evidence-based protocols & best practices & draft practice guideline.	Check & adjust AIM statement & pathway (3 times) until the process is standard.	Develop training, education materials,	Metrics monitoring
	Engage subject matter experts (clincal, front line, quality)	Conduct root cause analysis to identify improvement opportunities & countermeasures based on research and current state.	Finalize Guideline/Pathway	Secure analytics support for automated measurement process.	Share and celebrate wins publically
		Prioritize improvements & countermeasures with AIM statement to drive outcomes.	Develop Order Sets/Education materials		

Guideline Approval

Key Deliverables

	Prioritize/ Establish Aims	Investigate	Development	Development/ Implementation	Stabilization
Key Deliverables	• SMART AIM statement for eache collaborative • Reporting needs identified	• Baseline data and current state process map. • Prioritization of specific opportunities for improvement related to AIM. • Draft practice guideline	• Care Guideline/Pathway • Final order sets	• Training plan & materials • Performance management plan • Education materials	• Monthly/quarterly report on outcome metrics • 3, 6, 9, 12 month follow up reports to assess and mitigate risks

Fig. 9.2 MultiCare Connected Care ACO's (MCC) five steps in guideline development and implementation. Copyright, 2016. Reprinted with permission

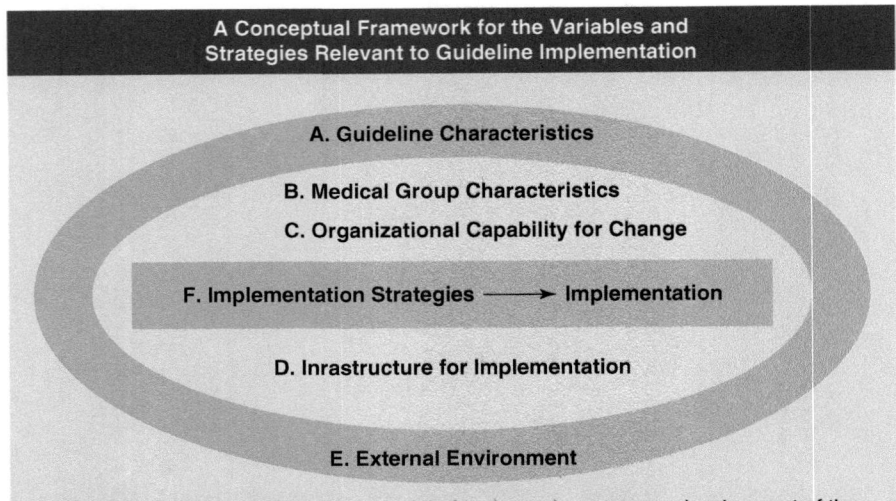

A. Guideline Characteristics: Factors related to the topic, nature, or development of the guideline itself.

B. Medical Group Characteristics: Factors associated with the nature or culture of the organization and only indirectly with guideline implementation.

C. Organizational Capability for Change: Factors directly associated with the organization's ability to understand and undertake desirable changes, including but not limited to guideline implementation.

D. Inrastructure for Implementation: Factors within the medical group that are designed to facilitate guideline implementation.

E. External Environment: Factors external to the medical group that can affect the desire of the group's leadership to undertake quality activities.

F. Implementation Strategies: Qualitatively different strategies to encourage behaviors that support guideline goals.

Fig. 9.3 Adapted from Conceptual Framework for the Variable and Strategies Relevant to Guideline Implementation. Godfrey MM, Melin CN, Muething SE, Batalden PB, Nelson EC. Clinical Microsystems, Part 3. Transformation of Two Hospitals Using Microsystem, Mesosystem, and Macrosystem Strategies. The Joint Commission Journal on Quality and Patient Safety. 2008 Oct;34(10):591–603. Copyright, 2008. Reprinted with permission

Capacity to Change

One of the first steps in implementing a new guideline is assessing the current climate for change and the perception of the change [17, 18]. For implementation to be successful, there should be a collective understanding of an identified gap from what is currently happening to what should be ideally happening. A common example of this might be hand hygiene adherence rates. If medical-surgical unit staff are dissatisfied with a rate of 50%, when it should be 100%, it provides a strong basis for change. This dissatisfaction may only come when there is a clear vision of the ideal state. A panel composed of experts in guideline implementation determined this readiness to change along with leadership support at all levels, to be an essential component [17]. Another important aspect that aligns and informs with leadership support is being transparent with data. This can be accomplished through the use of dashboards or simple displays on a unit. One such tool, Kamishibai cards (K cards), is gaining popularity. An example of this was described by Jureko et al. with their work at Helen DeVos Children's Hospital in Grand Rapids, Michigan; within 9 months of implementing these on various units, they accumulated over 3468 observations from their harm prevention bundles, from frontline leadership to executive involvement. They have since shared their approach with a pediatric hospital engagement network for spread [19].

Guideline Context

Once a gap or problem has been quantified, or there is a clinical need identified for a guideline, one must take the context into account before deploying and implementing. In the development phase, it is paramount to engage key stakeholders. These stakeholders can be clinicians, families or patients, information technologists, administrators, or even external sources such as corporations who may be large purchasers of health care. Forming a collaboration of these groups is more effective than any one in isolation. The benefits of including these groups include more effective training materials and education, effective analytic support, inclusion of priority focus areas, and a better basis for dissemination.

Institutional Culture

An indirect but equally important aspect of implementation is taking the cultural contexts of an organization into account. There is likely overlap with the previously described capacity to change, in terms of culture. There will have to be degrees of buy in and ownership as well as an understanding within the governance structure of an organization if these efforts are to be successful. Focus in this includes characteristics of the target group adopting the change, influence of technology, and incentives to reward behavior.

Characteristics of Adopters

When a change is introduced, there have been five categories of adopters that have been described [14]. It starts with a very small group called innovators, who generally push the boundaries and are not risk averse. Second and most important are the early adopters. This slightly larger group are individuals who adopt change first. One example of this group is electronic health record (EHR) "superusers." When an EHR is implemented in an organization, these superusers might be the first ones to adopt, celebrate the change, and assist others in learning the benefits and details of using this new technology. They are generally respected and well integrated into an institution, and there should be an ongoing investment in this group. One of the other key factors in developing the early adopter group is to make their work transparent to the rest of the organization. This may also involve granting time to connect their work to others in the organization through personal communication or formal presentations. Once this group influences the latter groups of the early and late majority, the largest of all the groups the momentum for change is usually set and will occur with some success. The last group, the laggards, is the last ones to adopt and may have a fondness of tradition and the past. Once a critical mass of around 15–20% change has occurred, there will be momentum in favor of implementation [14].

Technology

Electronic health records present an opportunity to integrate guidelines and can guide providers in many ways. Four of these have been described as decision support, process support, task support, and documentation support. Most are familiar with decision and documentation support; these support decision-making based on the current available clinical data and templates to facilitate documentation, respectively. Not as familiar, process support may involve supporting a sequence of recommended steps. An example of this may be support in classifying the severity of an asthmatic which then could translate into decision support for ordering medications and tests. Finally, task support can be represented by having guideline recommendations or links to pertinent guidelines or other checklists within the electronic record [20]. Many of these are used concurrently to support a guideline. A few critical factors have been identified in the uptake of using computerized support: usefulness, attitudes toward computerized support, social influence, and organizational support [21].

Incentives

In the near future, payment reform is going to require a shift from fee-for-service (FFS) to more global payment based upon quality, experience, and utilization of health care by populations or in essence value. Incentives will need to be aligned with institutional initiatives that advance value. Providers can be seen as change agents in this process if incentives and salary are aligned with guideline implementation as well as outcome improvement [22]. There is a nonmonetary example of an incentive system at Stanford that provides time and services. For example, time spent on a committee may earn credits that then translate into time-saving rewards such as finding housekeeping or assistance with grant writing [23]. Either way, alignment will need to occur as payment reform accelerates.

Strategy

No one strategy will maximize implementation efforts. It has been found that a multifaceted approach is most effective [24]. Common approaches include passive dissemination, education, reminders, audit with targeted feedback, and incentives. Least effective is the idea of "clinical serendipity." That is the passive dissemination of guidelines with the expectation that individuals or groups will start adhering to them [17]. Provider education, namely, through CME, has been found to increase provider knowledge, but this has not translated to clinical outcomes [25]. Clinician reminders can take on many different approaches. Common are automated reminders, alerts or decision support tools that alert a provider that a needed step is required, or consideration should be given to a specific decision. These can be welcome if they enhance or are integrated into the normal workflow in an ambulatory or acute care setting. A recent study looking at acute gastroenteritis and admission did not find any correlation between improved outcomes and the use of clinical decision tools; similar findings have been found in the adult literature as well [26]. Next, providing transparent data to providers allows for performance or adherence to a guideline change based upon real-time feedback. This would also potentially allow for targeted improvement efforts if a specific gap is identified. The other benefit to providing audit or performance data is that the individual physician or provider will inherently know whether the information is accurate or not. Lastly, incentives have not always been effective ways to increase performance, especially if there is not some intrinsic value to the provider. In a recent article in how ten of the leading health-care systems compensate providers, all but three linked between 5–42% of compensation to performance. All had some element of quality or outcomes associated with them [22]. These ten health-care systems also make performance data transparent to all providers.

Barriers to implementation of evidence	Example
Individual or local practice pattern	Different doses and frequencies of albuterol for status asthmaticus across one health-care system emergency departments. No consensus or agreement on best approach
Lack of resources	Lack of clinical nurse educators or specialists. Lack of personnel to do audits or observations of care
Misaligned leadership priorities	Different objectives and priorities at different levels of the organization that do not allow for full support, resource deployment, and incorporation into daily work
Provider autonomy	Guidelines do not take into account the "art" of medicine. Might decrease independent decision-making and increase "being told what to do"
Misinformation	Declining vaccines because of information that indicates unfounded potential harm to children. Antibiotics for viral infection

Sidebar. Examples of barriers to implementing evidence into practice [20]

Structure to Implement

As important as strategy is having a standard organizational approach to guideline implementation. This means creating and agreeing upon a quality improvement methodology, examples of which are Lean, Six Sigma, or the before-mentioned IHI model for improvement. Many of these methods may be complementary and can be used together. Robeznieks described implementation of lean methodologies through engagement of multidisciplinary teams achieving reduction in surgical costs by standardizing surgical supply trays. The trays were customized according to the surgeon needs. This work resulted in daily nurse walking distance by 750 miles per day, allowing for more time at the bedside [27]. Other important structural elements to be aware of are change management resources, data and information architecture, informatics, and accountability. Below is one example of an organization that has created a structure to support guideline development through a collaborative approach.

Collaborative Structure

One organization previously mentioned has created a structure to address this very issue, the creation and implementation of care guidelines. MultiCare Health System, in Tacoma, Washington, is a six-hospital, integrated health-care system with a children's hospital as one of its facilities. They have commissioned seven clinical collaborative groups across disciplines that have multidisciplinary participation and are led by physicians, nurses, and administrators. These groups were created in 2011, in an effort to tie together the desire to standardize, improve cost and quality, use information derived from the EHR in a meaningful way, and disseminate that knowledge into best practice with ongoing performance monitoring.

Each group is resourced with an executive sponsor; a medical (physician), operational, and clinical (nurse) leader; an informatics representative; an information or analytic consultant; and support from collaborative leadership, who also has a role in the accountable care organization (ACO). There are five main phases guidelines will go through development of an aim, investigation of evidence using methodologies previously discussed, development of tools such as electronic order sets and performance dashboards, educational materials, implementation, and finally stabilization. The PDSA cycles that were previously discussed can occur either in the development phase or the implementation phase. It is helpful to have all the tools at your disposal while testing, since some will need adjustment. Some initial results from this effort include reductions in adult sepsis mortality rates by 65%. In pediatrics there are focused workgroups in neonatal, ambulatory, and acute care medicine as well as patient safety and harm reduction [28].

External Influences

External influences also play an important role in the development of guidelines. Examples of these influences can be large purchasers of health who expect certain outcomes for their populations, regional alliances who set benchmarks in a certain geographic region, or multidisciplinary collaboratives within a state that are looking to decrease variation in care provided to its citizens. These influences are generally driven on the premise of increasing value-based care. They may drive the guideline context, especially if there is a defined gap or problem described.

Two examples of external influences are the Health Transformation Alliance, a nonprofit organization that is comprised of 20 major corporations that account for more than $14 billion in health-care costs. They have a vested interest in making sure their employees get the best outcomes per dollar spent. Another example is the Washington State Bree Collaborative, established by the state legislature in 2011. This group has many of the same aims as the previously described alliance but is made up of a variety of stakeholders across health care including physicians, third-party payers and the state. Each year this group selects conditions where there is a high degree of variation and brings together key stakeholders, as described above, to create clinical care guidelines. To date 17 guidelines have either been created or endorsed by this group [29].

Policies and Procedures

Policies and procedures are the official rules that dictate what should be happening with regard to a specific operational task. There may also be some that dictate governance as well. They may differ from guidelines in that there is less room for judgment and interpretation. As described above for guidelines, there may be internal or external contexts that create the need for a policy or procedure. Some examples of internal needs may be a procedure for central line placement and maintenance care, administration of a specific drug that carries a higher level of risk, such as intravenous magnesium, or cardiopulmonary monitoring for specific populations. External drivers may be infection control practice, environment of care standards, and employee safety.

Implementing policies and procedures may follow a different trajectory than a clinical guideline. Depending on the level of the institution where they are created, administrative, department, or even a specific unit may dictate which committees approve and who is affected by the rule being put into place. Implementation may not differ much from that described for guidelines and may provide a powerful platform for accountability, especially in the presence of a just culture.

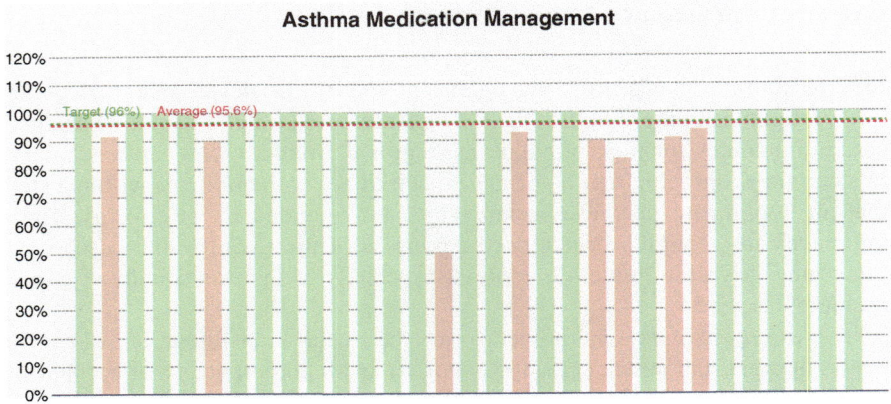

Fig. 9.4 Example of a provider performance dashboard denoting controller medication usage in persistent asthmatics. Each bar would denote provider performance in a specified time frame. Reprinted with permission

Sustaining Change

Once a guideline is successfully implemented, it signals a time for celebration and recognition to the staff that went through the process. Once implemented, sustaining change will be as challenging if not more so. One imperative will be getting staff to own the process, a slight difference from the idea of "buy in." There will need to be a mechanism to measure performance and provide feedback when needed. The context from which the guideline was created may need to be revisited on a somewhat frequent basis, for instance, every 2–3 years. Evidence will also need to be reviewed at similar regular intervals and guidelines updated or revised. Dashboards and run charts may be simple and helpful tools to keep the outcome and process data in front of clinicians and administrators as time goes on with adjustments highlighted that have been made (Fig. 9.4).

Conclusion

In the past 100 years, we have been on a journey in health care that has witnessed great advances in science and technology and more recently the idea of gathering evidence and putting that knowledge into practice consistently. Systems have been created, to evaluate evidence, ask the critical questions, compare outcomes, and assess the relative strength of that evidence in comparative populations of patients so that practice is better informed. More recently, there has been an emphasis on assessing rapid cycle improvement and assessing the effects implementing evidence has on systems and patients. Implementing evidence in a health-care organization can come in a few different forms:

clinical guideline and institutional policies and procedures. Although the latter portion of the chapter focused on guidelines, the concepts can be translated across different documents that will dictate how care is delivered to specific populations. It is important to assess the capacity to change, context in which the evidence will be translated into practice, institutional culture, strategy to deploy, the resources available to support implementation, and the external influences that are either driving or will support success. Once implementation takes place, having a system of transparent data feedback will be critical to inform and improve as time passes from the initial "go live" date.

References

1. Perry S. Book review: technology in the hospital: transforming patient care in the early twentieth century. N Engl J Med. 1996;334:128–9.
2. Zimerman AL. Evidence-based medicine: a short history of a modern medical movement. Am Med Assoc J Ethics. 2013;15(1):71–6.
3. Sackett DL, Rosenberg WM, Gray J, Haynes R, Richardson W. Evidence based medicine: what it is and what it isn't. BMJ. 1996;312(7023):71–2.
4. Fernandez A, Sturmberg J, Lukersmith S, Madden R, Torkfar G, Colagiuri R, Salvador-Carulla L. Evidence-based medicine: is it a bridge too far? Health Res Policy Syst. 2015;13(1):1–9.
5. White B. Making evidence-based medicine doable in everyday practice. Fam Pract Manag. 2004;11(2):51–8.
6. Langley GJ, Moen RD, Nolan KM, Nolan TW, Norman CL, Provost LP. The improvement guide: a practical approach to enhancing organizational performance. San Francisco, CA: Jossey-Bass; 2009.
7. Glasziou P, Ogrinc G, Goodman S. Can evidence-based medicine and clinical quality improvement learn from each other? BMJ Qual Saf. 2011;20:i13–7.
8. Shojania KG, Grimshaw JM. Evidence-based quality improvement: the state of the science. Health Aff. 2005;24(1):138–50.
9. McGlynn EA, Asch SM, Adams J, Keesey J, Hicks J, DeCristofaro A, et al. The quality of health care delivered to adults in the United States. N Engl J Med. 2003;348(26):2635–45.
10. Plsek P. Complexity and the Adoption of Innovation in Health Care. Accelerating Quality Improvement in Health Care Strategies to Speed the Diffusion of Evidence-Based Innovations. 2003 Jan [cited 2016 Feb 5] [18 pp]. Available from: http://www.nihcm-old.com/pdf/Plsek.pdf.
11. Irving A. Policies and Procedures for Healthcare Organizations: A Risk Management Perspective. PSQH [Internet]. 2014 Oct [cited 2016 Feb 5] [6 pages]. Available from: http://psqh.com/september-october-2014/policies-and-procedures-for-healthcare-organizations-a-risk-management-perspective.
12. Godfrey MM, Melin CN, Muething SE, Batalden PB, Nelson EC. Clinical microsystems, part 3. Transformation of two hospitals using microsystem, mesosystem, and macrosystem strategies. Jt Comm J Qual Patient Saf. 2008;34(10):591–603.
13. Solberg L, Brekke ML, Fazio CJ, Fowles J, Jacobsen DN, Kottke TE, et al. Lessons from experienced guideline implementers: attend to many factors and use multiple strategies. Jt Comm J Qual Patient Saf. 2000;26(4):171–88.
14. Berwick DM. Developing and testing changes in delivery of care. Ann Intern Med. 1998;128(8):651–6.
15. Institute of Medicine. Crossing the quality chasm. A new health system for the 21st century. Washington, DC: National Academy Press; 2001.
16. Brili RJ, Allen S, Davis JT. Revisiting the quality chasm. Pediatrics. 2014;133(5):763–5.

17. Parston G, McQueen J, Patel H, Keown OP, Fontana G, Kuwari HA, et al. The science and art of delivery: accelerating the diffusion of health care innovation. Health Aff. 2015;34(12):2160–6.
18. Berwick DM. Disseminating innovations in health care. JAMA. 2003;289(15):1969–75.
19. Jurecko L. Lean Tools Help Prevent Hospital Acquired Infections. [Internet]. Children's Hospital Association; 2015 [Updated July 20, 2015; cited Feb13, 2016]. Available from: https://www.childrenshospitals.org/newsroom/childrens-hospitals-today/summer-2015/articles/lean-tools-help-prevent-hospital-acquired-infections.
20. Lyng KM. From clinical practice guidelines, to clinical guidance in practice-Impacts for computerization. Int J Med Inform. 2013;82(12):e358–63.
21. Hsiao JL, Chen RF. Critical factors influencing physicians' intention to use computerized clinical practice guidelines: an integrative model of activity theory and the technology acceptance model. BMC Med Inform Decis Mak. 2016;16(16):1–15.
22. Khullar D, Kocher R, Conway P, Rajkumar R. How 10 leading health systems pay their doctors. Healthcare. 2015;3(2):60–2.
23. Clarke N. Can a time bank beat physician burnout? Stanford thinks so. [Internet]. Advisory Board; 2015 [Updated September 30th, 2015; cited Feb 27, 2016]. Available from: https://www.advisory.com/research/medical-group-strategy-council/practice-notes/2015/september/stanford-time-bank-program.
24. Shojiana KG, Grimshaw JM. Evidence-based quality improvement: the state of the science. Health Aff. 2005;24(1):138–50.
25. Grimshaw JM, Shirran L, Thomas R, Mowatt G, Fraser C, Bero L, et al. changing provider behavior: an overview of systematic reviews of interventions. Med Care. 2001;39(8):II-2–II-45.
26. Bahm A, Freedman SB, Guan J, Guttman A. Evaluating the impact of clinical decision tools in pediatric acute gastroenteritis: a population-based cohort study. Acad Emerg Med. 2016;23(5):599–609.
27. Robeznieks A. Prospering by standardizing processes and improving the patient experience. [Intenet]. Modern Healthcare; 2014 [Updated Jan 11, 2014, cited March 9, 2016]. Available from: http://www.modernhealthcare.com/article/20140111/MAGAZINE/301119950.
28. Landi H. At Tacoma's MultiCare, Leaders Pursue Core Patient Safety Improvement. [Internet]. Healthcare Informatics; 2016 [Updated March 14, 2016, cited March 19, 2016]. Available from: http://www.healthcare-informatics.com/article/tacoma-s-multicare-leaders-pursue-core-patient-safety-improvement.
29. Washington State Bree Collaborative. [Internet]. [Cited September 4, 2016]. Available from: http://www.breecollaborative.org.

Chapter 10
Chemotherapy and Medication Safety

Sylvia Bartel, Audrea H. Szabatura, and Colin Moore

Background/Overview

The use of antineoplastic agents provides substantial benefits to pediatric patients with cancer, but also come with significant risk as these medications have high toxicity profiles and narrow therapeutic indexes. The pediatric population is at particular risk due to the complexity of regimens, need for frequent dose changes, and age- and weight-based dosing. Although the literature regarding chemotherapy error rates in the outpatient pediatric oncology setting is limited, one study reported that 18.8% of pediatric visits were associated with a medication error, and 4.3 (95% CI, 2.3–4.2) per 100 visits were associated with a chemotherapy error specifically [1].

Causes for medication errors are multifactorial and can be attributed to communication defects; information gaps; confusion related to drug names, labels, directions, and packaging; competency; and education (staff and patients) among others. They can occur at any step of the medication use process of prescribing, preparing, dispensing, and administration. The medication use process is complex, involving multiple interacting clinical systems, staff from different disciplines, and work environments that are stressful with many interruptions. When determining what changes should be implemented to improve the safety of the medication use process, it is important to utilize a systems approach and look at the entire process instead of responding only to single events. The analysis of patterns/trends and vulnerabilities in the medication use process are essential to eliminate or minimize

S. Bartel (✉) • A.H. Szabatura
Dana-Farber Cancer Institute, Boston, MA 02215, USA
e-mail: Sylvia_Bartel@dfci.harvard.edu; Audreah_szabatura@dfci.harvard.edu

C. Moore
Johns Hopkins All Children's Hospital, Johns Hopkins University School of Medicine, Baltimore, MD 21205, USA
e-mail: Colin.Moore@jhmi.edu

© Springer International Publishing AG 2017
C.E. Dandoy et al. (eds.), *Patient Safety and Quality in Pediatric Hematology/Oncology and Stem Cell Transplantation*, DOI 10.1007/978-3-319-53790-0_10

risks of errors reaching the patient. This chapter will outline strategies for measurement, improvement strategies, and sustainability to ensure safe chemotherapy and medication practices and processes.

Measurement

Introduction

Quality expert H. James Harrington stated that "measurement is the first step that leads to control and eventually to improvement. If you can't measure something, you can't understand it. If you can't understand it, you can't control it. If you can't control it, you can't improve it" [2]. In all forms of quality improvement, it is extremely difficult to create solutions to a problem until you truly understand its scope. Measuring medication errors as they relate to chemotherapy is critical in identifying areas that are in need of safety improvements. The measurement of these errors, however, remains a difficult field that is clouded by issues of nomenclature and the nature of reporting systems. This section of the chapter will focus on outlining the components that contribute to a medication error and how these components can be captured in order to allow for analysis and appropriate implementation of safe practices. All of the reviewed methods have distinct advantages and disadvantages, and no study has shown the clear advantage of one stand-alone system. The impetus is then placed on each hospital and patient care setting to find the best combination of these methods that maximize identifying serious preventable medication events while efficiently allocating resources. Ensuring proper measurement techniques will ultimately allow for trending medication errors after implementation of system changes and aid in creating sustainability for patient safety regarding chemotherapy and other medications.

Classification of Severity of Medication Errors

The World Health Organization (WHO) has adopted the definition of a medication error as "a failure in the treatment process that leads to, or has the potential to lead to, harm to the patient" [3]. An adverse drug event (ADE) is defined as any injury resulting from medical interventions related to a drug [4]. A key component in understanding medication errors is identifying the severity of the incident [5]. For the most efficient use of resources, many organizations focus their efforts on identifying those errors with the greatest potential harm to the patient as the most important to drill down and understand processes that could be improved. This can be accomplished by designating categories of severity for chemotherapy errors. The National Coordinating Council for Medication Error Reporting and Prevention (NCC MERP) has established an index that helps better define the severity of medication errors (Fig. 10.1) [6]. This severity index can be applied to all medication

NCC MERP Index for Categorizing Medication Errors

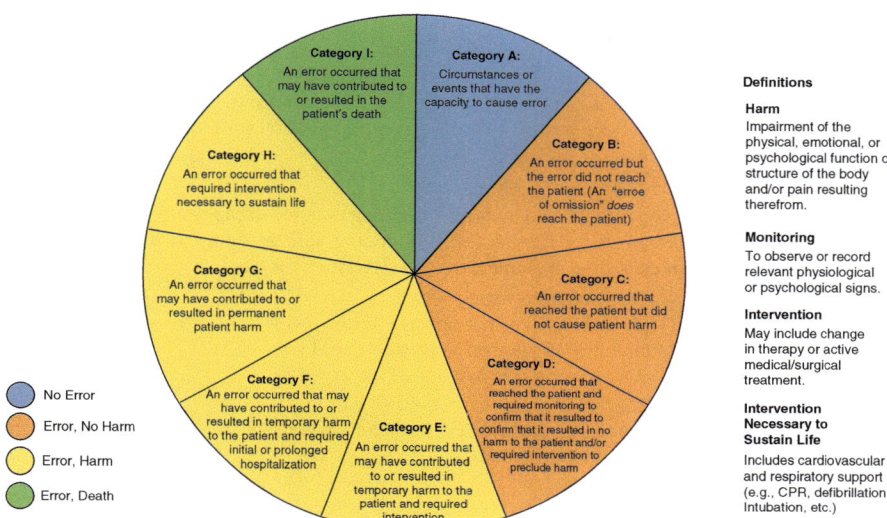

Fig. 10.1 Severity index for categorizing medication errors from NCC MERP (Used with permission. © 2001 National Coordinating Council for Medication Error Reporting and Prevention)

errors involved in the care of hematology and oncology patients including both chemotherapy and supportive care medications. Many other severity indexes are available, and institutions can tailor which index helps them discover and address their ADEs in the most efficient manner.

Classification of Processes Involved in Medication Errors

The processes that lead to medication errors related to chemotherapy mimic those involved in general medication errors. With the unique complexity and toxicity of these medications, however, the risk to the patient can increase greatly when an error does occur [7]. The areas in which chemotherapy medication errors can occur include the time of prescribing, preparing, dispensing, administering, and monitoring a medication (e.g., see Table 10.1). In many chemotherapy errors, there are numerous processes at play that contribute to the ultimate error taking place. Even within one location, there may be many issues that contribute to an error. With respect to prescribing errors, many medical facilities continue the practice of ordering chemotherapy via paper utilizing handwritten orders as opposed to computerized physician order entry (CPOE). This process can lead to numerous potential errors that may have been caught and otherwise eliminated by utilizing the process checks built into CPOE such as elimination of hand-writing interpretation errors

Table 10.1 The processes where errors can occur while a patient receives chemotherapy and common errors associated with each procedure

Error location	Examples of errors
Prescribing	Wrong dosing weight and height are used while calculating chemotherapy dose (mg/m^2 vs. mg/kg)
	Wrong unit of measure utilized (milligram vs. microgram)
	Incorrect or absent dose adjustment based on prior toxicity
Preparing	Incorrect diluent selected
	Prepared with wrong volume
Dispensing	Product labeled incorrectly (wrong patient, wrong drug)
	Lack of verification that correct drug, diluent, and dose have been prepared by chemotherapy pharmacist
Administration	Administered to wrong patient
	Infused over incorrect time (IV push vs. 3-h infusion)
	Administered via inappropriate route (IV vs. IT)
	Infusion pump is programmed incorrectly
Monitoring	Failure to identify toxic levels of a drug
	Inappropriate monitoring for acute toxicities after administration of a drug (e.g., anaphylaxis)

and utilities such as dose calculators [8]. Coupled with severity classification, identifying and appropriately labeling the various processes involved in each error can help ensure accurate measurement and subsequent interpretation of the events that lead to a chemotherapy error.

Medication Error Measuring Systems

In 1999, the Institute of Medicine published a report that outlined significant patient safety concerns through the medical system in the United States and outlined recommendations on how to measure and address these concerns [9]. The report elucidated that voluntary reporting systems have the best means to focus on patient safety improvement in the field of medication safety. These types of systems usually evaluate errors that resulted in minimal or no harm to patients, and analyzing these errors can lead institutions to identify and address vulnerabilities in their systems before harm occurs [9, 10]. Following the release of this report, there was a large growth and advancement in medication error reporting systems. One recent review cited over 12 various types of medication error reporting systems available [11]. Since that time with the help of technological advances within electronic medical record (EMR) information systems, automated medication event reporting systems have been implemented as well. With the many variations on measuring and reporting systems, medical institutions are now burdened with identifying which systems can help provide a balance between resources available and identifying patient safety concerns. Outlined in the following sections are the most commonly used reporting systems and analysis of the benefits and potential concerns of each.

Incident Reporting Systems

Incident reporting systems utilize structured data collection to input medication error information. These systems are all confidential and can vary from anonymous to non-anonymous reporting strategies. [12] Incident reporting systems are the most commonly utilized measurement system, and numerous reporting systems exist in healthcare in both local hospital systems and nationally [13]. Several countries have developed national adverse medication event systems, such as the UK's National Reporting and Learning System (NRLS), which have allowed findings to be applied to a wider system and have a national affect [14]. On average over 1.5 million incident reports are submitted each year to the NRLS. In the United States, the Patient Safety and Quality Improvement Act of 2005 established a voluntary reporting system that utilizes patient safety organizations through the Agency for Healthcare Research and Quality in an attempt to standardize and nationalize incident reporting [15]. The benefits and concerns of these varied reporting systems can be applied fairly universally. These systems have been identified as being relatively easy to implement and are generally of low cost to a health system [11]. This system allows frontline staff who were directly involved in the incident to input data in a structured format that is submitted to be reviewed via the hospital systems' designated review structure. Examples of standardized systems include MEDMARX and the MedWatch program from the US Food and Drug Administration (FDA) [16, 17]. Table 10.2 outlines the components required for documentation of an incident report using the MedWatch system from the FDA.

While this type of measurement system may be easily implemented at relatively low cost, there exist several concerns regarding its stand-alone efficacy. Volunteer incident reporting systems can be impacted significantly by reporter bias [12, 18, 19]. They have been shown to identify only a small percentage of target problems

Table 10.2 Components required in documentation of incident report as outlined from MedWatch from the US FDA

Category	Details
Patient information	Patient identifier (MRN/FIN), age, sex, height, weight, ethnicity/race
Type of event	Adverse event, product defect
Outcome	Death, life-threatening, hospitalization—initial or prolonged, other serious, required intervention to prevent permanent impairment/damage, disability or permanent damage, congenital anomaly/birth defects
Chronology/location	Date, time, location/hospital unit
Event description	Free text area for thorough event description
Relevant tests/laboratory data	Any additional testing necessary secondary to the event that would not have been obtained otherwise
Suspected medication	Name, dose, route, frequency, length of infusion time
Indication for use	Diagnosis or problem indicated for use of medication

and are dependent upon the involved parties accurately filling out details that are
critical for analysis of the event [19]. An additional concern is that physicians have
relatively low error reporting rates. One study which surveyed over 1600 hospitals
reported that at 86% of hospitals, physicians submitted few or no incident reports
[18]. With the complexities of chemotherapy and biotherapies in the practice of
pediatric hematology/oncology and bone marrow transplant, physician contribution
to error reporting is critical. While these concerns can overlap with many of the
other reporting systems, a more specific concern is that events are reported without
clearly identifying the total numbers of patients at risk for such an event [19]. This
may allow for analysis of trends of error types over time, but does not allow for
assessment of which populations are at most risk and who would benefit the most
from intervention based on incident report review. Medication error measurement
via incident report submission and review involves having a structured review process. Often multidisciplinary teams are involved in the review process, identification of potential preventable errors, and creation of subsequent system changes.
This system of a review and subsequent feedback loop to correct and prevent errors
is a critical element of all measurement systems.

Chart Review

Utilizing chart review as a form of medication error measurement builds upon many
of the processes involved with incident report creation. Chart review does this in a
retrospective manner in surveying patient's medical records prior to an error being
reported and attempting to identify issues in a timely manner [11, 20]. The process
of chart review often involves evaluating many components of the medical record
including medication administration record (MAR) review and identifying any specific signals or triggers that might be concerning for an error. While reviewing the
patient's MAR, the orders are screened for the appropriate inclusion of important
details such as legibility, medication name, dosage form, route of administration,
dose, dosage unit, frequency of administration, duration of therapy, number of doses
to be dispensed, and directions or warnings for use [21, 22]. Data reviewers are vigi-
lant for certain changes in patient status (e.g., transfer to the intensive care unit), and
new diagnostic or laboratory tests that can indicate where errors may have occurred
(e.g., abnormal echocardiogram, elevated liver enzymes). The data is collected on
forms, and when errors are identified, further drill down occurs. This is a labor- and
resource-intensive process that requires dedicated teams for review and usually
necessitates daily review of charts to have effective real-time identification of errors
and interventions.

In comparison to incident reports alone, more detailed data is generally gathered
from prospective chart review [11, 23]. This system can be an effective tool at identifying errors during the prescribing, administration, and monitoring of medications
[11, 22, 23]. As chart review identifies errors that have not yet been voluntarily
reported, there have been concerns that the seriousness of problems detected via this

method is often associated with lower clinical significance [23]. While a higher number of errors may be identified, fewer error reviews that would lead to system changes have been observed in some studies [22, 23]. The significant time and resources needed to have a large-scale prospective chart review for medication error must also be considered when evaluating this as a medication error measurement tool and often preclude this from being a viable solution for most institutions.

Trigger Tools

In 1999, the Institute for Healthcare Improvement's expert panel on patient safety devised a trigger tool methodology that utilizes identifying key triggers in patient records during review that prompt medication error detection [24].The IHI Global Trigger Tool is incorporated by utilizing a team of three or more reviewers evaluating randomly selected charts and searching for triggers to adverse events in six modules: cares, medication, surgical, intensive care, perinatal, and emergency department [25].Within the medication module, triggers have been identified that are often included when a medication error occurs such as diphenhydramine administration, partial thromboplastin time (PTT) greater than 100 s, and vitamin K administration. The use of this trigger-focused review expands on the concept of chart review and allows for a more streamlined approach that has been shown to be an effective and reproducible form of medication error detection [24, 25]. Many of the components that are manually evaluated in trigger tool-focused chart review can be automated by utilizing the ever-expanding technology of the EMR information systems. Automated adverse event detection or trigger tools have been developed to allow the prospective gathering of data via specific signals or triggers. Several EMR trigger tools have been implemented and reviewed in the general pediatric setting [26–28] and in the pediatric hematology and oncology subspecialty setting as well [29]. These trigger tools focus on discrete events that occur in the EMR, and reports can be created that prompt further investigation into potential medication errors. Several multi-institutional collaborations have been formed, such as the Automated Adverse Event Detection Collaborative (AAEDC), with the goal of improving the detection, collection, and analysis of medication events among groups of academic pediatric hospitals [26]. The triggers utilized by the AAEDC cover a wide range of medication and laboratory values and are summarized in Table 10.3.

These triggers can be utilized in a wide variety of EMR information systems and utilized as both retrospective auditing tools and real-time interventions to prevent an error before it occurs. A more specific tool for the automated detection of medication errors in pediatric hematology oncology has been developed and evaluated at St. Jude Children's Research Hospital (SJCRH) with a focus on supportive care and chemotherapy-related medications including protamine, vitamin K, sodium polystyrene, naloxone, flumazenil, and hyaluronidase [29]. This trigger tool noted that when one of the listed medications was ordered and administered

Table 10.3 Triggers utilized by the Automated Adverse Event Detection Collaborative

Medication administration	Laboratory results
Digoxin immune fab	Anti-Xa > 1.5
Flumazenil	aPTT > 100 s
Hyaluronidase	Bilirubin > 25 mg/dL
Sodium polystyrene	Creatinine doubling
Naloxone	Glucose < 50 mg/dL
Protamine	INR > 4.0
Acetylcysteine	Potassium > 6 mmol/L
Glucagon	
Vitamin K	

to a patient, it was logged and the data could be extracted into a report. These triggers for potential medication errors were reviewed by both a pharmacist and physician. After review, if a medication event was truly linked to the trigger, data was collected regarding the event similar to that of an incident report. Trigger tools like the one developed at SJCRH can be developed within most existing EMR information systems and help automate the process of medication error detection. As with chart review and other forms of measurement, the data from these triggers must be then reviewed and classified in order to identify interventions to prevent future errors [26, 29].

Electronic trigger tools build upon the medication error capturing of a chart review in a quicker and automated process. This tool can allow for decreased sampling bias that can be seen with manual trigger identification via chart review. As with chart review, it allows for near real-time detection of medication errors which can help facilitate timelier investigations. Several studies have shown this tool to be a valuable addition to traditional measurement options as it has shown minimal overlap (1.9–7.8%) with voluntary incident reporting systems [26–28]. A major limitation in automated trigger tools are the lack of fully validated trigger events specifically related to chemotherapy, such as the use of methylene blue in ifosfamide neurotoxicity or timing of leucovorin administration following high-dose methotrexate infusion. Many of the validated trigger tools focus on identifying errors of supportive care medicines or hematology-related medications such as anticoagulants. As institutions continue to evaluate new chemotherapy-related triggers, it is important that these triggers proceed through an important validation phase. If the trigger tool has been validated appropriately, it can be as sensitive as chart review and more sensitive than incident report review at identifying medication errors [11].

During the validation process, it is important for hospital systems to evaluate the positive predictive value of each medication trigger. For example, during the validation study of the SJCRH trigger tool, no events were detected associated with the use of vitamin K. The study concluded that if the tool had been restricted to the use of patients only with known concurrent use of warfarin, that data may have been more helpful for review. It is therefore important that when a trigger tool is implemented, that there be a process of internal review to identify the predictive value of errors based on trigger to ensure continued measurement will be beneficial. There can be significant financial investments in the development and implementation of a trigger tool, but once implemented many studies have shown trigger tools to require the least resources to continually review medication errors [20, 30, 31]. As more tools are developed and validated, this field will continue to expand as a complimentary and potentially primary medication error measurement tool.

Direct Observation

Direct observation refers to real-time evaluation techniques throughout the medication process. This technique is one of the oldest methods of detecting medication errors and has been studied since the 1960s [32]. This measurement technique involves real-time auditing of the practices of prescribing, preparing, dispensing, administration, and monitoring of medications [11, 33]. Direct observation of nursing by review teams has been the backbone of direct observation, and over time this has been expanded to include both provider and pharmacist observation as well. Examples of observations include on the prescriber level of ensuring double provider signatures for chemotherapy ordering, on the pharmacy level by selecting correct diluents for medications, and on the nursing level of appropriate administration rates and times. Errors are noted in real time and data is collected for analysis.

This measurement tool has been considered the gold standard of identifying medication errors. A systematic review of medication safety assessment practices showed that direct observation revealed the highest number of error reports, in some studies up to 400-fold the number of reports compared with incident report review, chart review, or trigger tool [11]. As with any scientific study, there are concerns as that observer influence can be involved and significant [11, 29, 33]. The review teams often include representatives from physician, pharmacy, and nursing staffs and can be resource demanding regarding the time needed for this ongoing observation [11, 33]. Some of the limitations of other measurement techniques are avoided as knowledge of the errors by subjects is not needed and willingness to report the errors is not required. As with all other measurement techniques reviewed, once the errors have been measured, an infrastructure must be in place to review and analyze the errors.

The measurement of medication errors is key to understanding the processes involved with the error and subsequently creating system changes to ensure prevention of future errors. Many studies have evaluated the costs and benefits of the individual measurement techniques. While the reviewed methods have distinct advantages and disadvantages, no study has shown the clear advantage of one stand-alone system. It is critical to understand that a multifaceted approach to measurement will be key when a healthcare organization approaches improvement strategies for patient safety regarding chemotherapy and other medications.

Improvement Strategies

Introduction

Organizational strategies for improving chemotherapy and medication safety should focus on the overall chemotherapy process including chemotherapy prescription, preparation, and administration [1, 7, 34, 35]. Institutions must ensure that safeguards are in place at each step and should place these strategically within the chemotherapy use process. A successful system design should account for psychological precursors and human factors and incorporate standardization, technology, patient input, and double checks to ensure that errors are prevented [1, 36].

Standardization

One of the most effective ways to minimize error is to standardize the process and tools used to prescribe, dispense, and administer chemotherapy. A lack of standardization can create an environment of confusion, misinterpretation, and variability in these processes. One way to improve the chemotherapy process is to evaluate each of these steps and implement evidence-based strategies that can minimize errors [7, 34, 37].

Prescribing

It is well known that incomplete, illegible, or incorrect chemotherapy orders can lead to ambiguity and misinterpretation, thereby putting patients at significant risks [1]. Patient care facilities should utilize standardized pre-printed or electronic order sets whenever possible and at least for commonly used regimens and treatments. This tool helps to simplify the ordering process in that much of the basic information is prefilled [7, 37, 38].

Best practice recommendations suggest that the basic elements of all chemotherapy orders should include patient demographic information and treatment plan, hydration orders if applicable, supportive care medications, and chemotherapy medications. The orders should be presented in a standard format, in the order which they will be administered and incorporate general medication safety principles (Table 10.4). Specific recommendations for each component of the order template include the following [1, 7, 38–42]:

1. Patient demographics:

    (a) At least two patient identifiers, including the patient's name
    (b) Patient-specific dosing parameters: Height (cm), weight (kg), and BSA (m^2)
    (c) Diagnosis

Table 10.4 General medication order safety principles

	Do	Correct example	Don't	Incorrect example
Drug name	Generic name Brand name in parenthesis (when appropriate) Tallman lettering	CISplatin Fluorouracil	Do not use unapproved abbreviations for drug names	CDDP SFU
Dosage	Planned treatment dose as function of patient-specific parameters and calculated dose Place a space between the dose and units Use commas when expressing numbers >999 Doses less than 1 should be preceded by a zero	CISplatin $36 \text{ mg} = 20 \text{ mg/m}^2 \times 1.8 \text{ m}^2$ Fluorouracil $1800 \text{ mg} = 1000 \text{ mg/m}^2 \times 1.8 \text{ m}^2$	Avoid trailing zeros	CISplatin $36.0 \text{ mg} = 80 \text{ mg/m}^2 \times 1.8 \text{ m}^2$ Fluorouracil $1800.0 \text{ mg} = 80 \text{ mg/m}^2 \times 1.8 \text{ m}^2$
Route	Clearly define administration routes and durations	IV over 30 min	Do not use bolus as administration instruction	IV Bolus
Schedule of administration	Frequency Number of doses Days to be taken Include total daily dose and total dose over total length of time for continuous infusions	CISplatin **Q24 h for** three doses on days **1, 2, 3** Fluorouracil $1000 \text{ mg/m}^2/\text{day}$ IV continuous over 24 h on days 1, 2, 3, 4 (total 4000 mg/m^2 continuous IV over 96 h)	Do not use hyphens used to express dosing schedules Avoid unapproved abbreviations, such as QD Avoid unclear expression of timing and frequency of administration	Oplatia **days 1–3** Fluorouracil 4000 mg/m^2 IV over 96 h 1000 mg/m^2 OD $\times$ 4 days

2. Treatment plan:

   (a) Name of treatment regimen and protocol number for research regimens
   (b) Treatment intent (optional)
   (c) Current day and cycle, cycle length, and total number of anticipated cycles

3. Hydration orders:

   (a) Solution type
   (b) Volume of solution
   (c) Route of administration
   (d) Duration of infusion

4. Supportive care medications (pre-chemotherapy)

   (a) Include default medication choices. These should be customized to the regimen given and meet evidence-based practice guidelines
   (b) Alternative or add-on options should be available for situations in which the patient does not respond appropriately to default medication choices. These options should also be based on clinical practice guidelines
   (c) Standardized full generic name, dose, route of administration, duration of infusion as applicable, and time of administration in relation to chemotherapy should be included.

5. Chemotherapy medications

   (a) Standardized full generic name of the chemotherapy agent.
   (b) Brand names should be included in situations of look-alike-sound-alike medication names.
   (c) Dosing unit (mg/m^2, mg/kg, etc.) and patient calculated dose.
   (d) Reasons for dose modifications.
   (e) IV solution and volume and duration of infusion as applicable.
   (f) Drug dosages and calculated doses should be expressed according to the "container" rule (i.e., the calculated dose is the amount prepared and administered from a single container).
   (g) Chemotherapy medications infused over multiple days (continuous infusions) should include total daily dose and total dose over total length of time (i.e., 1200 mg/m^2/day IV continuous over 24 h on days 1 and 2 (2400 mg/m^2 IV over 48 h).
   (h) Solution types, volume, and duration of infusion should be standardized for each chemotherapy medication.
   (i) The administration schedule, including frequency of administration and days on which each dose is to be given within a treatment cycle or course, should be specified.

6. Supportive care medications (post chemotherapy)

   (a) Growth factor support
   (b) Anaphylaxis control
   (c) Prescriptions for post chemotherapy emesis control

7. Provider signature, date, and time

Standardized chemotherapy order forms and electronic templates should be developed by designated multidisciplinary teams who prescribe, prepare, and administer chemotherapy medications. Practitioners involved in this process should draft the template content which should then undergo formal independent review and approval by each discipline (a physician, advanced practice providers, pharmacist, and nurses). Review and approvals should be completed in a quiet area. The information from the creation, review, and approval process should be retained for future reference. The standardized order set templates should be reviewed on a regular basis. A maintenance schedule should also be established. Reviewing the templates on a standard frequency (i.e., annually or every 2 or 3 years) will help ensure that the templates are up-to-date in terms of evidence-based clinical practice guidelines and formulary changes [7, 38, 40].

The institution should consider restricting who is allowed to order chemotherapy. Be sure to consider all situations. For example, you may want an emergency room physician to be able to order chemotherapy for a patient who is admitted into the emergency room with blast crisis; however, you may not want a fellow or other trainee ordering chemotherapy without an attending co-signature.

Preparation/Dispensing

Chemotherapy orders should be reviewed by an oncology pharmacist. The value of a pharmacist's review has been well documented in playing a pivotal role in identifying prescribing errors. Although the use of standardized order templates minimizes the need to reverify predefined elements of medication orders, certain treatment aspects are not captured by order templates. A pharmacist's review should consist of the following [7, 38]

(1) Patient-specific parameters: including height (cm), weight (kg), BSA (m²), and significant changes in these parameters.
(2) Drug allergies and current medications for potential drug interactions.
(3) Treatment plan is appropriate for the patient and treatment indication (i.e., evidence supports the use of the regimen in the disease being treated).
(4) Relevant laboratory test and physical assessment values have been taken, and results are within appropriate limits for treatment.
(5) Dose and dose calculations are correct according to patient-specific parameters.
(6) Doses, cycle number, and day of treatment are consistent with treatment history, and the appropriate treatment interval has elapsed.

Orders should be compared with a primary reference, and if an investigational agent is used, the research protocol should be referenced to verify the appropriateness of the orders for the patient. Tools such as checklists or chemotherapy

Pt_____ MRN:_____ Appt time_____ RN:_____

♦ Verify the following:
Height:_____cm   Weight:_____kg   BSA_____m2
Allergies_____ ☐ Consent   Diagnosis:_____

☐ The following are appropriate per protocol #_____, standard, or exception order:
   ☐ Drug
   ☐ Dose
   ☐ Schedule

☐ Review patient's treatment history and verify:
   ☐ Drugs and doses Cycle_____ Day_____ Time elapsed since last dose:_____

☐ Criteria to treat has been assessed
   Labs: ANC:_____ PLTs:_____ T.Bill:_____ Scr:_____ Others:

☐ Hydration is appropriate

☐ Supportive Care is appropriate:

Dexamethasone	Palonosetron	Famotidine	Others:
Ondansetron	Acetaminophen	Hydrocortisone	
Aprepitant/Fosaprepitant	Diphenhydramine	Methylprednisolone	

Notes:

Fig. 10.2 Chemotherapy order checklist example

drug work cards can be used to help ensure that all elements of chemotherapy orders have been verified. An example of a chemotherapy order checklist is provided (Fig. 10.2).

Standardizing the preparation process is another component of minimizing medication errors. Standardized guidelines for the reconstitution, dilution, packaging, and labeling of chemotherapy admixtures [7, 37] should be established. These guidelines should be readily available to all practitioners involved in verification, drug preparation, and drug preparation checking processes. Commercially available products should also be used whenever possible but are often not available for chemotherapy. Thus, when admixing these medications, it has been recommended that direct observation of product preparation be used whenever possible. Ideally, two individuals should independently verify the drug, diluents, administration containers, and volume measurements before the drug dose is transferred into the final administration container. Other post hoc verification methods, such as the syringe pull-back method, in which the syringe plunger is pulled back to demonstrate the volume of drug that was injected into the container, have been described. However, it is recommended that this should not be used alone as a verification method. Other practices include drawing up the volume to be administered and marking the syringe before transferring the medication into the final container, using specific gravity information to confirm doses [7]. At the completion of preparation, all original medication vials,

Order/Label Information:	Drug Preparation

Review the following:
  Patient
  Drug
  Dose
Ingredients scanned and Quantity:
  Drug
  Base
  Warnings fired during preparation and actions taken
	Drug:
	    Drug vials are correct
	    Expiration is within date
	    Volume (dose) used to prepare product is correct
	    (*marked syringe volume)
	
	Reconstitute:
	    Type is appropriate
	    Expiration is within date
	    Volume used is correct
	    Caution:verify concentration of IV versus SQ preps

Final Preparation
Total volume is correct
Expiration date/time (if <24 hours) is indicated on bag
Attachments are correct-red cap versus PhaSeal, etc
Tubing type is correct (regular vs taxol tubing vs syringe tubing, etc)
Attachments/tubing is secure-clamps are clamped, etc
Tubing is primed
	Base:
	    Type of Base is correct
	    Expiration is within date
	    Volume is correct
	
	Dose (_ mg) = drug conc (_mg/ml) × syr vol (_mls)

Fig. 10.3 Pharmacy preparation checklist example

diluents, syringes, and transfer devices should be presented for final product verification. At this point, a pharmacist should verify label/order information, drug reconstitution, and final product preparation. Checklists or chemotherapy drug work cards can serve as useful tools to aid in these processes as well (Fig. 10.3).

Administration

Nurses often have the last opportunity for error recognition and intervention in the medication use process. It is therefore necessary to institute administration practices that will allow nurses to easily identify and intercept errors to prevent potentially lethal consequences. Similar to a pharmacist's order review, nurses should also verify order and patient-specific elements prior to drug administration. They should assess the patient for previous chemotherapy-related toxicity, confirm treatment plans for the day, and counsel patients on expected toxicities and how to manage symptoms. Prior to drug administration, recommendations indicate that two nurses should compare the pharmacy product to the original order and assess the medication's integrity [7, 35, 37] Infusion pumps should be used to administer chemotherapy. The infusion rate and pump settings should be entered and then independently reviewed by another individual prior to the start of administration. Ideally, this should occur at the bedside where the two practitioners can also validate the patient's identity to ensure that the correct drug is given to the correct patient [7, 35].

Errors in administration have been documented to account for 13% of errors in one study of hospitalized pediatric patients [19]. Institutions can minimize the incidence of these errors by following recommended practices: chemotherapy should be administered on designated units or floors where chemotherapy competent nurses are located; cutoff times for nonurgent chemotherapy administration should be established to ensure adequate pharmacy and nursing staffing; the institution should determine whether chemotherapy agents should be infused as a primary or secondary infusion. Another important component to the medication administration process includes documentation of administration.

Treatment flow sheets can serve as a useful tool to outline information regarding a patient's treatment history, especially when a standardized format of documentation is employed, including patient's name; medical record number and/or date of birth (two patient identifiers); drug name, dosing unit, and calculated dose; administration rate, route, duration of infusion, time infusion started and ended, and date of administration; and information regarding tolerance.

Technology

Implementing the use of technology at various points in the medication use process can improve communication and structure workflow and aid in clinical decisions. By eliminating handwritten orders and providing clinical decision support, prescribers can gain significant ordering advantages through the use of computerized order entry. Bar code scanning technology can prevent medication mix-ups at the point of preparation, and infusion pump guardrails can ensure that medications are administered at the appropriate rates.

Computerized Order Entry

The Institute of Medicine recommends that all medication orders be written electronically [43]. Although the benefit of its use is well established, institutions should recognize that the implementation of these systems can introduce new errors. Experience from various institutions indicates that each step of the existing and proposed medication use process should be compared for potential gaps and failure points. Failure modes and effects analysis (FMEA; see also Chap. 20) and failure modes, effects, and critical analysis (FMECA) have been successfully used for this purpose [44–47]. These proactive risk assessment methods allow institutions to evaluate risks and design chemotherapy processes accordingly.

The positive impact of computerized physician order entry (CPOE) on error reduction serves as a primary motivation to implement its use in the pediatric chemotherapy setting. Depending on how CPOE is designed, it can reduce the likelihood of improper dosing, incorrect dosing calculations, and missing cumulative dose calculations, among others. To maximize the benefits of CPOE, several concepts should be considered [7, 37, 48–51]

1. Workflow: Display data in CPOE consistent with the chemotherapy use process. Chemotherapy orders should be entered first, followed by pharmacy verification, product preparation, nursing verification, medication administration, and documentation.
2. Verification: The number and type of checks should be placed strategically in the medication use process. Consider the capabilities of CPOE, which can restrict

provider privileges, automate calculations, apply forcing functions, and provide drug interaction checking.

3. Information access: Ensure that all providers have access to patient information including demographics, laboratory values, notes, treatment plans, consents, past medication administration history, etc. This information should display in a manner that encourages that appropriate clinical decisions and verifications are made during each step of the chemotherapy use process.

4. Clinical decision support: Automated safety checks should be instituted wherever possible. A few examples include:

(a) Automated dose calculations and dose rounding
(b) High-dose warnings
(c) Dose caps
(d) Cumulative dose calculations
(e) Interaction and allergy alerts

Bar Code Verification

Linking the manufacturer's bar code, the National Drug Code (NDC) number to respective medications ordered for a particular patient in a CPOE system can allow bar code verification to prevent wrong patient and medication mix-ups at the point of administration. During preparation, systems allow each ingredient of a preparation to be checked against the components of an order and can fire warnings or hard stops to guide drug selection. These systems have been particularly helpful in preventing look-alike-sound-alike drug errors. Some intelligent systems can also direct the amount of drug used to prepare the product, alerting the preparer if too many or too little drug packages have been scanned to complete the ordered dose.

"Smart" Pumps

Infusion pumps which incorporate medication safety software ("smart pumps") can prevent errors in administration rates. This software has a comprehensive drug dictionary with limits for dosing, dosing units, concentration, and duration of infusion. These dictionaries should be customized to the institution's established drug preparation and administration guidelines and utilize the following functions [7, 48]:

(1) Customize different profile settings for different patient populations and locations (pediatric vs. adult; NICU vs. general pediatric unit or clinic).
(2) Incorporate soft and hard limits strategically.
(3) Use nomenclature that mirrors medication orders in CPOE and pharmacy labels.
(4) Provide drug-specific clinical advisory alerts (i.e., infusion tubing or filter needs).

Patient and Family Involvement

Although a survey by the National Patient Safety Foundation revealed that only 10% of patients had taken an active role in ensuring their own safety, patients and families can play an integral part in the medication use process [51]. Healthcare providers, patients, and families share responsibility to ensure that this happens.

Healthcare providers should present patients and families with information important to their care including their treatment course, medications, expected side effects, and when to call the provider's office. They should do this with clear and complete instructions at a level that the patient and family can understand. Medical jargon should be avoided; pictures can be used if needed and information should be repeated. An underutilized method of teach-back is an effective practice to ensure that the information was received and interpreted in the manner intended. The pediatric setting offers additional intricacies to this task. Patients are often young and may have limited abilities to fully participate in their own care. Thus, patient and family dynamics need to be greatly considered since multiple people may be involved in the child's care. It is important that all family members involved receive education and are coordinated in their roles.

It is imperative that patients and families ask questions about their care. They should speak up if something is unclear or does not seem right. Patients and parents should verify all medications given. When picking up a prescription from the pharmacy, they should read labels and compare the information on the bottles to what the doctor told them. Patients and families should be encouraged to review the prescription bottle for patient name, medication name, and directions for use and read about possible side effects. Since children's medications are often in liquid form, the pharmacist should be asked to demonstrate how to use the oral syringe to measure and administer the dose prescribed. Patients and parents should also keep records of all medications, including over-the-counter medications and record information regarding missed doses, side effects, etc. This information should be reported back to all providers so that treatment plans can be adapted accordingly.

Institutions should also incorporate patients and families into their chemotherapy use policies and processes. They can be involved at a global level, participating in institutional quality improvement and safety initiatives as well as granular levels and verifying their name and date of birth prior to medication administration. Their input is invaluable in identifying ways to ensure that care is tailored to patient needs.

Overall Chemotherapy Use Process and Double Checks

Evaluating the overall chemotherapy process in addition to the individual steps of the process is essential in determining if gaps persist. It is helpful to outline the overall chemotherapy use process and respective checks and balances used within

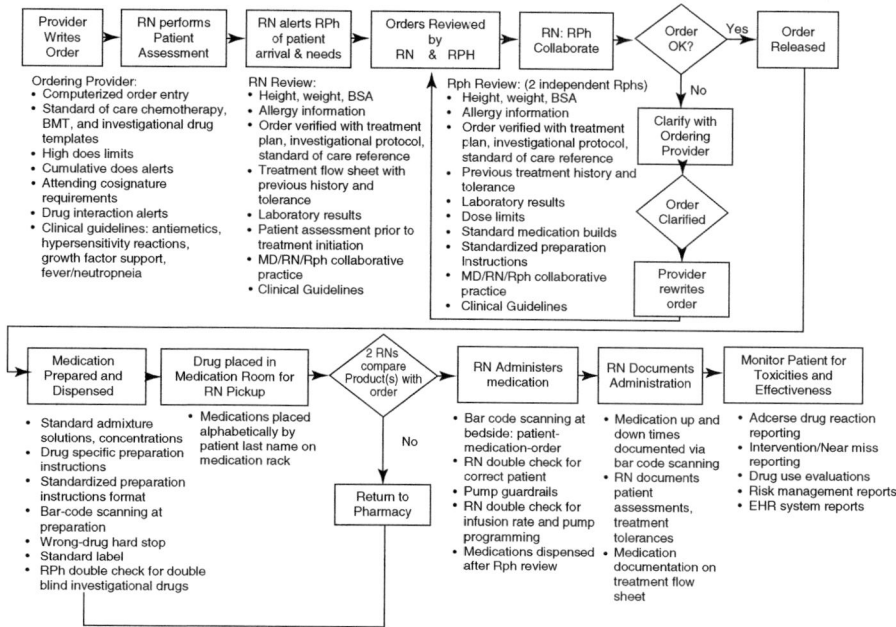

Fig. 10.4 Chemotherapy use process map example

each step [7, 34, 35, 37] (Fig. 10.4). It may be noted that technology is used in various process aspects and is successful in preventing errors; however, it cannot prevent all and can even introduce new issues. For example, the CPOE system may autocalculate doses based on height and weight, but if the incorrect parameter is entered into the system, then the dose will inevitably be wrong. It is imperative that everyone in the process asks themselves if the information at hand makes sense. The CPOE system may also be effective in alerting providers to drug allergy or drug-drug interaction checking, but if patient allergies are not entered or medications are not reconciled, these interactions may go unrecognized. In other cases, alert fatigue can cause significant interactions and contraindications to slip through. This speaks to the importance of carefully designed process double checks. One common strategy used is the double check.

Various studies have demonstrated the effectiveness of double checks when they are conducted appropriately [52, 53]. It is important to note that the double check must be performed independently, meaning that a second practitioner verifies the work process that a first practitioner has verified, but does this separately. This minimizes the risk of confirmation bias. When performed in this manner, double checks can detect up to 95% of errors [52]. Although this error prevention method can be quite effective, it should be used purposefully and should not replace system fixes when they are needed. Developing policies which standardize when double checks should be conducted will help ensure consistency. Additionally, tools to support double checks can improve error detection rates by making it easier for practitioners to complete checks without relying on memory. One study showed that the use of a checklist increased the detection of wrong patient errors by 433% [54]. Tools should provide specific direction. For example, leave space to allow practitioners to enter information related to the aspect that should be checked. (Fig. 10.2) Maximizing the design can improve the effectiveness of the tool itself, increasing error detection rates from 45% to 60% [54]. Overall, their use can be quite successful. However, double checks should be layered among other risk reduction strategies to minimize error risks.

Clinical practice is a continuously evolving field in which new chemotherapies and treatment regimens are proven and new providers join the healthcare team regularly. Reassessment of the chemotherapy use process using methods to measure and sustain its effectiveness is an ongoing process.

Strategies for Sustainability

A systems approach should be utilized to drive improvements in the medication use process. As improvements are made, it is critical that these changes become integrated into daily workflow, processes, and systems. Sustainability of improvements in the medication use process is dependent on establishing and maintaining an organizational culture of safety, utilization of a quality improvement process including ongoing process monitoring, data collection and analysis, and the redesign of systems and workflow.

Culture of Safety

Establishing and maintaining an organizational culture of safety are the foundation for achieving improvements in medication safety as well as sustaining improvements [55, 56]. The American Society of Health-System Pharmacists (ASHP) definition of culture is as follows: "A just culture is one that has a clear and transparent process for evaluating errors and separating events arising from flawed system design or inadvertent human error from those caused by reckless behavior, defined as a behavioral choice to consciously disregard what is known to be a substantial or unjustifiable risk" [57]. An organizational culture of safety is one where leadership has prioritized safety, created an environment where weaknesses in the medication use process can be openly discussed through ongoing learning and education, promoted inclusion of frontline staff, and include the participation of patients and families (Fig. 10.5). The engagement of leadership, including the board of trustees, is critical in order to keep the organization focused on safety. Leadership must prioritize safety, establish specific safety culture principles, and make these visible to the frontline staff [58]. The prioritization of safety involves the inclusion of specific safety goals in the organization's annual goals. The organizational safety goal can then be incorporated into the various departments' goals and initiatives.

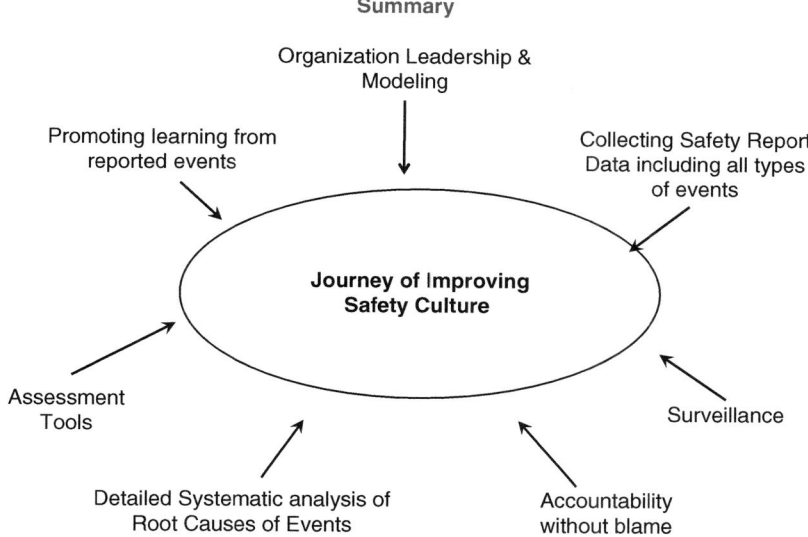

Fig. 10.5 Summary of components to improving safety culture and sustainability

It is equally important that leadership establish safety culture principles that address the balance between individual accountability and system failures, support transparent discussion of actual and potential safety issues and risks, support implementation of specific system or workflow changes, and include patients and families in open discussions of weaknesses in the medication use process [59]. These principles are important not only for creating an organizational safety culture but also serve as a guide during event and process evaluations and improvement initiatives. An additional principle that is important to integrate into the safety culture especially when guiding specific improvement initiatives is safety over convenience or efficiency. Leadership has a key role in communicating these principles to staff and modeling appropriate safety culture behavior in order to sustain safe medication use processes instead of focusing on short-term fixes in response to single events.

Data Collection, Surveillance, and Analysis

To identify the medication-related risks, it is important to collect data from a variety of sources. As discussed previously in the measurement section, these include voluntary staff incident reporting, detailed analysis of specific errors or events, proactive review of the medication use process, and health information record review. Data collection from the various measurement modalities allows for root cause analysis and failure mode effects analysis, which provide critical underlying reasons for the occurrence of the adverse event or near miss. These are analytical approaches based on information provided by automated trigger tools or staff that have been involved in the event or workflow process. Based on the information that is gathered, there are specific recommended actions to ensure the event does not occur in the future.

An additional data collection tool is proactive risk assessments. This includes routine literature review from peer-reviewed journals and Institute for Safe Medication Practices Safety Alerts. The use of self-assessments, such as the ISMP International Medication Safety Self Assessment for Oncology [60], is another way to obtain proactive information regarding key components of an institution's medication use systems. Executive leadership walk-rounds and management meetings where staff are able to discuss safety concerns, policies/procedures that are challenging to adhere to, and technology or other system defects are very good sources of information about vulnerabilities or defects that are in the medication use process. The use of national guidelines, standards, and practice recommendations such as the ASCO/ONS Chemotherapy Administration Safety Standards, and the American Society of Health-System Pharmacists guidelines on preventing medication errors with chemotherapy and biotherapy can serve as a tool for organizations to review their current chemotherapy medication systems. These proactive risk assessments can be used as a starting point for organizations to prioritize current focus areas as well as serve as a road map for future initiatives.

An additional data source is from technology such as the computerized order entry system, pharmacy system, bar coding during drug preparation and administration, and smart pumps. This includes data on alerts clinicians receive during the drug ordering, preparation, and administration processes.

The ISMP has identified targeted medication safety best practices for 2014–2015 and now 2016–2017 [61, 62]. These are best practices of specific safety issues that continue to result in patient harm and should be adopted by hospitals. This is a way for hospitals to review their own practices and focus their medication safety efforts on strategies that have been successfully implemented in other organizations. Implementing these best practices allows organizations to reduce vulnerabilities and sustain improvements in reducing patient harm.

In 2016, the ISMP has identified selected safety risks that might not be identified as a risk unless an adverse event happens [63, 64]. These ten risks and their management can be used by organizations to review their associated workflows and processes, focus their efforts, and be proactive before an adverse event occurs. This approach is also important so that organizations can begin to look at the entire medication use process as a system instead of focusing on single-event improvements.

System Redesign

The sustainability of improvements in medication safety depends on the redesign of systems, workflows, and processes based on the data that has been gathered and its analysis. In order to accomplish the redesign, it is important to have the support of leadership, a multidisciplinary team—including patients and/or families—and identified project managers and timeline. The system redesign includes technology and ensuring they contain specific safety features. These safety features include the appropriate and significant alerts and warnings, presentation of information on the computer screens and printed information, and the availability of information across disciplines or applications. Working with the technology vendors is critical in being able to achieve computer system changes.

The redesign of workflows and processes should include the utilization of techniques and principles such as Lean Six Sigma that have been successful in improving the safety in other industries. It is important to have a formal process improvement methodology that is utilized in an organization to ensure the new workflow or processes will have the best positive impact. Leadership is essential in supporting the redesign and assisting in the change management process.

The sustainability of the improvements in medication safety requires a culture of patient safety, an identified process improvement tool, current data on the risk areas in the medication use process, and a culture of transparency and continuing learning. It should be expected that institution's systems and workflows will be continuing to change and evolving as new systems and information and knowledge are gained. Therefore, it is essential to continue to keep medication safety as a top priority in our organizations and work.

References

1. Walsh KE, Dodd KS, Seetharaman K, et al. Medication errors among adults and children with cancer in the outpatient setting. JCO. 2009;27(6):891–986.
2. Levy J. In my opinion: if measurement is critical to business success, why don't executives measure the things that matter? CIO Enterprises, Sept 1999. 1992.
3. Aronson JK. Medication errors: definitions and classification. Br J Clin Pharmacol. 2009 Jun;67(6):599–604. doi:10.1111/j.1365-2125.2009.03415.x.
4. Edwards IR, Aronson JK. Adverse drug reactions: definitions, diagnosis, and management. Lancet. 2000;356(9237):1255–9.
5. Nebeker JR, Hurdle JF, Hoffman J, Roth B, Weir CR, Samore MH. Developing a taxonomy for research in adverse drug events: potholes and signposts. In: Proceedings of the AMIA Symposium. 2001. pp. 493–497.
6. National Coordinating Council for Medication Error Reporting and Prevention (NCC MERP). Taxonomy of Medication Errors; Available at http://www.NCCMERP.org. Accessed 25 Mar 2016.
7. Goldspiel B, Hoffman JM, Griffith NL, Goodin S, DeChristoforo R, Montello CM, Chase JL, Bartel S, Patel JT. ASHP guidelines on preventing medication errors with chemotherapy and biotherapy. Am J Health Syst Pharm. 2015 Apr 15;72(8):e6–e35. doi:10.2146/sp150001.
8. Voeffray M, Pannatier A, Stupp R, Fucina N, Leyvraz S, Wasserfallen JB. Effect of computerization on the quality and safety of chemotherapy prescription. Qual Saf Health Care. 2006 Dec;15(6):418–21.
9. Institute of Medicine (IOM). In: Kohn LT, Corrigan JM, Donaldson MS, editors. To err is human: building a safer health system. Washington, DC: National Academy Press; 2000.
10. Classen DC, Metzger J. Improving medication safety: the measurement conundrum and where to start. Int J Qual Health Care. 2003 Dec;15(Suppl 1):i41–7.

11. Meyer-Massetti C, Cheng CM, Schwappach DL, Paulsen L, Ide B, Meier CR, Guglielmo BJ. Systematic review of medication safety assessment methods. Am J Health Syst Pharm. 2011;68(3):227–40. doi:10.2146/ajhp100019.

12. Phillips MA. Voluntary reporting of medication errors. Am J Health Syst Pharm. 2002;59(23):2326–8.

13. Thomas EJ, Petersen LA. Measuring errors and adverse events in health care. J Gen Intern Med. 2003;18(1):61–7.

14. Williams SK, Osborn SS. The development of the National Reporting and Learning System in England and Wales, 2001–2005. Med J Aust. 2006;184(10 Suppl):S65–8.

15. The Patient Safety and Quality Improvement Act of 2005. Overview, 2008. Agency for Healthcare Research and Quality, Rockville. http://www.ahrq.gov/qual/psoact.htm.

16. MEDMARX. Quantros, Inc. Available at: https://www.medmarx.com. Accessed 25 Mar 2016.

17. MedWatch: The FDA Safety Information and Adverse Event Reporting Program. US Food and Drug Administration, Center for Drug Evaluation and Research. http://www.fda.gov/medwatch/. Accessed 25 Mar 2016.

18. Farley DO, Haviland A, Champagne S, Jain AK, Battles JB, Munier WB, Loeb JM. Adverse-event-reporting practices by US hospitals: results of a national survey. Qual Saf Health Care. 2008;17(6):416–23. doi:10.1136/qshc.2007.024638.

19. Shojania KG. The frustrating case of incident-reporting systems. Qual Saf Health Care. 2008;17(6):400–2. doi:10.1136/qshc.2008.029496.

20. Jha AK, Kuperman GJ, Teich JM, Leape L, Shea B, Rittenberg E, Burdick E, Seger DL, Vander Vliet M, Bates DW. Identifying adverse drug events: development of a computer-based monitor and comparison with chart review and stimulated voluntary report. J Am Med Inform Assoc. 1998;5(3):305–14.

21. Kaushal R, Bates DW, Landrigan C, McKenna KJ, Clapp MD, Federico F, Goldmann DA. Medication errors and adverse drug events in pediatric inpatients. JAMA. 2001;285(16):2114–20.

22. Kaushal R. Using chart review to screen for medication errors and adverse drug events. Am J Health Syst Pharm. 2002;59(23):2323–5.

23. Manias E. Detection of medication-related problems in hospital practice: a review. Br J Clin Pharmacol. 2013;76(1):7–20. doi:10.1111/bcp.12049. Review

24. Classen DC, Lloyd RC, Provost L, Griffin FA, Resar R. Development and evaluation of the Institute for Healthcare Improvement Global Trigger Tool. J Patient Saf. 2008;4(3):169–77.

25. Griffin FA, Resar RK. IHI global trigger tool for measuring adverse events, IHI innovation series white paper. 2nd ed. Cambridge: Institute for Healthcare Improvement; 2009. Available on www.IHI.org

26. Stockwell DC, Kirkendall E, Muething SE, Kloppenborg E, Vinodrao H, Jacobs BR. Automated adverse event detection collaborative: electronic adverse event identification, classification, and corrective actions across academic pediatric institutions. J Patient Saf. 2013;9(4):203–10. doi:10.1097/PTS.0000000000000055.

27. Ferranti J, Horvath MM, Cozart H, Whitehurst J, Eckstrand J. Reevaluating the safety profile of pediatrics: a comparison of computerized adverse drug event surveillance and voluntary reporting in the pediatric environment. Pediatrics. 2008;121(5):e1201–7. doi:10.1542/peds.2007-2609.

28. Kilbridge PM, Noirot LA, Reichley RM, Berchelmann KM, Schneider C, Heard KM, Nelson M, Bailey TC. Computerized surveillance for adverse drug events in a pediatric hospital. J Am Med Inform Assoc. 2009;16(5):607–12. doi:10.1197/jamia.M3167. Epub 2009 Jun 30

29. Call RJ, Burlison JD, Robertson JJ, Scott JR, Baker DK, Rossi MG, Howard SC, Hoffman JM. Adverse drug event detection in pediatric oncology and hematology patients: using medication triggers to identify patient harm in a specialized pediatric patient population. J Pediatr. 2014;165(3):447–52.e4. doi:10.1016/j.jpeds.2014.03.033. Epub 2014 Apr 25

30. Hope C, Overhage JM, Seger A, Teal E, Mills V, Fiskio J, Gandhi TK, Bates DW, Murray MD. A tiered approach is more cost effective than traditional pharmacist-based review for classifying computer-detected signals as adverse drug events. J Biomed Inform. 2003;36(1–2):92–8.

31. Dormann H, Muth-Selbach U, Krebs S, Criegee-Rieck M, Tegeder I, Schneider HT, Hahn EG, Levy M, Brune K, Geisslinger G. Incidence and costs of adverse drug reactions during hospitalisation: computerised monitoring versus stimulated spontaneous reporting. Drug Saf. 2000;22(2):161–8.
32. Barker KN, McConnell WE. The problems of detecting medication errors in hospitals. Am J Hosp Pharm. 1962;19:360–9.
33. Barker KN, Flynn EA, Pepper GA. Observation method of detecting medication errors. Am J Health Syst Pharm. 2002;59(23):2314–6.
34. David BA, Rodriguez A, Marks SW. Risk reduction and systematic error management: standardization of the pediatric chemotherapy process. In: Henriksen K, Battles JB, Keyes MA, et al., editors. Advances in patient safety: new directions and alternative approaches (Vol 2: Culture and Redesign). Rockville: Agency for Healthcare Research and Quality (US); 2008.
35. Fisher DS, Alfano S, Knobf MT, Donovan C, Beaulieu N. Improving the cancer chemotherapy use process. J Clin Oncol. 1996;14:3148–55.
36. Leape L. Error in medicine. JAMA. 1994;272(23):1851–7.
37. ASHP. Guidelines on Preventing Medication Errors in Hospitals.
38. Institute for Safe Medication Practices. Guidelines for Standard Order Sets 2010. Available from http//www.ismp.org/Tools/guidelines/StandardOrderSets.pdf. Accessed 23 Mar 2016.
39. Miller MR, Robinson KA, Lubomski LH, Rinke ML, Pronovost PJ. Medication errors in paediatric care: a systematic review of epidemiology and an evaluation of evidence supporting reduction strategy recommendations. Qual Saf Health Care. 2007;16:116–26.
40. Dinning C, Branowicki P, O'Neill JB, Marino BL, Billet A. Chemotherapy error reduction: a multidisciplinary approach to create templated order sets. J Pediatr Oncol Nurs. 2005;22(1):20–30.
41. Kohler DR, Montello MJ, Green L, et al. Standardizing the expression and nomenclature of cancer treatment regimens. Am J Health-Syst Pharm. 1998;55:137–44.
42. Healthcare Human Factors. Guidelines for developing ambulatory chemotherapy preprinted orders. Centre for Global eHealth Innovation, University Health Network: Toronto, Ontario, Canada. Available from: http://www.capca.ca/wp-content/uploads/PPO-Guidelines-FINAL-Jan-9-20111.pdf. Accessed 28 Mar 2016.
43. Committee on Identifying and Preventing Medication Errors. Board on Health Care Services. Philip A, Wolcott JA, Bootman JL, Cronenwett LR, editors. Preventing medication errors. Washington, DC: Institute of Medicine of the National Academies. The National Academies Press.
44. Kaushal R, Shojania KG, Bates DW. Effects of computerized physician order entry and clinical decision support systems on medication safety. A systematic review. Arch Intern Med. 2003;163(12):1409–16.
45. Bonnabry P, Cingria L, Ackermann M, Sageghipour F, Bigler L, Mach N. Use of a prospective risk analysis method to improve the safety of the cancer chemotherapy process. Int J Qual Health Care. 2006;18(1):9–16.
46. Robinson DL, Heigham M, Clark J. Using failure mode and effects analysis for safe administration of chemotherapy to hospitalized children with cancer. Jt Comm J Qual Patient Saf. 2006;32(2):161–6.
47. Baker DK, Hoffman JM, Hale GA, et al. Advances in patient safety: new directions and alternative approaches (Vol. 2: Culture and redesign). In: Analysis of patient safety: converting complex pediatric chemotherapy ordering processes from paper to electronic systems. Rockville: Agency for Healthcare Research and Quality (US); 2008.
48. Cohen MR. Medication errors. 2nd ed. Washington, DC: American Pharmacists Association; 2007.
49. Bonnabry P, et al. A risk analysis method to evaluate the impact of a computerized provider order entry system on patient safety. J Am Med Inform Assoc. 2008;15:453–60.
50. Shulman LN, et al. Principles of safe practice using an oncology EHR system for chemotherapy ordering, preparation, and administration, part 2 of 2. J Oncol Pract. 2008;4(5):254–7.

51. Louis Harris and Associates. Public opinion of patient safety issues: research findings. Prepared for National patient safety foundation at AMA. September 1997. Available at: www.npsf.org/download/1997survey.pdf.
52. Institute for Safe Medication Practices (ISMP). Independent double checks: Undervalued and misused: selective us of this strategy can play an important role in medication safety. ISMP Medication Safety Alert. June 13, 2013. Available at the ISMP website under newsletters.
53. ISMP. Safety Bulletin, Canada. Lowering the risk of medication errors: independent double checks. 2005;5(1). Available at the ISMP website under newsletters.
54. White RE, Trbovich PL, Easty AC, et al. Checking it twice: an evaluation of checklists for detecting medication errors at the bedside using a chemotherapy model. Qual Saf Health Care. 2010;19(6):562–7.
55. Conway J, Nathan D, Benz E, et al. Key learning from the Dana-Farber Cancer Institute's 10-year patient safety journey. J Clin Oncol. 2006;1092–9118:615–9.
56. National Patient Safety Foundation. Free from harm accelerating patient safety improvement fifteen years after *To Err is Human*. December 2015. Available at: www.npsf.org/free-from-harm.
57. ASHP Policy 1021 Just Culture and Reporting Medication Errors available at: http://www.ashp.org/import/practiceand policy/policypostionsguidelinesbestpractices.aspx.
58. Conway J. Taking it to the Top. Hospital and Health Networks. March 2000; p. 100.
59. Connor M, Duncombe D, Barclay E, et al. Creating a fair & just culture: one institutions path toward organizational change. J Qual Patient Safety. 2007;33(10):617–24.
60. ISMP International Medication Safety Self-Assessment for Oncology. 2012; Available at: http://mssa.ismp-canada.org/oncology.
61. ISMP. Targeted medication safety best practices for hospitals. 2014:19(1). 2014–2015. Available at the ISMP website under newsletters.
62. ISMP. Targeted medication safety best practices for hospitals. 2016:21(3). 2016–2017. Available at the ISMP website under newsletters.
63. ISMP medication safety alert—selected medication safety risks to manage in 2016 that Might Otherwise Fall off the Radar Screen—part 1. 2016:21(2). 2016–2017. Available at the ISMP website under newsletters.
64. ISMP medication safety alert—selected medication safety risks to manage in 2016 that Might Otherwise Fall off the Radar Screen—part II. 2016:21(3). 2016–2017. Available at the ISMP website under newsletters.

Chapter 11
Healthcare-Associated Infections in Pediatric Hematology-Oncology

James M. Hoffman, Chris I. Wong Quiles, Ashley Crumby, and Elisabeth E. Adderson

In the last decade, advances in cancer therapy have led to improved survival in children and adolescents with malignant disorders. As cure rates improve, treatment-related toxicity, especially infections, accounts for a greater proportion of morbidity and mortality. Pediatric hematology and oncology patients are often highly susceptible to infection. Those with medical devices, such as indwelling central catheters, and those with intermittent or chronic neutropenia are particularly at high risk of healthcare-associated infections (HAIs) such as central line-associated bloodstream infections (CLABSI), *Clostridium difficile* infections (CDIs), ventilator-associated pneumonia (VAP), catheter-associated urinary tract infections (CAUTI), and respiratory viral infections. In the past, infectious complications of therapy for oncological and hematological disorders were regarded as largely unavoidable. It is now recognized that many, although not all, of the most common infections in this population are preventable. Collaborative quality improvement efforts have led to effective strategies to reduce rates of HAI and improved outcomes in these populations.

J.M. Hoffman
Department of Pharmaceutical Sciences, St. Jude Children's Research Hospital, Memphis, TN, USA
e-mail: james.hoffman@stjude.org

C.I. Wong Quiles
Dana-Farber Cancer Institute, Harvard Medical School, Boston, MA, USA
e-mail: chris_wong@dfci.harvard.edu

A. Crumby
Department of Pharmacy Administration, University of Mississippi, Oxford, MS, USA
e-mail: ashley.crumby@stjude.org

E.E. Adderson, MD, Msc (✉)
Department of Pediatric Infectious Diseases, St. Jude Children's Research Hospital, Houston, TX, USA

Department of Pediatrics, University of Tennessee Health Sciences Center, Memphis, TN, USA
e-mail: elisabeth.adderson@stjude.org

© Springer International Publishing AG 2017
C.E. Dandoy et al. (eds.), *Patient Safety and Quality in Pediatric Hematology/Oncology and Stem Cell Transplantation*, DOI 10.1007/978-3-319-53790-0_11

Healthcare-Associated Infections

Central Line-Associated Bloodstream Infections (CLABSI)

Central lines, or central venous catheters, have proved invaluable in the management of children with cancer. Indeed, the National Healthcare Safety Network (NHSN) reported that the highest permanent central line utilization rates in 2013 were in pediatric general hematology-oncology and hematopoietic stem cell transplant (HSCT) wards [1]. These units also reported substantial temporary central line use. CLABSI, however, are the most common healthcare-associated infection (HAI) affecting pediatric hematology-oncology patients. Table 11.1 lists the relative rates of CLABSI observed across different patient populations and catheter types. As in adults, these contribute significantly to mortality, hospital length of stay, and costs [1, 2].

Microorganisms colonize most central lines, often in as a little as a day, by (a) migration from the skin insertion site along the external surface of the catheter, (b) introduction into the hub lumen during manipulation of the catheter or by exposure to contaminated infusates, or (c) hematogenous spread from a focal infection [3]. Thrombin covering the intravascular portion of the catheter and the biofilm produced by many microbial pathogens promotes the adhesion of pathogens. The risk of subsequent bloodstream infection is dependent on both the number of organisms and their intrinsic virulence. Host, underlying disease, and treatment characteristics also contribute to the risk of CLABSI [4, 5].

Many institutions in the United States monitor rates of inpatient central line infections and assess the effectiveness of prevention efforts through the Centers for Disease Control and Prevention's NHSN, and these data are publically reported in many states. These surveillance strategies have also been applied to infections in ambulatory pediatric hematology and oncology patients [4, 6]. Specific criteria for bloodstream infections developed by the CDC Prevention Healthcare Infection Control Practices Advisory Committee (Table 11.2) distinguish between a CLABSI, an infection occurring in a patient who has had a central line in place for >2 days, and a catheter-related bloodstream infection (CRBSI), a CLABSI for which specific laboratory testing has identified the central line as the source of the infection [7]. Practically, it is sometimes not possible to implicate or exclude the catheter because the appropriate laboratory test was not feasible (e.g., if the central line is not removed and cultures of the catheter tip, therefore, not possible) or not obtained (e.g., simultaneous blood cultures from both the central line and a peripheral vein for comparison of time to positivity). The simpler definition of CLABSI has, therefore, been used for NHSN surveillance although it is recognized that it is less specific than desirable.

Figure 11.1 the successes of early efforts to track, report, and prevent CLABSI over the last decade led to the emergence of a "zero tolerance" attitude toward CLABSI, with many organizations setting a goal of eliminating all infections through a series of interventions that include strict adherence to hand hygiene, asepsis during catheter insertion, adherence to a maintenance bundle, and the use of an appropriate dressing [8]. More recently, it has been recognized that many bloodstream infections in persons with cancer or severe neutropenia from other causes, or who have undergone HSCT, are not CRBSI, but result

Table 11.1 Pooled means of laboratory-confirmed permanent and temporary central line bloodstream infections, by type of unit

Location	Overall pooled mean CLABSI	Pooled mean CLABSI—permanent central line days	Pooled mean CLABSI—temporary central line days
Adult general medical/surgical inpatient	0.8	NA	NA
Adult medical/surgical ICU	0.8–1.1[a]	NA	NA
Adult general hematology-oncology ward	NA	1.4	2.0
Adult HSCT ward	NA	2.6	3.0
Pediatric general medical/surgical inpatient	0.9	NA	NA
Pediatric medical/surgical ICU	1.2	NA	NA
Pediatric general hematology-oncology ward	NA	2.1	2.1
Pediatric HSCT ward	NA	2.4	2.2

HSCT hematopoietic stem cell transplant, *ICU* intensive care unit, *NA* not available
[a]Rates vary by unit size and teaching status
National Patient Safety Network 2013 [1]

Table 11.2 Criteria for catheter and mucosal barrier injury laboratory-confirmed bloodstream infections

Laboratory-confirmed bloodstream infection (LCBI)	(1) A recognized pathogen identified from ≥1 blood cultures (2) Fever, chills, or hypotension in association with the same common commensal bacteria being obtained from ≥2 blood cultures drawn on separate occasions (3) Fever, hypothermia, apnea, or bradycardia in a patient ≤1 year of age in association with the same common commensal bacteria being obtained from ≥2 blood cultures drawn on separate occasions In each case, the organism identified from blood should not be related to an infection at another site (i.e., the infection represents a primary bacteremia), and criterion elements must take place 3 days before to 3 days after the collection date of the first positive blood specimen
Central line-associated bloodstream infection (CLABSI)	A LCBI that develops in a patient with a central line in place for >2 days before the onset of the infection

Catheter-related bloodstream infection (CRBSI)	A LCBI with additional laboratory evidence that identifies the central line as the source of the bloodstream infection (e.g., differential time to positivity of blood cultures)

Mucosal barrier injury LCBI	A LCBI:
	(1) That meets LCBI criteria 1 and ≥1 blood specimen is positive for a select group of recognized intestinal organisms, in association with:
	   a. A history of allogeneic HSCT within 1 year and Grade III or IV gastrointestinal GVHD) or ≥1 liter diarrhea (≥20 mL/kg in patients <18 years of age) in a 24-h period on or ≤7 days before the collection date of the first positive blood specimen
	   b. A history of ≥2 days of an ANC or WBC <500 cells/mm^3 on or within 3 days of the collection date of the first positive blood specimen
	(2) That meets LCBI criteria 2 and ≥1 blood specimen is positive for viridans group streptococci only, in association with:
	   a. A history of allogeneic HSCT within 1 year and Grade III or IV gastrointestinal GVHD or ≥1 liter diarrhea (≥20 mL/kg in patients <18 years of age) in a 24-h period on or ≤7 days before the collection date of the first positive blood specimen
	   b. A history of ≥2 days of an ANC or WBC <500 cells/mm^3 on or within 3 days of the collection date of the first positive blood specimen
	(3) A patient ≤1 year of age who meets LCBI criteria 3 and ≥1 blood specimen is positive for viridans group streptococci only, in association with:
	   a. A history of allogeneic HSCT within 1 year and Grade III or IV gastrointestinal GVHD or ≥1 liter diarrhea (≥20 mL/kg in patients <18 yrs. of age) in a 24-h period on or ≤7 days before the collection date of the first positive blood specimen
	   b. A history of ≥2 days of an ANC or WBC <500 cells/mm^3 on or within 3 days of the collection date of the first positive blood specimen

ANC absolute neutrophil count, GVHD graft versus host disease, HSCT hematopoietic stem cell transplant, LCBI laboratory-confirmed bloodstream infection, WBC white blood cell count
National Patient Safety Network 2013

from the translocation of gastrointestinal microorganisms to the bloodstream, particularly in patients with severe neutropenia or who have gastrointestinal graft versus host disease [9]. Use of CLABSI as a surveillance definition in these populations, therefore, overestimates the proportion of bloodstream infections that are attributable to central lines and has implications for whether or not these infections may be prevented by traditional approaches or, indeed, if these infections are preventable at all [10]. In 2013, the NHSN introduced a new surveillance definition of "mucosal injury-associated laboratory-confirmed bloodstream infection" (MBI-LCBI, Table 11.2). Additional studies of the impact of distinguishing MBI-LCBI from CLABSI in high-risk pediatric and adult populations are ongoing.

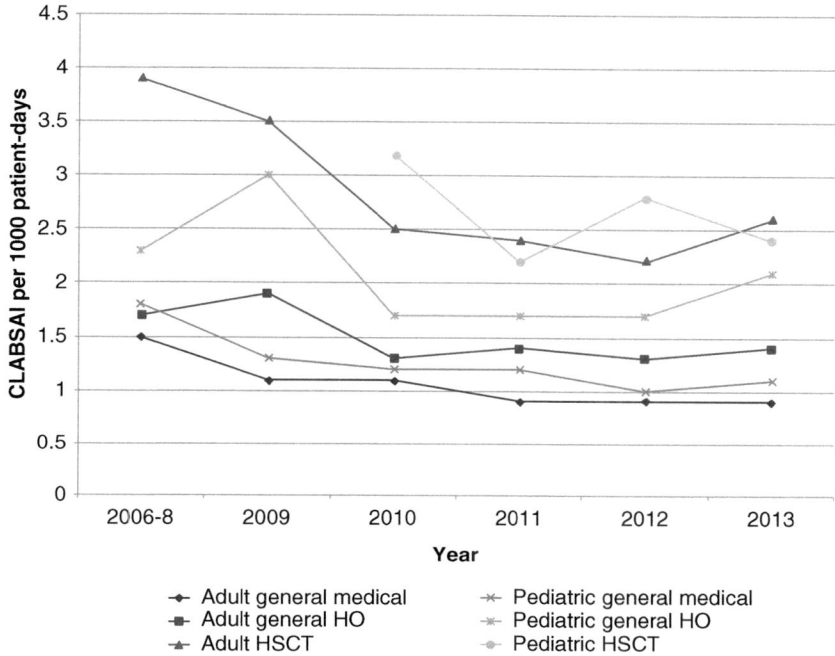

Fig. 11.1   Pooled mean rates of permanent central line-associated bloodstream infections (number of infections per 1000 patient-days) in hospitalized adults and children 2006–2013, by care unit. Data from the National Healthcare Safety Network, available at: http://www.cdc.gov/nhsn/data-stat/index.html

Clostridium difficile *Infection (CDI)*

C. difficile is the single most common organism causing HAI in the United States, with an estimated incidence of 95.3 infections per 100,000 persons overall and 6.3 per 100,000 children under 18 years of age [11, 12]. *C. difficile* is a Gram-positive, anaerobic, spore-forming bacillus. Intestinal colonization occurs when infectious spores, which may persist for long periods in the environment, are ingested. Some strains elaborate two homologous exotoxins, toxin A and toxin B, which bind to and damage intestinal epithelial cells and incite strong inflammatory responses [13]. North American pulsed-field gel electrophoresis type 1 (NAP1) PCR ribotype 027 strains of toxogenic *C. difficile*, which express more toxin A and B than other strains and an additional binary toxin, emerged in the early 2000s. Now commonly found in North America, these strains are associated with more severe disease in adults, but it is not yet clear whether they are more pathogenic in either children or cancer patients [14].

   In order for CDI to occur, patients must be colonized with toxogenic *C. difficile* and undergo some alteration in the gastrointestinal microbiome that promotes decreased microbial diversity [13]. The most commonly recognized risk factor for

CDI is antibiotic use; others include antineoplastic chemotherapy, the use of proton pump inhibitors, gastrointestinal surgery, inflammatory bowel disease, and immunocompromising conditions [15]. Adults with cancer and recipients of HSCT are at significantly greater risk of CDI than the general hospital population, with rates ranging from 3.4% to 27% [16]. Disease manifestations range from mild diarrhea to fulminant pseudomembranous colitis. Complications such as toxic megacolon, bowel perforation, and sepsis are responsible for an estimated fatality rate of up to 15% in adults [12]. Malignancy is also a strong predictor of recurrent CDI. Most children with healthcare-associated CDI have underlying medical comorbidities, with malignancy being the most common. Up to 25% of cases of CDI in hospitalized children occur in those with cancer, a rate tenfold higher than that observed in children without cancer [17, 18]. Boyle reported 17% of pediatric HSCT recipients older than 1 year of age developed CDI within 100 days of transplant (20/10,000 patient days), significantly higher than that the rate observed in adult recipients [19]. Severe and complicated disease appear to be less common in children than adults, but more frequent in children with cancer than those without malignancy [15, 16, 20].

The NHSN defines healthcare-associated CDI as a positive test for toxin-producing *C. difficile* in an unformed stool specimen and/or gross anatomic or histopathological evidence of pseudomembranous colitis, with disease beginning >3 days after admission to a healthcare facility [21]. This and other clinical and surveillance definitions have significant limitations that may affect estimates of the incidence of CDI in pediatric oncology patients. Over half of young children, especially those <2 years of age, and almost a third of pediatric oncology patients may be asymptomatically colonized by *C. difficile*, often for long periods of time [22–24]. Some investigators have suggested that sensitive molecular diagnostic tests, such as nucleic acid amplification of toxin A and B genes, are more likely to overestimate the incidence of CDI than older assays because these are more likely to identify the clinically inconsequential carriage of *C. difficile* [22]. Viruses and other gastrointestinal co-pathogens are also detected in as many as 80% of children, including immunocompromised children with CDI, making it difficult to judge the contribution of each potential pathogen to diarrheal disease [25, 26]. Importantly, however, patients who are colonized with toxogenic *C. difficile* may still represent a source of environmental shedding and transmission of infectious spores. Judicious use of antimicrobials, infection prevention precautions, and environmental cleaning are the mainstays of CDI prevention in healthcare settings.

Ventilator-Associated Pneumonia (VAP)

The NHSN surveillance definition for pneumonia incorporates the results of diagnostic imaging, clinical signs and symptoms, and laboratory tests [27]. A specific algorithm is available for immunocompromised patients (Table 11.3). Ventilator-associated pneumonia (VAP) is defined as pneumonia that occurs >2 calendar days after a patient is placed on mechanical ventilation; the ventilator must have been in place on the day that the first criterion for the diagnosis of VAP was met or on the previous day.

Table 11.3 National Hospital Safety Network surveillance definition for pneumonia in immunocompromised patients

Evidence	Definition
Diagnostic imaging	≥2 serial chest imaging studies at a ≤ 7-day interval demonstrating at least one of: • New or progressive and persistent infiltrate(s) • Consolidation • Cavitation • Pneumatoceles in infants ≤1 year of age In patients without underlying pulmonary or cardiac disease, a single unequivocal chest imaging study is acceptable
Clinical findings	At least one of: • Fever (>38.0 °C) • New onset of purulent sputum, change in character of sputum, increased respiratory secretions, or increased suctioning requirements • New onset or worsening cough, dyspnea, or tachypnea • Crepitations or bronchial breath sounds • Hemoptysis • Pleuritic chest pain
Laboratory tests	At least one of: • Positive blood culture not related to another source of infection • Positive pleural fluid culture • Positive quantitative culture from minimally contaminated lower respiratory tract specimen • 5% BAL-obtained cells with intracellular bacteria on Gram stain • Positive quantitative culture of lung tissue • Histopathological evidence of abscess formation or intra-alveolar/bronchiolar accumulation of PMNs For viral and fastidious bacterial (e.g., *Legionella*) pneumonias: • Positive culture from respiratory secretions • Positive nonculture diagnostic test from respiratory secretions • Fourfold rise in paired acute and convalescent serum antibody titers • Detection of *Legionella* antigen in urine For fungal infection: • Matching positive blood and sputum/ET aspirate cultures with *Candida* spp. • Evidence of fungi from minimally contaminated LRT specimen by direct microscopic examination and culture or nonculture diagnostic test

Adapted from [27]

The precise incidence and clinical outcomes of VAP have been difficult to establish because studies have used diverse diagnostic criteria and inconsistently applied these criteria and because diagnostic definitions for VAP, including those reported by the NHSN, have limited sensitivity and specificity [28]. The signs and symptoms of VAP, for example, may overlap with other infections, such as tracheobronchitis, and with noninfectious pulmonary disorders [29]. Reactivation of latent pulmonary or systemic infection, such as cytomegalovirus or tuberculosis, in oncology and transplant patients, including children, may be indistinguishable from VAP. Some features of the current NHSN surveillance definition make its application to children problematic. Respiratory specimens, for example, must be obtained by methods that limit contamination, such as bronchoalveolar lavage, that may have

Table 11.4 CAUTI rates [1]

Location	Pooled mean CAUTI
Adult general medical/surgical inpatient	1.3
Adult medical/surgical ICU	1.3–2.7[a]
Adult general hematology-oncology ward	2.1
Adult HSCT ward	2.2
Pediatric general medical surgical inpatient	1.4
Pediatric medical/surgical ICU	2.5
Pediatric general hematology-oncology ward	3.0
Pediatric HSCT ward	0.0

[a]Rates vary by unit size and teaching status

technical limitations and greater risks in young patients [30]. Recognizing the limitation of VAP surveillance definitions, NHSN surveillance began to assess a broader range of ventilator-associated events, including VAP, in adults in 2015 [31]. A pediatric-specific algorithm for VAP is not yet available, but one study that applied adult definitions retrospectively to PICU patients receiving mechanical ventilation suggests that this strategy may be useful [32].

Obstacles to diagnosis notwithstanding, VAP are the second most common HAI in pediatric and neonatal intensive care units. In the United States in 2012, there were 0.7 VAP per 1000 ventilator days in pediatric medical/surgical units [33]. Overall, between 3% and 10% of ventilated PICU patients develop VAP, a rate that is approximately threefold lower than that of adults (Table 11.4) [34]. Data are limited, but have suggested that VAP in children, as in adults, is associated with longer duration of mechanical ventilation and PICU stay, greater hospital costs, and increased mortality [35, 36]. The specific rates and characteristics of VAP in pediatric oncology patients have not been reported, but it is plausible that immunosuppression might predispose to infection and increase the rate and severity of VAP in this population.

The pathogenesis of VAP has not been completely elucidated. VAP may, like conventional pneumonia, result from the inhalation of infectious aerosols or complicate hematogenous bacteremia or fungemia. The presence of the same microorganisms in the oropharynx and in endotracheal aspirates, however, suggests that a frequent and potentially preventable cause of VAP is the aspiration of microorganisms colonizing the endotracheal tube (ET), oropharynx, or stomach [37]. Micro-aspiration of upper airway secretions around the uncuffed ET commonly used in infants and children or through channels formed by folds in low-pressure high-volume cuffed ET may be exacerbated by the impairment of mucociliary clearance and pooling of secretions in the subglottic airway. Risk factors for VAP in children include a prolonged duration of mechanical ventilation, prior antimicrobial exposure, and the use of immunosuppressing drugs, particularly corticosteroids [38]. Additional contributing elements may include the replacement of the usual microbiological flora of the oropharynx and stomach by more virulent species (such as *Staphylococcus aureus* and Gram-negative bacilli), the contamination of suction equipment (particularly associated with the use of open systems and nonsterile solutions), and the presence of a naso-gastric tube, enteral feeding, poor oral hygiene, gastric distension, and positioning (with the semirecumbent position associated with a lower risk of VAP than the supine position). The contribution of each of these elements to the pathogenesis of VAP in pediatric hematology-oncology patients has not been studied; most prevention strategies target multiple risk factors for infection.

Catheter-Associated Urinary Tract Infections (CAUTI)

Overall, urinary tract infections (UTI) are the fourth most common HCA infection in the United States [39]. Almost all are related to catheterization or other instrumentation. Short-term indwelling urinary catheterization may be necessary because of acute urinary retention or obstruction, or the need to monitor urinary output (especially perioperatively, during critical illness, or if receiving large volumes of fluid or diuretics). More prolonged use may be required to promote healing of sacral or perineal wounds or incisions, in incontinent patients or for comfort during end of life care.

The NHSN defines CAUTI as a UTI that occurs >2 calendar days after a urinary catheter is placed and <1 day after the catheter has been removed, if applicable [39]. Rates are generally higher in children than in adults (Table 11.4), but little has been reported on outcomes in children outside of the intensive care setting or in specific populations such as pediatric hematology-oncology and transplant recipients. CAUTI are associated with secondary bloodstream infections, increased hospital stay and costs and, in adults, increased mortality [40, 41].

Most CAUTI are ascending in origin. Uropathogens that colonize the periurethral area adhere to fibrinogen that accumulates on the catheter, multiplying and forming biofilm [41]. Thereafter, bacteria may colonize the bladder, often within days, releasing toxins and proteases that damage urinary epithelium and promote ascension to the kidney and hematogenous dissemination. Up to a third of infections may occur from contamination of the urinary collecting system from exogenous sources, such as the hands of healthcare providers [42]. Efforts to prevent CAUTI have focused on reducing the duration of catheter use and the contamination of drainage systems.

Respiratory Viral Infections

Most respiratory viruses are spread by indirect contact, droplet, or airborne transmission. Sources of infection include other patients, caregivers or visitors, and healthcare providers, who may be asymptomatic or symptomatic, and contaminated environmental sources [43]. Patient factors that increase the likelihood of healthcare-associated respiratory viral infections in pediatric hematology-oncology and transplant patients include their frequent close physical contact with caregivers, young age, lack of previous natural infection or immunization and subsequent acquired immunity, and the presence of primary or secondary immunodeficiency. In the ambulatory healthcare setting, patients may be cared for in extended periods in common areas; the risk of infection is increased when infectious persons are not immediately recognized and when environmental cleaning is inadequate because of time constraints.

Strategies to reduce healthcare-associated respiratory viral infections include transmission-based infection, prevention, precautions, and vaccination. Institutions must provide infection prevention staff, clinical microbiology support, and the supplies and equipment necessary to assess and correct remediable causes of healthcare-associated respiratory viral infections. Risk assessment should inform the development of processes for the surveillance for and management of endemic, epidemic (e.g., influenza), and emerging (e.g., Middle East respiratory syndrome-coronavirus) respiratory infections.

Respiratory hygiene/cough etiquette strategies designed to facilitate the prompt recognition of respiratory illness in patients and caregivers have been developed with the intention of incorporating these into infection prevention standard precautions (Table 11.5) [43]. Transmission-based precautions should be implemented for hospitalized patients with any signs or symptoms of respiratory viral infections pending diagnostic tests. A single patient room with toilet and hand hygiene facilities is preferred. If this is not feasible, spatial separation of >3 ft and the use of curtains or other room dividers are recommended. Other strategies, such as cohorting patients with the same organism or the same symptoms or cohorting providers, should be considered in outbreak or other special circumstances, in consultation with infection preventionists. When patients are transferred to other facilities or departments, the presence of a potentially communicable disease and current infection prevention precautions should be communicated to the receiving providers. Viral shedding may persist for weeks to months in immunocompromised patients. Discontinuing transmission-based precautions in this population, therefore, must consider host factors, disease epidemiology, and the results of diagnostic tests.

Few high-quality randomized clinical trials have addressed the effectiveness of masks for the prevention of transmission of respiratory viruses. Existing evidence suggests, however, that both medical masks and respirators are effective. The CDC and other agencies recommend the use of these devices to protect patients and healthcare providers against seasonal influenza and tuberculosis. Clinical trials suggest that face masks provide compliance-dependent protection against

Table 11.5 Respiratory hygiene and cough etiquette components

1. Education of staff, patients, and visitors regarding respiratory hygiene and cough etiquette
2. Posted signs instructing patients and caregivers to make healthcare personnel aware of symptoms of respiratory illness
3. Provision of materials for source control (e.g., tissues, alcohol-based hand rub or supplies for handwashing after contact with respiratory secretions)
4. Masking and spatial separation of persons with respiratory symptoms from others in common waiting areas (ideally in a single room, a minimum of 3 ft from others)
5. Observance of droplet and standard precautions by healthcare providers when examining patients with symptoms of a respiratory infection

Adapted from [43]

infection in the community [44]. For healthcare providers, respirators appear to provide superior protection, but the choice of respiratory protection should be based on availability, etiology of illness, comfort, and the degree of risk.

Healthcare providers should refrain from working when ill with symptoms of a communicable respiratory infection; management policies should support and not discourage this practice. Likewise, visitors with respiratory illnesses should be discouraged from entering healthcare facilities unless this is unavoidable.

Seasonal influenza vaccination of healthcare providers reduces hospital-acquired influenza infections in cancer patients, and most evidence suggests that this practice decreases employee morbidity and absenteeism [45–47]. The Centers for Disease Control and Prevention Advisory Committee on Immunization Practices (ACIP) recommends that, unless medical contraindications exist, all healthcare personnel should be vaccinated annually to protect themselves, their families, and their patients against influenza [48]. Similar recommendations exist for the use of tetanus-diphtheria-acellular pertussis (Tdap) vaccine for the prevention of pertussis [49]. These recommendations direct organizations to provide vaccine as part of employee health programs and to make efforts to reduce administrative and financial barriers to immunization [50]. Personnel refusing influenza vaccination for reasons other than a documented medical contraindication should sign a written declination that outlines the risks of vaccine refusal. Influenza immunization of HCP is tracked by the NHSN. During the 2014–2015 season, 88.6% of employees and 84.5% of all healthcare personnel in acute care hospitals received seasonal influenza vaccination, representing a significant increase over historical rates of compliance with vaccine recommendations [51, 52]. Successful strategies to improve compliance with vaccination policies have included education and incentive-based (i.e., reward) systems, but the most effective approaches have been mandatory vaccination policies that require the use of protective face masks or antiviral prophylaxis for the duration of the influenza season or result in the suspension or termination of unvaccinated workers [53]. Some states have enacted legislation to increase healthcare provider immunization rates [54].

Measurement

Both process (important data elements related to patient care activities) and outcome data must be systematically collected to prevent HAI. Ongoing process and outcome data collection can inform the development of more effective prevention strategies or lead to the modification of suboptimal processes. The latest CDC surveillance definitions should be used to identify the occurrence and rates of HAI within an institution [6]. If ongoing surveillance reveals a sharp increase in infections, standard epidemiological investigation techniques must be used to investigate the outbreak; these methods are beyond the scope of this chapter [55]. Organizations should remain open to reevaluating and improving measures for HAI based on new knowledge. For example, the recently developed definition for MBI-LCBI, clearly differentiating these infections from other CLABSI, is a relatively new outcome measurement that has substantial importance to the pediatric hematology-oncology population.

Table 11.6 Prevention bundle elements for CLABSI, CAUTI, and VAP[a]

Bundle	Standard Elements
CLABSI—insertion	Hand hygiene
	CHG scrub
	No iodine treatment
	Prepackaged or filled insertion cart, tray, or box
	Insertion checklist with staff empowerment to stop non-emergent procedure
	Full sterile barrier for providers and patients
	Insertion training for all providers
CLABSI—maintenance	Daily discussion of central line necessity, functionality, and utilization including bedside and medical care team members
	Regular assessment of dressing to assure clean/dry/occlusive
	Standardized access procedure
	Standardized dressing cap and tubing change procedures/timing
CLABSI—recommended element	Utilize a system approach to review all hospital-acquired CLABSI
CAUTI—insertion	Use aseptic technique for insertion
	Avoid unnecessary catheterization
CAUTI—maintenance	Maintain a closed drainage system
	Maintain hygiene
	Keep bag below level of bladder
	Maintain unobstructed flow of urine
	Remove catheter when no longer needed
CAUTI—recommended element	Secure catheter
VAP	Readiness to extubate—assess readiness to extubate daily
	Head of bed elevation—elevate head of bed to 30–45 degrees
	Minimize distribution of the circuit—inspect ventilator circuit for gross contamination daily, and if present, change circuit
	Oral hygiene—perform oral hygiene minimally every 12 h

[a]Adapted from SPS Bundle Elements [57]

When considering process data collection, it is important to identify the methods utilized by institutions to prevent the occurrence of HAI. A common approach to infection prevention is the "prevention bundle," designed to provide a list of elements that should be routinely implemented to prevent HAI. One identified authority for information on prevention bundles is the Children's Hospitals' Solutions for Patient Safety (SPS), which is an international network of over 90 hospitals that aims to reduce patient harm, including HAI, in children's hospitals [56]. SPS provides a document that includes prevention bundle information for CLABSI, CAUTI, and VAP infections [57]. Listed in Table 11.6 are examples of elements included in these bundles that focus on standards for both insertion and maintenance of devices for CLABSI and CAUTI and important processes for the prevention of VAP. Of note, the insertion bundle elements were developed for bedside insertion in the ICU, not for line placement in an operating room. Bundle elements are stratified based on their level of evidence to provide hospitals with guidance for prioritizing their efforts.

The SPS document lists standard and recommended bundle elements and provides tools for assessing the reliability of these bundles, such as protocols for audits of performance on all SPS Prevention Bundle Standard elements [57, 58]. Institutions can choose to include additional elements if they desire to gather data on other processes, but SPS suggests limiting these to five or fewer so that healthcare staff are not overwhelmed or confused by the number of interventions [57]. For CLABSI and CAUTI, it is recommended that insertion and maintenance bundles be measured separately. SPS recommends performing a minimum of 20 audits per month in order to obtain data frequently enough to rapidly identify barriers to compliance and to make changes in the processes to eliminate these barriers [57]. A 90% compliance rate for bundle data is a common goal within SPS. Organizations using sophisticated electronic health records (EHR) with capabilities to discretely document and subsequently retrieve data may be able to gather some or all data electronically. However, this approach may not be feasible in all settings, and direct observation of bundle elements may identify additional opportunities for improvement that may not be revealed through automated retrieval of data documented in the EHR.

Recommended practices include structured investigation, data collection, and analysis of all episodes of infection. These efforts may be referred to by various names, depending on the organization [e.g., mini root cause analyses (RCA) or line rounds]. Many institutions use this approach, documented most commonly for CLABSI, to retrace every step leading up to the infection and thereby identify improvement opportunities. The goal of this approach is to allow institutions to learn from each and every infection and implement improvements based on these findings. For example, Rinke et al. used a RCA approach to systematically investigate all CLABSI in hospitalized pediatric oncology patients [59]. When a positive blood culture was reported, a multidisciplinary team interviewed care providers and analyzed 13 patient and system factors that could have contributed to the CLABSI. A similar approach was used by Bundy et al. in a multicenter quality improvement collaborative that included the implementation of a standardized bundle as well as CLABSI survellience. This approach resulted in significant reductions in CLABSI rates among 32 pediatric hematology-oncology centers [60]. In both instances, the use of this RCA approach provided vital data elements that could then be used for system changes and the implementation of improvement strategies.

When comparing the evidence base for the prevention bundles discussed in this chapter, the most detailed and convincing data in the pediatric hematology-oncology and transplant population are available for CLABSI prevention [60]. CAUTI and VAP bundles have data supporting their effectiveness in other populations [61, 62]. Formal SPS Prevention Bundles for CDI have not been developed, and, without this guidance, other approaches must be utilized to reduce the number of these infections. One example is the guideline provided by the Society for Healthcare Epidemiology of America (SHEA); this includes strategies for prevention of CDI in adults, but can be adapted for pediatric hematology-oncology patients [63, 64]. A list of recommendations can be found in Table 11.7. Evaluating and monitoring each of these practices can provide institutions with compliance data as well as identifying areas for improvement, much like the approaches taken using the SPS bundles. If analysis is done using these approaches and the CDI incidence remains higher than the institution's goal, SHEA also provides special approaches for preventing CDI in high-risk settings [63].

Table 11.7 Basic practices for prevention and monitoring of CDI: recommended for all acute care hospitals and ambulatory care settings [63, 64]

1. Encourage appropriate use of antimicrobials
2. Initiation of contact precautions for patients with signs and symptoms consistent with CDI, single-patient room preferred
3. Implement a laboratory-based alert system to provide immediate notification about newly diagnosed CDI patients
4. Education of healthcare personnel, environmental service personnel, and hospital administration about CDI, specifically the importance of handwashing with soap and water and the use of personal protective equipment
5. Educate patients and their families about CDI as appropriate, including hand hygiene and the cleaning of cell phones and other personal effects.
6. Cleaning and maintenance of reusable medical devices according to the manufacturer's instructions and institutional policies; do not reuse single-use devices
7. Establish policies and procedures for routine cleaning and disinfection of environmental surfaces in both inpatient and ambulatory care facilities, including placing emphasis on surfaces that are most likely to be contaminated with pathogens and the use of EPA-registered detergents/disinfectants; assess adequacy of cleaning
8. Notify receiving caregivers of CDI within and outside of facility upon transfer
9. Conduct CDI surveillance and analyze and report CDI data
10. Measure compliance with CDC or WHO hand hygiene and contact precautions

Improvement

When data indicate deviations in bundle performance data, an increase in infections, or other opportunities for improvement, various actions must be taken. A wide variety of causes and contributing factors must be considered, including staff, patient, and family practices, equipment and supply changes, the environment of care, and others. Similar to other areas of patient safety, actions must focus on high leverage changes that provide fundamental and lasting changes in the process of care. Simple actions such as education and policy changes may provide value in some situations, but rarely provide lasting change and improvement. Iterative, ongoing improvements will often be needed to embed lasting change into practice, and leaders must be nimble and responsive to promote changes in practice.

Participation in formal collaborations across children's hospitals focused on reducing HAI has become a core technique. The Quality Transformation Network, managed by the Children's Hospital Association (CHA), unified pediatric hospitals to work together in order to deliver high-quality, reliable, and safe care for pediatric patients [56]. Initial collaborative efforts to prevent HAI in children's hospitals were focused on CLABSI in the pediatric intensive care unit (PICU). The successful PICU work prompted CHA to expand these efforts to inpatient pediatric hematology-oncology units in 2009, and to the ambulatory setting in 2011, by creating the Hematology-Oncology CLABSI Collaborative, later renamed the Childhood Cancer and Blood Disorders Learning Network (CCBDN) [56, 60, 65]. Recently, the CHA collaborative has worked with SPS [56]. SPS now collects data on inpatient

CLABSI for pediatric oncology/hematology units, and CCBDN has concentrated efforts on reducing CLABSI in ambulatory patients with cancer and blood disorders, recognizing that the majority of these children and adolescents receive much of their care outside the hospital and that CLABSI occur more than twice as frequently in the ambulatory setting than in hospitalized children in this population [56, 65, 66].

Ultimately, preventing HAIs is a team effort that requires sustained involvement and engagement across the entire healthcare team as well as patients and families. For example, the entire team should routinely discuss the continuing need for intravenous and urinary catheters. In the pediatric hematology-oncology population, however, care may require a central venous catheter for months to years at a time. Further, to reduce line accesses, nurses and physicians will need to work together to bundle lab draws, and nurses, pharmacists, and physicians will need to work together to switch from intravenous to oral therapy. All of this ongoing communication must occur in an environment with a positive patient safety culture that encourages team members and families to speak up to make changes for patient care.

Sustainability

Sustaining the improvements achieved after reducing healthcare-associated infections is necessary to continue to obtain successful outcomes in pediatric hematology-oncology patients, given the high rates of infections in this population and the associated morbidity and mortality [2, 67–69]. Although sustainability has been recognized as a key practice in quality improvement and safety work, including the reduction of HAI in pediatric hematology-oncology patients, it does not occur automatically [70]. The Institute for Healthcare Improvement refers to sustainability as locking in the progress that groups have made already and continually building upon it [71]. In pediatric hematology-oncology patients, sustaining reductions in HAI implies adoption and long-term implementation of the established evidence-based practices that are known to result in infection rate reductions, such that these become the norm within a group and ideal adherence is accomplished (i.e., strict compliance with the central line care bundle to reduce CLABSI). The goal is to develop a change to reduce pediatric HAI with enduring impact, even after the initiative is no longer the top priority for a group, and it begins to function without additional dedicated resources. Yet, maintaining a positive change long-term is known to have a high rate of failure, and only limited reports exist of sustained healthcare improvements [72].

Some of the factors associated with difficulty achieving sustainable change are not specific to efforts aiming to reduce HAI in pediatric hematology-oncology patients, but certainly apply. These include incorporation of new staff unaware and/or untrained in best practice and the development of new projects that create distraction or shift the focus away from infection reduction, complacency, and the commonality of emergencies and complex cases in this group of patients, which can at times justify the lack of adherence to best practice [73]. Therefore, a specific focus on sustainability is necessary in order to hold on to the gains achieved.

Strategies for sustainability must be incorporated early on and embedded into the process as it occurs, such that it is inseparable from the process of designing, testing, and implementing change. Some of the improvement strategies utilized to achieve reductions in HAI can also lead to sustainability independently, but a formal focus on this aspect through careful planning increases the chances of maintaining improvements. A number of approaches to foster sustainability after change based on high reliability principles have been described in other chapters of this book and elsewhere [71]. Many of these are applicable to preserving the changes after reductions in pediatric hematology-oncology HAI are obtained, but limited evidence exists that is unique to sustainability in this particular area. Rather, efforts have primarily been concentrated on achieving improvements and reducing HAI in this vulnerable population, rather than on upholding gains.

Organizing children's hospitals around the United States into large-scale pediatric collaborative improvement networks has been an overarching principle in successful and sustainable pediatric quality improvement and safety efforts. These efforts have paved the way for additional healthcare improvement and safety initiatives in pediatric hospitals. These, in turn, have led to sustainable reductions in patient harm, including fewer pediatric HAI [47, 49, 54]. The first visible success story in sustainable improvements specific to pediatric cancer and blood disorder patients resulted from the CHA CCBDN effort to reduce inpatient CLABSI in pediatric hematology-oncology patients; this has successfully achieved and maintained an inpatient CLABSI rate reduction of approximately 28% for years [60].

Collaboration has been central in sustaining reductions in CLABSI rates in pediatric hematology-oncology patients and spreading change. Hospitals collaborating in networks are being encouraged to share success stories and helpful tools and strategies in achieving and maintaining reductions in CLABSI rates. In addition, networking provides a platform for spread and expansion. The success of networking and collaboration is based on providing a common forum to work, learn, and improve together [60, 74].

The collaborative success in pediatric hematology-oncology CLABSI reduction highlights a number of strategies that are central in sustaining change within this complex population. These can be summarized into three categories: People, Process, and Place (the three Ps).

People

Similar to the importance it has in achieving improvement, a strong leadership that is visible and effective is central to sustaining change. The collaborative has provided this at a high level, but individual institutions also require the presence of strong leaders locally in order to maintain the changes achieved. A large majority of successful efforts in reducing CLABSI in pediatric hematology-oncology patients have emphasized the importance of a dedicated team with direct leadership, central to maintaining hospital-wide support even after the goal has been achieved, such that efforts can be continued [60, 68, 75].

One of the main strategies of sustaining a change that is primarily reliant on staff consistently performing all aspects of a bundle, as is as the case with many pediatric HAI prevention efforts, is ensuring formalized ongoing staff education and training of newcomers on best practice. This requires high-quality training of staff, where multidisciplinary teamwork and communication are key to successfully holding on to the gains achieved [73]. Formal competency testing processes are essential. One recommended approach is to have ongoing formal competency testing through fidelity simulation, which has been associated with assuring competency in care delivery of aspects such as central line care [70, 71].

Process

Standardization and spreading of change are both key aspects to sustainability [71]. These aspects were also observed as a result of the large-scale collaboration to reduce CLABSI in pediatric hematology-oncology patients. Participating children's hospitals across the nation were required to continuously report rates of infection and compliance with the central line care bundle [60]. The collaborative reproduced detailed data about CLABSI and bundle compliance rates for participating centers, allowing for transparency, visibility, and the ability to generate benchmarking data facilitating comparison among centers. Furthermore, the process of monitoring and reporting continued even after a reduction in CLABSI rates was observed, thus serving as a main strategy in sustaining gains. Monitoring and reporting of infection rates incentivizes adherence to best practice and, therefore, leads to sustained reductions in rates. Similarly, connecting teams at other hospitals reduces trial and error to find effective solutions. Also central to sustainability is the fact that these initiatives were expected to be long term and were built to persist until goals were achieved and quality improvement was maintained [60, 66, 67].

In pediatric hematology-oncology CLABSI reduction, the collaborative's use of self-audit not only served as a measurement tool but also as a reminder to staff regarding best practices when caring for central lines. This strategy encourages strict compliance with evidence-based practice, standardization, ongoing monitoring of performance, and incorporation into the daily routine, all of which are aspects central to maintaining change [60, 74]. Other strategies that have been used include the development of processes to learn from outstanding scenarios by RCA and identifying local barriers through methodology such as failure modes and effects analysis, a strategy used to prospectively identify areas of risk. One group specifically described the importance of ongoing monitoring of infection rates and the need to have a process in place to respond to unexpected changes in the face of an observed rise in CLABSI rates. Their strategies included preemptively identifying patients with CLABSI-specific risk factors, identification of variables associated with increased CLABSI rates directly from frontline staff, and the evaluation of variables associated with increased micro-system stress [76].

Place

Embedded in every improvement process that is meant to last is the need to promote culture change [71]. In pediatric hematology-oncology, reducing HAI has required both a national and international focus that has helped identify the severity of the problem and concluded that improvements are achievable. The large-scale collaboration that has led to sustainable reductions in pediatric hematology-oncology CLABSI both directly and indirectly contributed to culture change [60, 66]. An emphasis on reducing HAI collectively led to increased awareness of the problem. This key step in developing culture change also indirectly led to increased attention to detail, and both contributed to a focus on safety culture and changes in belief systems [60, 66, 71].

In summary, attitudes toward infectious complications of pediatric hematology-oncology care have evolved over the past decade from the belief that these illnesses were largely inevitable to the understanding that, with diligent adherence to best practices, the incidence of many common infections in pediatric hematology-oncology patients and transplant recipients can be significantly reduced. The efforts of individual institutions are critical to identifying risks for infection in these populations and new strategies for infection prevention and ensuring that the organization itself maintains compliance with standards. Large-scale collaborations have provided forums for testing of new interventions; for disseminating standardized, evidence-based infection prevention methods; and for developing measurement and monitoring processes and benchmarks for improvement. Although still a relatively new effort, the systematic incorporation of quality improvement strategies has already demonstrated great promise in reducing the morbidity and mortality associated with infection in children and adolescents with cancer and improving disease outcomes.

References

1. Dudeck MA, Edwards JR, Allen-Bridson K, Gross C, Malpiedi PJ, Peterson KD, et al. National Healthcare Safety Network report, data summary for 2013, device-associated module. Am J Infect Control. 2015;43:206–21.
2. Wilson MZ, Rafferty C, Deeter D, Comito MA, Hollenbeak CS. Attributable costs of central line-associated bloodstream infections in a pediatric hematology/oncology population. Am J Infect Control. 2014;42:1157–60.
3. Raad II, Hanna HA. Intravascular catheter-related infections: new horizons and recent advances. Arch Intern Med. 2002;162:871–8.
4. Hord JD, Lawlor J, Werner E, Billett AL, Bundy DG, Winkle C, et al. Central line associated blood stream infections in pediatric hematology/oncology patients with different types of central lines. Pediatr Blood Cancer. 2016;63:1603–7.
5. Dandoy CE, Haslam D, Lane A, Jodele S, Demmel K, El-Bietar J, et al. Healthcare burden, risk factors, and outcomes of mucosal barrier injury laboratory-confirmed bloodstream infections after stem cell transplantation. Biol Blood Marrow Transplant. 2016;22:1671–7.
6. Rinke ML, Bundy DG, Chen AR, Milstone AM, Colantuoni E, Pehar M, et al. Central line maintenance bundles and CLABSIs in ambulatory oncology patients. Pediatrics. 2013;132:e1403–12.

7. O'Grady NP, Alexander M, Burns LA, Dellinger EP, and the Healthcare Infection Control Practices Advisory Committee. 2011 Guidelines for the prevention of intravascular catheter-related infections. http://www.cdc.gov/hicpac/BSI/BSI-guidelines-2011.html (2011). Accessed 18 Dec 2015.
8. Miller SE, Maragakis LL. Central line-associated bloodstream infection prevention. Curr Opin Infect Dis. 2012;25:412–22.
9. See I, Iwamoto M, Allen-Bridson K, Horan T, Magill SS, Thompson ND. Mucosal barrier injury laboratory-confirmed bloodstream infection: results from a field test of a new National Healthcare Safety Network definition. Infect Control Hosp Epidemiol. 2013;34:769–76.
10. Metzger KE, Rucker Y, Callaghan M, Churchill M, Jovanovic BD, Zembower TR, et al. The burden of mucosal barrier injury laboratory-confirmed bloodstream infection among hematology, oncology, and stem cell transplant patients. Infect Control Hosp Epidemiol. 2015;36:119–24.
11. Lessa FC, Mu Y, Bamberg WM, Beldavs ZG, Dumyati GK, Dunn JR, et al. Burden of Clostridium difficile infection in the United States. N Engl J Med. 2015;372:825–34.
12. Cohen SH, Gerding DN, Johnson S, Kelly CP, Loo VG, McDonald LC, et al. Clinical practice guidelines for Clostridium difficile infection in adults: 2010 update by the Society for Healthcare Epidemiology of America (SHEA) and the Infectious Diseases Society of America (IDSA). Infect Control Hosp Epidemiol. 2010;31:431–55.
13. Monaghan TM. New perspectives in Clostridium difficile disease pathogenesis. Infect Dis Clin North Am. 2015;29:1–11.
14. Warny M, Pepin J, Fang A, Killgore G, Thompson A, Brazier J, et al. Toxin production by an emerging strain of Clostridium difficile associated with outbreaks of severe disease in North America and Europe. Lancet. 2005;366:1079–84.
15. Samady W, Pong A, Fisher E. Risk factors for the development of Clostridium difficile infection in hospitalized children. Curr Opin Pediatr. 2014;26:568–72.
16. Nicholson MR, Osgood CL, Acra SA, Edwards KM. Clostridium difficile infection in the pediatric transplant patient. Pediatr Transplant. 2015;19:792–8.
17. Kim J, Smathers SA, Prasad P, Leckerman KH, Coffin S, Zaoutis T. Epidemiological features of Clostridium difficile-associated disease among inpatients at children's hospitals in the United States, 2001-2006. Pediatrics. 2008;122:1266–70.
18. de Blank P, Zaoutis T, Fisher B, Troxel A, Kim J, Aplenc R. Trends in Clostridium difficile infection and risk factors for hospital acquisition of Clostridium difficile among children with cancer. J Pediatr. 2013;163:699–705. e1
19. Boyle NM, Magaret A, Stednick Z, Morrison A, Butler-Wu S, Zerr D, et al. Evaluating risk factors for Clostridium difficile infection in adult and pediatric hematopoietic cell transplant recipients. Antimicrob Resist Infect Control. 2015;4:41.
20. Kim J, Shaklee JF, Smathers S, Prasad P, Asti L, Zoltanski J, et al. Risk factors and outcomes associated with severe clostridium difficile infection in children. Pediatr Infect Dis J. 2012;31:134–8.
21. Centers for Disease Control and Prevention. Multidrug-resistant organism & Clostridium difficile infection (MDRO/CDI) module. 2016. In: National healthcare safety manual [internet]. Atlanta, GA; [12.1–42]. http://www.cdc.gov/nhsn/pdfs/pscmanual/pcsmanual_current.pdf.
22. Sammons JS, Toltzis P. Pitfalls in diagnosis of pediatric Clostridium difficile infection. Infect Dis Clin North Am. 2015;29:465–76.
23. Guerrero DM, Becker JC, Eckstein EC, Kundrapu S, Deshpande A, Sethi AK, et al. Asymptomatic carriage of toxigenic Clostridium difficile by hospitalized patients. J Hosp Infect. 2013;85:155–8.
24. Dominguez SR, Dolan SA, West K, Dantes RB, Epson E, Friedman D, et al. High colonization rate and prolonged shedding of Clostridium difficile in pediatric oncology patients. Clin Infect Dis. 2014;59:401–3.
25. Stockmann C, Rogatcheva M, Harrel B, Vaughn M, Crisp R, Poritz M, et al. How well does physician selection of microbiologic tests identify Clostridium difficile and other pathogens in paediatric diarrhoea? Insights using multiplex PCR-based detection. Clin Microbiol Infect. 2015;21:179. e9–15.

26. Gu Z, Zhu H, Rodriguez A, Mhaissen M, Schultz-Cherry S, Adderson E, et al. Comparative evaluation of broad-panel PCR assays for the detection of gastrointestinal pathogens in pediatric oncology patients. J Mol Diagn. 2015;17:715–21.
27. Centers for Disease Control and Prevention. Device-associated module, Pneumonia (Ventilator-associated [VAP] and non-ventilator-associated Pneumonia [PNEU] event). 2016. In: National healthcare safety manual [internet]. Atlanta, GA:[6.1–17]. http://www.cdc.gov/nhsn/pdfs/pscmanual/pcsmanual_current.pdf.
28. Kalanuria AA, Zai W, Mirski M. Ventilator-associated pneumonia in the ICU. Crit Care. 2014;18:208.
29. Klompas M. The paradox of ventilator-associated pneumonia prevention measures. Crit Care. 2009;13:315.
30. Venkatachalam V, Hendley JO, Willson DF. The diagnostic dilemma of ventilator-associated pneumonia in critically ill children. Pediatr Crit Care Med. 2011;12:286–96.
31. Centers for Disease Control and Prevention. Device-associated module, Ventilator-associated event (VAE). 2016. In: National Healthcare Safety Manual. Atlanta, GA: [10.1–49]. http://www.cdc.gov/nhsn/pdfs/pscmanual/pcsmanual_current.pdf.
32. Mariki P, Rellosa N, Wratney A, Stockwell D, Berger J, Song X, et al. Application of a modified microbiologic criterion for identifying pediatric ventilator-associated pneumonia. Am J Infect Control. 2014;42:1079–83.
33. Patrick SW, Kawai AT, Kleinman K, Jin R, Vaz L, Gay C, et al. Health care-associated infections among critically ill children in the US, 2007-2012. Pediatrics. 2014;134:705–12.
34. Foglia E, Meier MD, Elward A. Ventilator-associated pneumonia in neonatal and pediatric intensive care unit patients. Clin Microbiol Rev. 2007;20:409–25.
35. Beardsley AL, Nitu ME, Cox EG, Benneyworth BD. An evaluation of various ventilator-associated infection criteria in a PICU. Pediatr Crit Care Med. 2016;17:73–80.
36. Gupta S, Boville BM, Blanton R, Lukasiewicz G, Wincek J, Bai C, et al. A multicentered prospective analysis of diagnosis, risk factors, and outcomes associated with pediatric ventilator-associated pneumonia. Pediatr Crit Care Med. 2015;16:e65–73.
37. Torres A, el-Ebiary M, Gonzalez J, Ferrer M, Puig de la Bellacasa J, Gene A, et al. Gastric and pharyngeal flora in nosocomial pneumonia acquired during mechanical ventilation. Am Rev Respir Dis. 1993;148:352–7.
38. Kusahara DM, Enz Cda C, Avelar AF, Peterlini MA, Pedreira ML. Risk factors for ventilator-associated pneumonia in infants and children: a cross-sectional cohort study. Am J Crit Care. 2014;23:469–76.
39. Centers for Disease Control and Prevention. Device-associated module, urinary tract infection (catheter-associated urinary tract infection [CAUTI] and non-catheter-associated urinary tract infection [UTI]) and other urinary system infection [USI]) events. 2016. In: National Healthcare Safety Manual [Internet]. Atlanta, GA: [7.1–16]. http://www.cdc.gov/nhsn/pdfs/pscmanual/pcsmanual_current.pdf.
40. Goudie A, Dynan L, Brady PW, Fieldston E, Brilli RJ, Walsh KE. Costs of venous thromboembolism, catheter-associated urinary tract infection, and pressure ulcer. Pediatrics. 2015;136:432–9.
41. Flores-Mireles AL, Walker JN, Caparon M, Hultgren SJ. Urinary tract infections: epidemiology, mechanisms of infection and treatment options. Nat Rev Microbiol. 2015;13:269–84.
42. Chenoweth CE, Gould CV, Saint S. Diagnosis, management, and prevention of catheter-associated urinary tract infections. Infect Dis Clin North Am. 2014;28:105–19.
43. Siegel JD, Rhinehart E, Jackson M, Chiarello L, and the Health Care Infection Control Practices Advisory Committee. 2007 Guideline for isolation precautions: preventing transmission of infectious agents in health care settings. Am J Infect Control. 2007;35:S65–164.
44. MacIntyre CR, Chughtai AA. Facemasks for the prevention of infection in healthcare and community settings. BMJ. 2015;350:h694.
45. Frenzel E, Chemaly RF, Ariza-Heredia E, Jiang Y, Shah DP, Thomas G, et al. Association of increased influenza vaccination in health care workers with a reduction in nosocomial influenza infections in cancer patients. Am J Infect Control. 2016;44:1016–21.

46. Van Buynder PG, Konrad S, Kersteins F, Preston E, Brown PD, Keen D, et al. Healthcare worker influenza immunization vaccinate or mask policy: strategies for cost effective implementation and subsequent reductions in staff absenteeism due to illness. Vaccine. 2015;33:1625–8.
47. Yassi A, Kettner J, Hammond G, Cheang M, McGill M. Effectiveness and cost-benefit of an influenza vaccination program for health care workers. Can J Infect Dis. 1991;2:101–8.
48. Grohskopf LA, Olsen SJ, Sokolow LZ, Bresee JS, Cox NJ, Broder KR, et al. Prevention and control of seasonal influenza with vaccines: recommendations of the Advisory Committee on Immunization Practices (ACIP) -- United States, 2014-15 influenza season. MMWR Morb Mortal Wkly Rep. 2014;63:691–7.
49. Kretsinger K, Broder KR, Cortese MM, Joyce MP, Ortega-Sanchez I, Lee GM, et al. Preventing tetanus, diphtheria, and pertussis among adults: use of tetanus toxoid, reduced diphtheria toxoid and acellular pertussis vaccine recommendations of the Advisory Committee on Immunization Practices (ACIP) and recommendation of ACIP, supported by the Healthcare Infection Control Practices Advisory Committee (HICPAC), for use of Tdap among health-care personnel. MMWR Recomm Rep. 2006;55:1–37.
50. Pearson ML, Bridges CB, Harper SA, Healthcare Infection Control Practices Advisory Committee, Advisory Committee on Immunization Practices. Influenza vaccination of health-care personnel: recommendations of the Healthcare Infection Control Practices Advisory Committee (HICPAC) and the Advisory Committee on Immunization Practices (ACIP). MMWR Recomm Rep. 2006;55:1–16.
51. Centers for Disease Control and Prevention. NHSN healthcare personnel influenza vaccination summary data tables by state, acute care hospitals, 2014–2015. 2015. http://www.cdc.gov/nhsn/pdfs/datastat/statehcp-influenzavaxdatatable_hospitals-2015.pdf.
52. Walker FJ, Singleton JA, Lu P, Wooten KG, Strikas RA. Influenza vaccination of healthcare workers in the United States, 1989-2002. Infect Control Hosp Epidemiol. 2006;27:257–65.
53. Lytras T, Kopsachilis F, Mouratidou E, Papamichail D, Bonovas S. Interventions to increase seasonal influenza vaccine coverage in healthcare workers: a systematic review and meta-regression analysis. Hum Vaccin Immunother. 2016;12:671–81.
54. Lin CJ, Nowalk MP, Raymund M, Sweeney PM, Zimmerman RK. Association of state laws and healthcare workers' influenza vaccination rates. J Natl Med Assoc. 2016;108:99–102.
55. Centers for Disease Control and Prevention. Principles of epidemiology in public health practice. An Introduction to applied epidemiology and biostatistics. 3rd ed. Atlanta: U.S. Department of Health and Human Services; 2012.
56. Children's Hospital Solutions for Patient Safety. About us: how it all started. 2016. http://www.solutionsforpatientsafety.org/about-us/how-it-all-started/.
57. Children's Hospital Solutions for Patient Safety. SPS prevention bundles. 2014. http://www.solutionsforpatientsafety.org/wp-content/uploads/SPS-Prevention-Bundles.pdf.
58. Resar R, Griffin FA, Haraden C, Nolan TW. Using care bundles to improve health care quality. 2012. http://www.IHI.org.
59. Rinke ML, Chen AR, Bundy DG, Colantuoni E, Fratino L, Drucis KM, et al. Implementation of a central line maintenance care bundle in hospitalized pediatric oncology patients. Pediatrics. 2012;130:e996–e1004.
60. Bundy DG, Gaur AH, Billett AL, He B, Colantuoni EA, Miller MR, et al. Preventing CLABSIs among pediatric hematology/oncology inpatients: national collaborative results. Pediatrics. 2014;134:e1678–85.
61. Davis KF, Colebaugh AM, Eithun BL, Klieger SB, Meredith DJ, Plachter N, et al. Reducing catheter-associated urinary tract infections: a quality-improvement initiative. Pediatrics. 2014;134:e857–64.
62. Muszynski JA, Sartori J, Steele L, Frost R, Wang W, Khan N, et al. Multidisciplinary quality improvement initiative to reduce ventilator-associated tracheobronchitis in the PICU. Pediatr Crit Care Med. 2013;14:533–8.
63. Dubberke ER, Carling P, Carrico R, Donskey CJ, Loo VG, McDonald LC, et al. Strategies to prevent Clostridium difficile infections in acute care hospitals: 2014 Update. Infect Control Hosp Epidemiol. 2014;35:628–45.

64. Centers for Disease Control and Prevention. Guide to infection prevention for outpatient settings: minimum expectations for safe care. Atlanta, GA; 2015. https://www.cdc.gov/HAI/settings/outpatient/outpatient-care-guidelines.html.
65. Miller MR, Griswold M, Harris 2nd JM, Yenokyan G, Huskins WC, Moss M, et al. Decreasing PICU catheter-associated bloodstream infections: NACHRI's quality transformation efforts. Pediatrics. 2010;125:206–13.
66. Childood Cancer & Blood Diseases Network. https://www.childrenshospitals.org/Programs-and-Services/Quality-Improvement-and-Measurement/Collaboratives/Cancer-and-Blood-Disorders
67. Allen RC, Holdsworth MT, Johnson CA, Chavez CM, Heideman RL, Overturf G, et al. Risk determinants for catheter-associated blood stream infections in children and young adults with cancer. Pediatr Blood Cancer. 2008;51:53–8.
68. Ibrahim KY, Pierrotti LC, Freire MP, Gutierrez PP, Duarte Ldo P, Bellesso M, et al. Health care-associated infections in hematology-oncology patients with neutropenia: a method of surveillance. Am J Infect Control. 2013;41:1131–3.
69. Kelly M, Conway M, Wirth K, Potter-Bynoe G, Billett AL, Sandora TJ. Moving CLABSI prevention beyond the intensive care unit: risk factors in pediatric oncology patients. Infect Control Hosp Epidemiol. 2011;32:1079–85.
70. Langley GJ, Moen R, Nolan KM, Nolan TW, Norman CL, Provost LP. The improvement guide: a practical approach to enhancing organizational performance. 2nd ed. San Francisco, CA: Jossey-Bass; 2009.
71. Institute for Healthcare Improvement. 5 million lives campaign. Getting started kit: sustainability and spread. How-to guide. 2008. http://www.ihi.org/education/IHIOpenSchool/Courses/Documents/CourseraDocuments/13_SpreadSustainabilityHowToGuidev14[1].pdf
72. Wiltsey Stirman S, Kimberly J, Cook N, Calloway A, Castro F, Charns M. The sustainability of new programs and innovations: a review of the empirical literature and recommendations for future research. Implement Sci. 2012;7:17.
73. Flodgren G, Conterno LO, Mayhew A, Omar O, Pereira CR, Shepperd S. Interventions to improve professional adherence to guidelines for prevention of device-related infections. Cochrane Database Syst Rev. 2013;3:CD006559.
74. Billett AL, Colletti RB, Mandel KE, Miller M, Muething SE, Sharek PJ, et al. Exemplar pediatric collaborative improvement networks: achieving results. Pediatrics. 2013;131:S196–203.
75. Dandoy CE, Hausfeld J, Flesch L, Hawkins D, Demmel K, Best D, et al. Rapid cycle development of a multifactorial intervention achieved sustained reductions in central line-associated bloodstream infections in haematology oncology units at a children's hospital: a time series analysis. BMJ Qual Saf. 2016;25(8):633–43.
76. Rinke ML, Milstone AM, Chen AR, Mirski K, Bundy DG, Colantuoni E, et al. Ambulatory pediatric oncology CLABSIs: epidemiology and risk factors. Pediatr Blood Cancer. 2013;60:1882–9.

Chapter 12
Outline: Pediatric Venous Thromboembolism

Julie Jaffray and Char Witmer

Introduction/Background

Venous thromboembolism (VTE) in hospitalized pediatric patients is a rapidly increasing problem, with an increase from 5.3 events per 10,000 hospital admissions in the early 1990s to a current estimate of 58 events per 10,000 hospital admissions [1–3]. VTE is currently considered the second most common contributor to harm in hospitalized pediatric patients secondary only to central line-associated infection [4]. The epidemiological pattern of VTE in pediatrics is bimodal, revealing a peak in the neonatal and then the adolescent age groups [3]. The resultant harms from VTE are numerous and include loss of venous access, pain at the site of thrombosis, pulmonary embolism, paradoxical emboli, infection, and post-thrombotic syndrome (PTS). The overall mortality rate associated with VTE is estimated at 2.2% [5].

Virchow's triad describes the three main risk factors for venous thrombosis formation including endothelial injury, circulatory stasis, and a hypercoagulable state. The pathogenesis of VTE in pediatric patients is commonly in the setting of multiple thrombotic risk factors. Ninety-five percent of VTE cases in children are related to an underlying disorder such as cancer, congenital heart disease, trauma, surgery, nephrotic syndrome, inflammatory bowel disease, or autoimmune disorders [6]. The presence of a central venous catheter (CVC) is the single most important risk factor for developing VTE in pediatric patients [2, 5, 7].

J. Jaffray (✉)
Division of Hematology/Oncology, Children's Hospital Los Angeles,
4650 Sunset Blvd, Mailstop #54, Los Angeles, CA 90027, USA
e-mail: jjaffray@chla.usc.edu

C. Witmer
Division of Hematology, The Children's Hospital of Philadelphia, Philadelphia, PA, USA
e-mail: witmer@email.chop.edu

© Springer International Publishing AG 2017
C.E. Dandoy et al. (eds.), *Patient Safety and Quality in Pediatric Hematology/Oncology and Stem Cell Transplantation*, DOI 10.1007/978-3-319-53790-0_12

Children with oncologic diagnoses represent a high-risk group for VTE with a reported incidence of symptomatic VTE ranging from 2.1% to 7.9% [8–10]. Studies utilizing screening for asymptomatic VTE with the placement of a central line have reported much higher rates of VTE at 44–50% [11, 12]. Older age and the type of cancer specifically, hematologic malignancies, (acute lymphoblastic leukemia and lymphoma) are associated with a higher risk of thrombosis [8]. Pediatric patients undergoing hematopoietic stem cell transplantation have additional unique VTE risk factors including endothelial damage from transplant conditioning regimens and inflammation from acute and chronic graft-versus-host disease [13, 14]. There is limited data regarding VTE incidence and pediatric bone marrow transplant, one small single-center study reported a VTE incidence of 5.4%, including patients with malignant, nonmalignant, and immune disorders [15].

There are also nonmalignant hematologic disorders with an increased incidence of VTE including sickle cell disease (SCD) and beta thalassemia. A large longitudinal US cohort study of patients age >15 years with SCD reported a VTE incidence of 5.2/1000 person years (95% CI 3.8–6.9) with a cumulative incidence of 11.3% [16]. Interestingly, the incidence of PE exceeded that of isolated DVT [16]. Beta thalassemia is also associated with a hypercoagulable state with an estimated incidence of both arterial and venous thrombosis of 1.65% and was more frequent in patients with beta-thalassemia major [17].

Determining Venous Thromboembolism Incidence

As previously reviewed, VTE incidence is on the rise in hospitalized pediatric patients and the first step in decreasing the occurrence of VTE is in the ability to accurately count and track VTE events. Accurate tracking will indicate whether quality improvement methods are successful or in need of adjustment. With the improved tracking of VTE incidence, be mindful that rates will likely initially increase due to improved detection methods.

A simple database should be created to record all VTEs events. At a minimum, information within the database should include patient demographics, such as age at VTE diagnosis, sex and past medical history, as well as details about a patient's VTE (type of thrombosis, veins involved in the VTE, if it was CVC related, hospital location of the patient at the time of VTE diagnosis). This will allow the ability to track the VTE incidence as well as create targeted prevention mechanisms based on patient characteristics.

A definition of VTE must be agreed upon and kept consistent over time. In general, VTE encompasses thrombosis within the deep (not superficial) veins, which includes the limbs, abdomen, cerebral sinuses, intracardiac, as well as thrombosis in the pulmonary arterial bed [pulmonary embolus (PE)]. The Children's Hospitals Solutions for Patient Safety defines a hospital-acquired VTE (HA-VTE) as a VTE, which occurs after 48 h of hospital admission (without previous signs of VTE), or 4 weeks after a previous hospital discharge [4]. Although a VTE associated with the placement of a new CVC during a hospitalization should be counted regardless of the time to development.

$$\text{Total VTE Rate per 1000 patient days} = \frac{\text{(all VTE events)}}{\text{Number of patient days}} * 1000$$

Fig. 12.1 Formula to calculate incidence of hospital-acquired venous thrombosis rate

To improve accuracy, multiple methods should be implemented to capture all diagnosed HA-VTE events. Using International Classification of Diseases, Ninth or Tenth Edition (ICD-9 or ICD-10) coding alone has shown to be insufficient in predicting the true incidence of VTE within a population [18]. Efforts should be implemented to use a combination of ICD 9/10 coding, hematology consults for VTE, automated pharmacological alerts for new orders of anticoagulation, or automated radiology report alerts when there is a new VTE diagnosis. Methods utilized will depend on what is available at individual centers.

When tracking the incidence of VTE, regardless of the method utilized, the same approach should be applied in order to keep consistency of data and metrics. For HA-VTE rates, the incidence can be calculated for the entire hospital or individual units (pediatric intensive care, hematology/oncology/BMT, etc.). The numerator should be the number of VTE events within the last month within the hospital or unit. Care should be taken to use the same day of each month and time of day when recording the rates. The denominator is the total number of patients assigned to a bed in the hospital or unit for each day of the included time period, referred to as patient days [19]. The incidence is then reported per 1000 patients (Fig. 12.1).

VTE incidence can also be tracked for CVC-associated VTE. CVCs have been shown to be the biggest risk factor for pediatric VTE (see section on risk factors), and thus some practices may want to report this incidence separately. The numerator is the number of CVC-associated VTE events within the last month, again taking care to report on the same day and time of the month. The denominator is the total number of central line days during the time period, which is the number of patients with one or more central lines of any type daily [20]. These rates can be separated out by line-type and hospital unit if desired.

Once clear definitions and tracking abilities have been established, VTE education should be provided to the clinical and medical staff, as well as to patients and families. Points that should be highlighted include the background and incidence of VTE in children as stated previously, diagnosing and treating VTE, as well as acute and long-term sequelae and practice improvement objectives (discussed later in this chapter). These educational opportunities should be repeated at appropriate intervals to keep the staff engaged in the QI project. Modalities for patient and family education can be in the form of pamphlets distributed prior to the placement of a central line (biggest risk factor for VTE), upon hospital admission or electronically through a patient television portal. When creating patient and family appropriate education, use simple, plain language [21].

A greater level of success will be obtained if there is buy-in from families, administration, and hospital staff [22]. Patients and families who have a better understanding of the healthcare risks and needs tend to have better outcomes [23]. Implementation of the techniques to identify, track and diagnose, as well as prevent

VTE within the practice requires money and time, thus educating the administration on the need for VTE prevention and treatment is important. Associated patient harms from VTE were previously discussed. In addition, pediatric patients with a HA-VTE are admitted 8.1 days longer and cost $25,000 more per hospital admission than those without a HA-VTE [24]. Thus, the expense of VTE treatment may outweigh the added expense for prevention therapies.

Risk Factors for VTE and Risk Assessments

Risk Factors

Understanding the risk factors for VTE is essential for safely targeting prevention techniques. As previously mentioned patients with cancer, both adults and children, have an increased risk of developing a VTE due to the malignancy itself, the chemotherapy treatment, and the presence of a CVC [1]. Additively, hematology/oncology/BMT patients have many of the same VTE risk factors affecting all children with VTE, including infection or inflammation, surgeries, immobility, intubation, intensive care unit admission, obesity, and inherited or acquired thrombophilias.

The most frequently identified risk factors for VTE in all pediatric patients are listed in Table 12.1. A systematic review of risk factors for children with HA-VTE revealed the presence of CVCs, intensive care unit stay, mechanical ventilation, and increased hospital length of stay to be the most predictive risk factors for pediatric VTE [25].

The presence of a CVC is the single biggest risk factor for pediatric VTE, most likely due to endothelial cell damage, vessel wall trauma caused by the insertion, as well as stasis of blood flow caused by an indwelling line [5, 28]. Indwelling CVCs are essential, life-saving devices that providing access for chemotherapy infusions, blood transfusions, medications, and frequent laboratory

Table 12.1 Clinical characteristics which have been shown to increase risk of pediatric venous thromboembolism

Clinical characteristics	Reference(s)
Active cancer/bone marrow transplant	[5, 26, 27]
Central venous catheter	[5, 11, 25, 28, 29]
Prolonged hospital admission	[25, 30]
Immobility	[25]
Estrogen	[31]
Asparaginase	[27, 32]
Thrombophilia (inherited or acquired)	[5, 33]
Intensive care unit admission	[25]
Obesity	[31, 34]
Infection/inflammation	[5, 28]
Nephrotic syndrome	[26]
Surgery	[5, 26]
Trauma	[5, 26, 35]

Table 12.2 Characteristics of central venous catheters that may cause an increased incidence of venous thromboembolism in children

CVC characteristic associated with increased VTE incidence	Study
External CVCs (vs. internal CVCs, such as port-o-caths)	[36]
CVCs placed in the femoral vein (vs. upper extremity)	[38]
CVCs placed on the upper left side, in the subclavian vein (vs. jugular), and percutaneous technique (vs. cutdown)	[39]
Peripherally inserted central catheters (vs. tunneled lines)	[37]
Increased time CVC is in place, especially over 4 years	[40]

CVC central venous catheter

blood draws. The incidence of CVC-associated VTE in pediatric cancer patients has been reported anywhere from 2% to 50% [11, 29, 36, 37]. The variability in incidence is due to many of the studies reporting incidental VTEs from surveillance imaging without clinical manifestations. Table 12.2 describes CVC characteristics that may lead to an increased VTE rate. Future studies are needed to determine if altering these VTE risk CVC characteristics could reduce thrombotic events.

Pediatric cancer patients, especially those with acute lymphoblastic leukemia (ALL), have a significantly increased VTE risk, most likely due to their chemotherapy treatment [26, 32]. Asparaginase is known to decrease the production of natural anticoagulants, such as antithrombin [41]. Patients receiving high-risk ALL therapy and older children, aged 7–16 years, have been shown to have significantly more symptomatic VTEs [27]. A retrospective study evaluating oncology patients aged 15–24 years using the Pediatric Hospital Information System (PHIS) data from 2001 to 2008, also found an increased VTE rate in the older cohort of patients [32].

Inherited and acquired thrombophilias are a known risk factor for pediatric VTE [33, 42]. These include Factor V Leiden mutation, prothrombin G20210G polymorphism, protein C deficiency, protein S deficiency, antithrombin deficiency, elevated lipoprotein a, elevated homocysteine, and antiphospholipid antibodies, including the lupus anticoagulant and anticardiolipin antibody. A review of thrombophilia in children with VTE found the prevalence varies greatly from 13% to 60% throughout the literature [43]. Children with a malignancy who are found to have a thrombophilia are at an even higher risk for VTE [44, 45]. The significance of VTE in a patient with a thrombophilia is still not well defined, and expert panels have provided contradictory recommendations on whether to test pediatric patients for a thrombophilia [46, 47]. Some recommend patients with an unprovoked or recurrent VTE should be considered, although testing can be quite costly and individual centers should determine the necessity.

Hematopoietic stem cell transplant patients have many risk factors for VTE, some of which includes infections, which are exceedingly common in this population, prolonged hospital stay, prolonged steroid use, obesity, total body irradiation, and a long-term CVC in place [48, 49]. GVHD has added risk of VTE due to vascular and endothelial injuries which may contribute to inflammation, a known risk factors for VTE.

Patients with sickle cell disease (SCD) are known to be in a hypercoagulable state due to endothelial dysfunction and damage as well as impaired blood flow. Many patients with SCD also have CVCs, multiple hospitalizations, infections, and need for surgeries, thus increasing their risk for VTE. Antiphospholipid antibodies, low protein C and S levels are commonly identified in patients with SCD [50].

Risk Assessments

Once targeted risk factors for VTE have been identified, a VTE risk assessment with risk stratification should be created. Risk assessments and risk-based prevention strategies are standard of care for adult patients who are hospitalized or have cancer [51]. Unfortunately, the best way to assess pediatric patients for risk and stratify them for VTE prophylaxis has not been determined. Approaches have been published that are either disease specific or for any hospitalized pediatric patient.

Mitchell et al. developed and validated a predictive model specifically for children with ALL [52]. Subjects were treated according to Berlin-Frankfurt-Münster (BFM) 90/95/2000, the Cooperative Acute Lymphoblastic Leukemia (COALL) 92/97 or the French Acute Lymphoblastic Leukemia (FRALLE) 2000 induction protocols. The risk assessment placed patients into either a low-risk or high-risk category, depending on steroid type and dosage, presence of a CVC and the presence of a thrombophilia, with a specificity of 96.2% and sensitivity of 63.2%. The risk assessment was initially tested on subjects treated per BFM 92/95 or COALL 92/97, yet the score was validated on subjects treated per BFM 2000 or FRALLE 2000. The protocols use varied doses and types of steroids (prednisone or dexamethasone) and varying doses of asparaginase, which may affect their VTE risk. Therefore, the validity of their risk assessment model may not be applicable to other protocols or other patient populations.

The Children's Hospital of Philadelphia (CHOP) and Riley Hospital for Children published their institutional guidelines for VTE risk assessment and prophylaxis [53, 54]. CHOP developed a VTE risk assessment for all hospitalized patients ≥14 years. With a goal to prevent non-line-associated VTE in adolescents with risk factors that are similar to adults. Patients are placed into three risk categories, "low risk", "at risk" and "high risk" for developing a VTE, many of which are in Table 12.2, with an emphasis on immobility as the greatest risk factor. Those "at risk" without contraindications were placed on mechanical thromboprophylaxis (sequential compression devices) and those at "high risk," without contraindications were placed on both mechanical and prophylactic anticoagulation (LMWH). At Riley Children's hospital, all hospitalized patients ≥12 years were assessed for VTE risk, with an emphasis on immobility and the presence of a CVC. Their guidelines used logistic regression to determine the strength of all risk factor variables, rather than weighing each variable equally. Patients were also placed into three risk

Table 12.3 Pediatric venous thrombosis risk assessment models

Study	Predictive variables for risk assessment	Sensitivity/specificity	Notes
[56]	Positive blood culture, CVC, ICU admission, hospital stay ≥7 days, immobilization >72 h & OCP	Three or more variables had a high risk of VTE with sensitivity of 70% and specificity of 80%	Model was validated with sensitivity of 57% and specificity of 88%
[30]	Mechanical ventilation, systemic infection and hospital stay ≥5 days	45% sensitive and 95% specific for in-hospital VTE, with a post-test probability of VTE of 3.1% hospital-wide and 0.95% in the PICU	Risk factor model is 45% sensitive and 95% specific with a post-test probability of VTE of 3.1%
[55]	CVC, infection, hospital stay ≥4 days	Presence of all 3 RFs, 12.5% risk for HA-VTE	Non-critically ill patients only

CVC central venous catheter, *ICU* intensive care unit, *OCP* oral contraceptive pill, *VTE* venous thromboembolism, *PICU* pediatric intensive care unit, *HA-VTE* hospital-acquired venous thromboembolism

categories, low, moderate, and high with similar rules as CHOP for mechanical thromboprophylaxis and anticoagulation.

Three single-institutional studies created VTE risk assessment models to predict VTE risk in all hospitalized pediatric patients [18, 55, 56], and the results are summarized in Table 12.3. Sharathkumar et al. developed their Peds-Clot clinical Decision Rule (PCDR) through a retrospective case-control study and validated it using a separate validation cohort. Six risk factors were determined to be predictive of a HA-VTE, which were used to create their risk score. Branchford et al. also created their risk prediction model through a retrospective case-control study. Three independent risk factors were found to be most predictive of a HA-VTE and were used to create their risk model. Atchison et al. evaluated VTE risk exclusively in non-critically ill patients using a retrospective case-control model. Three VTE risk factors, which differed slightly from Branchford et al., were found to be most predictive of a HA-VTE and used to create their risk model.

A risk assessment model can then be created, using the above published studies as a guide, depending on your hospital's patient population and their known VTE risk factors. After creating a risk assessment, a determination must be made as to whom will best complete the assessment as well as implement the prevention strategies. Ideally, bedside nurses and frontline clinicians will be the best choice with the use of the electronic medical record (EMR) as a support tool. The risk assessment should be implemented slowly until reliability to the assessment is 80% or higher before expanding to other parts of the hospital. Education should be provided to the entire clinical team before implementation into a particular unit, and feedback should be encouraged. During the pilot stage, the risk assessment could be a paper form, with the goal of imbedding it into your institution's EMR when finalized. Once the assessment is placed in the EMR, many aspects should be populated automatically, such as age, if a CVC is present, problem lists, current medications, and body mass index (BMI). Simplifying the risk assessment form as much as possible will increase the completion compliance.

Implementing Prevention Techniques: Mechanical and Pharmacologic

When a hospitalized patient is determined to be at risk for VTE, appropriate prophylactic measures need to be instituted. There are two broad categories of VTE prevention strategies including mechanical and/or pharmacological prophylaxis. As previously discussed, different published guidelines have instituted degrees of intervention based on the risk severity. With moderate-risk patients receiving mechanical prophylaxis and the highest risk patients receiving both mechanical and pharmacologic interventions. The decision for pharmacologic intervention needs to be considered carefully against the risk of hemorrhage.

Mechanical prophylaxis includes the use of either intermittent pneumatic compression devices (IPC) or graduated compression stockings (GPS). GPSs provide circumferential pressure that gradually decreases from the ankle to the thigh. IPCs utilize intermittent inflation and deflation of a "sleeve" to increase venous return from the lower extremities mimicking that action of the calf muscles. These mechanical interventions are thought to decrease venous stasis addressing one of the pivotal VTE risk factors. In addition, IPCs have been demonstrated to activate systemic fibrinolysis which could theoretically promote clot dissolution [57–63]. Contraindications to mechanical prophylaxis include the device does not fit the patient, extremity trauma, or pain with compression (i.e., extremity veno-occlusive pain in a patient with SCD). Currently, there are no pediatric trials assessing the effectiveness of mechanical prophylaxis. Adult studies support the efficacy of mechanical interventions in preventing DVT and PE in many different clinical situations including post-trauma, postsurgical, and the medically ill hospitalized patient [64–68].

Until recently, questions remained regarding the efficacy of IPCs versus GPS. A recent prospective study of adult ICU patients compared the incidence of VTE in those patients receiving either IPC or GPS mechanical prophylaxis. Only IPC, and not GCS, was associated with a lower VTE incidence as compared with controls [0.45 (95% CI 0.22–0.95)] [64]. In addition a large meta-analysis in hospitalized medical patients also supports the finding that IPC is superior to GPS in the prevention of DVT [67]. It appears that IPC is more effective then GPS and should be used preferentially for VTE prevention.

What if a patient is receiving anticoagulation for thromboprophylaxis, is there still a role for compression therapy? A recent meta-analysis in adult patients revealed that combined IPC with pharmacologic prophylaxis was more effective than using IPC alone. Demonstrating an additive effect of VTE risk reduction with the use of both modalities for thromboprophylaxis. If a patient is at high risk for VTE, both modalities should be considered unless there is a contraindication.

There are limited studies addressing efficacy and safety of anticoagulation (pharmacologic prophylaxis) for VTE prevention in pediatric patients. The 2012 Chest guidelines provide recommendations for therapeutic ranges for prophylactic anticoagulation (warfarin INR 1.3–1.9 or LMWH anti-Xa 0.1–0.3 units/mL) [47]. They do not comment on indications for VTE prophylaxis in hospitalized pediatric patients [47]. Much of what is currently used in pediatric patients is extrapolated from the adult literature, especially as it pertains to the adolescent patient with VTE risk factors that are similar to that of adults. There are numerous adult studies that have demonstrated efficacy of medical anticoagulation for reducing hospital-acquired VTE and PE in both surgical and nonsurgical adult patients, and it is considered standard of care [66, 69]. Prophylactic dosing of enoxaparin for patients >60 kg is either 30 mg subcutaneously twice a day or 40 mg once daily. There should be a strong consideration for 30 mg twice daily in orthopedic surgery patients, which is what is used in adults. For patients <60 kg 0.5 mg/kg/dose subcutaneous, twice a day is recommended.

Unlike in adults, for pediatric patients, the most important risk factor for VTE is the presence of a CVC. Currently, data regarding the effectiveness of anticoagulation to prevent central line-associated thrombotic events in pediatric patients is lacking. The 2012 CHEST guidelines recommend against primary prophylaxis after the placement of a central venous line [47]. There are three randomized clinical trials that studied primary CVC prophylaxis in pediatric patients using prophylactic dosing of either low-molecular-weight heparin (anti-Xa goal 0.1–0.3), unfractionated heparin (10 units/kg/h), or warfarin (INR goal 1.3–1.9) [70–72]. None of these trials were able to demonstrate a difference in thrombotic events between the two treatment arms, although these studies were generally underpowered. A recent systematic review and meta-analysis of thromboprophylaxis in children was unable to find evidence that thromboprophylaxis reduced the risk of CVC-related thrombosis [73]. Ongoing research is needed to determine the most effective way to prevent CVC-associated thrombosis.

Detecting and Diagnosing VTE's

When a VTE event occurs, the first step toward making the diagnosis is in the ability to recognize the clinical symptoms of a VTE. Signs and symptoms of VTE are dependent on the site and degree of venous occlusion. When an extremity is affected, the clinical signs are consistent with venous obstruction and include swelling and pain of the affected extremity. If there is embolization of the clot to the lungs, the symptoms can include a sudden onset of pleuritic chest pain, shortness of breath, and persistent tachycardia. A large PE can present as acute respiratory and cardiac failure. In a patient who is intubated and unable to report symptoms it could present as an acute respiratory decompensation. For those patients who have an abnormal connection between the right and left side of the heart, a venous embolism could cause a paradoxical emboli with resultant stroke, gut ischemia, renal infarcts or limb ischemia. Signs and symptoms of a stroke in a pediatric patient can be challenging depending on their age and level of awareness. Symptoms can include seizure, altered mental status, or other focal neurologic deficits.

Additional sites of VTE will have specific symptoms associated with the location of the thrombotic event. Renal vein thrombosis most commonly presents with hematuria and a decrease in renal function. Portal vein thrombosis may present with alteration in liver function tests. Cerebral sinus venous thrombosis can present with vomiting, persistent headache, change in mental status, seizure, or focal neurologic changes if there is a venous infarct. Superior vena cava (SVS) thrombosis will present with SVC syndrome with marked swelling of the head.

Clinicians should have a high index of suspicion for thrombotic complications with CVCs. A thrombotic complication of a CVC can be associated with the line tip and/or vessel wall in different combinations, from isolated tip occlusion to partial or full vessel occlusion. This results in a wide range of clinical symptoms from no symptoms to catheter malfunction with a swollen extremity. A link with CVC thrombosis and bacteremia has been reported. In the setting of persistent bacteremia, CVC thrombosis should be considered.

It is imperative that bedside providers, patients, and family members be aware of how a thrombotic event presents since they will likely be the first to notice VTE symptoms. In addition a high index of suspicion on the frontline clinician's part will ensure that the adequate test is ordered when a concern for VTE is raised. When VTE is suspected, the imaging modality selected is dependent on the site of thrombosis (Table 12.4). Historically, venography was the gold standard, but it has increasingly fallen out of favor, being replaced by other imaging modalities like ultrasonography or CT or MR venography. The D-dimer has not been validated in pediatric clinical trials for the diagnosis of VTE, making interpretation difficult in this population. In addition, other conditions can elevate the D-dimer including newborn infants, recent surgery, malignancy, connective tissue disorders, and sickle cell disease [74].

Treatment of VTE in Hematology/Oncology/BMT Patients

Anticoagulation

In the setting of a thrombotic event, anticoagulation therapy is initiated to prevent thrombosis extension and pulmonary embolism. Large studies have not been conducted in children to determine the best anticoagulant for the hematology/oncology/BMT population. Generally, children with malignancies or undergoing HSCT are on multiple medications, many of which fluctuate weekly, and have multiple invasive procedures. The best choice for anticoagulation agents are ones with limited drug interactions and a short half-life, such as unfractionated heparin (UH), low-molecular-weight heparin (LMWH) or the synthetic heparin mimic (fondaparinux). Vitamin K antagonists (VKA) have many drug interactions as well as issues with diet variation and a prolonged half-life. Thus, choosing a VKA is less desirable

Table 12.4 Signs and symptoms of venous thrombosis and imaging

Site of thrombosis	Signs and symptoms	Imaging modality
Limb	Unilateral swelling and pain of the affected limb	*Lower extremity*: Compression US with Doppler imaging. If the proximal extent of the DVT cannot be determined consider a venography, CT, or MRV *Upper extremity*: Compression ultrasound with Doppler imaging. *The US has limited visualization of the subclavian vein. If the US is negative but there remains a high clinical suspicion for thrombosis, proceed to another form of imaging (venography, CT or MRV)*
Superior vena cava	Swelling of face, neck, and upper extremities	Echocardiography, CT, or MRV
Jugular vein	Asymptomatic or neck swelling and pain	Compression US with Doppler imaging *If proximal extent cannot be determined with US than a MRV should be performed to assess for CSVT*
Inferior vena cava	Bilateral lower extremity swelling and pain	Doppler ultrasound in infants Older children may require CT or MRV
Portal vein	Asymptomatic or abdominal pain	Doppler ultrasound
Renal vein	Flank pain, hematuria	Doppler ultrasound
Pulmonary embolism	Pleuritic chest pain, shortness of breath, tachycardia	Spiral CT Ventilation-perfusion scan
Cerebral sinuses	Headache, vomiting, depressed mental status, seizures	MRI with MRV most sensitive and specific (CT can miss up to 40% of cases)

US ultrasound, *CT* computed tomography, *MRV* magnetic resonance venography, *CSVT* cerebral sinus venous thrombosis

in this population, unless the patient is outpatient, without medication variation, or fluctuating platelet counts, has a stable diet, and does not require frequent procedures. Platelet counts should be monitored in pediatric cancer patients while on anticoagulation therapy, with possible dose adjustments based on counts to minimize the risk of bleeding.

UH is a continuous intravenous infusion and generally used when there is a higher bleeding risk due to its short half-life and ability for complete reversal with protamine. LMWHs (enoxaparin and dalteparin) can also be used as first-line therapy for the treatment of VTE in pediatric patients, and they are the primary choice for outpatient therapy. These medications are administered subcutaneously twice daily. They can be held 12–24 h prior to procedures such as lumbar punctures or bone marrow aspirations [47, 75, 76]. The CHEST guidelines for pediatrics recommends LMWH as the treatment of choice for VTE in children with cancer for 3 months or until the precipitating factor has resolved, such as completion of asparaginase therapy or removal of the CVC [47].

Studies are currently being conducted on using the new oral anticoagulants, the non-vitamin K antagonist anticoagulants (NOACs) in children. They are ideal for cancer patients due to their limited drug interactions and short half-life, but there is limited data. For adult cancer patients, the CHEST guidelines continue to recommend using LMWH [77]. There are ongoing clinical trials in adult patients with cancer.

Thrombolysis

Catheter directed or systemic thrombolysis with tissue plasminogen activator (TPA) is usually restricted to serious situations that are life or limb threatening such as a massive PE causing cardiopulmonary collapse, phlegmasia cerulea dolens where complete venous obstruction compromises arterial flow or a large (>2 cm) mobile atrial thrombi. A multidisciplinary team, including an intensivist, hematologist, and interventional radiologist who are comfortable with pediatric TPA must be available. Systemic TPA is given as a short-term continuous infusion followed by standard duration anticoagulation.

Alternatives to Anticoagulation

Due to bleeding risk, some patients are unable to receive anticoagulation. These patients should have close monitoring of their VTE, both clinically and with serial imaging, and anticoagulation should be initiated as soon as it is safe. Mobility, either active or passive, should be encouraged, as well as the use of sequential compression devices in the unaffected limb to prevent any new VTEs. In a select group of patients, clinicians should consider a temporary vena cava filter for those with a lower extremity DVT and contraindication for anticoagulation with a high risk of PE. Due to size restraints, they cannot be placed in children <10 kg. The temporary IVC filter itself is a nidus for thrombosis and should be removed as soon as the contraindication to anticoagulation resolves.

Morbidity Associated with VTE

PTS, which is chronic limb swelling, tingling, and pain secondary to venous insufficiency of the limb affected by the VTE, is found in 12% of pediatric VTE cases [5]. Over 50% of ALL patients with DVT of their limb were found to have PTS [78]. Unfortunately, prevention techniques for PTS have not been determined, in either the adult or pediatric patients, besides preventing the VTE itself. Elastic compression stockings, which can reduce edema and venous hypertension, may help PTS symptoms. Studies have shown conflicting results, some have shown improvement

Table 12.5 Recommended signs and symptoms to evaluate in pediatric patients at risk for post-thrombotic syndrome [81, 82]

Elements of PTS assessment
Signs
• Skin color changes • Ulceration • Dilated collateral vessels • Increased limb circumference • Edema • Venous ulcer • Varicosities
Symptoms
• Pain with aerobic activity • Pain with activities of daily living • Pain at rest

PTS Post-thrombotic syndrome

in symptoms, while others have shown no affect in adult patients [79]. There have not been any pediatric studies to evaluate PTS prevention techniques.

Pediatric patients are not routinely followed for signs of PTS alone, although due to the high incidence, especially in patients without DVT resolution, this may need to be reevaluated. Pediatric hematology/oncology/BMT patients are a unique group where long-term follow-up is established due to their primary diagnosis, thus implementing screening for PTS in patients with a history of CVC or extremity DVT should be considered. The Villalta scale is a reliable assessment instrument, which was created to diagnose PTS in adults [80]. Pediatric PTS assessment instruments have also been established, but they are not standardized [81, 82]. Key subjective and objective signs from these pediatric assessments should be evaluated in patients at risk for PTS (Table 12.5).

Process Measures

Monitoring and Measuring the Reliability of Risk Assessment Implementation

Full integration of the VTE risk assessment into the daily workflow of the nursing staff and frontline clinicians will ensure a higher likelihood of implementation success. This should be a shared assessment process between nurses and physicians and should be ongoing throughout the hospitalization since VTE risk can change over time. While education of staff is imperative by itself, it is not enough to sustain adherence. Support systems built into the EMR that will fully assist nurses and frontline clinicians in making VTE risk assessment and ordering of thromboprophylaxis will be the most successful. In addition, tracking of adherence will be easier if documentation is required through the EMR.

Monitoring and Measuring the Reliability of Mechanical and Pharmacologic Prevention Techniques

Overall, the goal of instituting thromboprophylaxis for those patients at high risk for VTE is to decrease the incidence of hospital HA-VTE. Ideally, excellent (>90%) adherence to VTE prevention interventions will result in a decreased incidence of HA-VTE, although proven prevention strategies in pediatric patients have not been determined. Adherence to these prevention processes should be tracked over time. How this is done will be based on your institution and available resources. It can be done manually with bedside review, but this can be timely. If utilizing the EMR, strongly consider requiring documentation of VTE risk assessment and the implementation of prevention strategies so these can be tracked electronically. Additionally, require documentation of contraindications to VTE prevention measures.

Side Effects from Mechanical and Medical Prophylaxis

With any intervention to prevent harm, it is imperative to monitor for any potential side effects. While in general, ICDs have little risk of harm, they can be uncomfortable for the patient, and there have been reports of skin abrasion; thus, these effects should be monitored. Patient discomfort can lead to nonadherence, which could have a significant impact on the efficacy of your VTE prevention strategy. Patient and family education regarding the importance of IPCs to prevent VTE could improve adherence with an inconvenient and uncomfortable intervention.

Prophylactic anticoagulation is associated with a risk of hemorrhage. A systematic review of the safety and efficacy of low-molecular-weight heparin in children reported a 2.3% rate of clinically relevant bleeding in those clinical trials implementing primary prophylaxis in children [83]. A single-center prospective cohort study reported the safety of anticoagulation for VTE prevention in 89 patients [84]. They reported 2.2% major and 5.6% minor bleeding events, which only occurred in patients who had undergone major orthopedic surgery. These event rates are similar to that in adults and are considered acceptable risks to prevent VTE.

To minimize the risk of hemorrhage from prophylactic anticoagulation, relative contraindications should be established and considered for every patient. In patients with cancer, thrombocytopenia is a common issue, and platelet thresholds for anticoagulation should be recommended. For example, consider holding prophylactic anticoagulation once the platelet count is <20,000 k/mcL. Avoid additional medications that could increase the patient's risk of bleeding like ibuprofen, aspirin, ketorolac, etc.

Tracking bleeding events related to anticoagulation can be a challenge, but it is imperative to ensure that this preventative measure is beneficial with limited unintended consequences. Institutional definitions of major bleeding should be established and tracked overtime. This could be completed through your pharmacy with an anticoagulation stewardship program that tracks all hospitalized patients on anticoagulation ensuring proper dosing for the indication, adequate monitoring, and associated harms. In addition, a major bleeding event should be considered a reportable safety event by nursing and frontline clinicians.

In summary, evaluating and preventing VTE involves many steps, which should include:

1. Implement multimodal VTE tracking mechanisms.
2. Creation of a database to house and track all cases of VTE.
3. Monitor VTE rates monthly, with consideration of separating out CVC-associated versus non-CVC VTE cases.
4. Determine the exact population of patients to focus VTE prevention.
5. Educate clinical staff, patients, and families about VTE.
6. Determine the relevant risk factors for your patient population and create a risk assessment model.
7. Consistently screen your patient population for their VTE risk using your risk assessment model.
8. Apply VTE prevention strategies to those patients determined to be at the highest risk (pharmacologic and/or mechanical).
9. Continuously monitor the compliance rate of risk assessment and prevention strategies with the VTE incidence within your practice and adjust prevention efforts as needed.

References

1. Andrew M, David M, Adams M, Ali K, Anderson R, Barnard D, Bernstein M, Brisson L, Cairney B, DeSai D, et al. Venous thromboembolic complications (VTE) in children: first analyses of the Canadian Registry of VTE. Blood. 1994;83:1251–7.
2. Massicotte MP, Dix D, Monagle P, Adams M, Andrew M. Central venous catheter related thrombosis in children: analysis of the Canadian Registry of Venous Thromboembolic Complications. J Pediatr. 1998;133:770–6.
3. Raffini L, Huang YS, Witmer C, Feudtner C. Dramatic increase in venous thromboembolism in children's hospitals in the United States from 2001 to 2007. Pediatrics. 2009;124:1001–8.
4. Zieker K. Children's hospitals' solutions for patient safety operational definitions. 2015. http://www.solutionsforpatientsafety.org/wp-content/uploads/sps-operating-definitions.pdf.
5. Monagle P, Adams M, Mahoney M, Ali K, Barnard D, Bernstein M, Brisson L, David M, Desai S, Scully MF, Halton J, Israels S, Jardine L, Leaker M, McCusker P, Silva M, Wu J, Anderson R, Andrew M, Massicotte MP. Outcome of pediatric thromboembolic disease: a report from the Canadian Childhood Thrombophilia Registry. Pediatr Res. 2000;47:763–6.
6. Macartney CA, Chan AK. Thrombosis in children. Semin Thromb Hemost. 2011;37:763–1.
7. Richardson MW, Allen GA, Monahan PE. Thrombosis in children: current perspective and distinct challenges. Thromb Haemost. 2002;88:900–11.
8. Athale U, Siciliano S, Thabane L, Pai N, Cox S, Lathia A, Khan A, Armstrong A, Chan AK. Epidemiology and clinical risk factors predisposing to thromboembolism in children with cancer. Pediatr Blood Cancer. 2008;51:792–7.
9. Lipay NV, Zmitrovich AI, Aleinikova OV. Epidemiology of venous thromboembolism in children with malignant diseases: a single-center study of the Belarusian Center for Pediatric Oncology and Hematology. Thromb Res. 2011;128:130–4.

10. Wermes C, von Depka Prondzinski M, Lichtinghagen R, Barthels M, Welte K, Sykora KW. Clinical relevance of genetic risk factors for thrombosis in paediatric oncology patients with central venous catheters. Eur J Pediatr. 1999;158(Suppl 3):S143–6.
11. Glaser DW, Medeiros D, Rollins N, Buchanan GR. Catheter-related thrombosis in children with cancer. J Pediatr. 2001;138:255–9.
12. Ruud E, Holmstrom H, Natvig S, Wesenberg F. Prevalence of thrombophilia and central venous catheter-associated neck vein thrombosis in 41 children with cancer—a prospective study. Med Pediatr Oncol. 2002;38:405–10.
13. Han Y, Zhu L, Sun A, Lu X, Hu L, Zhou L, Ren Y, Hu X, Wu X, Wang Z, Ruan C, Wu D. Alterations of hemostatic parameters in the early development of allogeneic hematopoietic stem cell transplantation-related complications. Ann Hematol. 2011;90:1201–8.
14. Zahid MF, Murad MH, Litzow MR, Hogan WJ, Patnaik MS, Khorana A, Spyropoulos AC, Hashmi SK. Venous thromboembolism following hematopoietic stem cell transplantation-a systematic review and meta-analysis. Ann Hematol. 2016;95(9):1457–64.
15. Azik F, Gokcebay DG, Tavil B, Isik P, Tunc B, Uckan D. Venous thromboembolism after allogeneic pediatric hematopoietic stem cell transplantation: a single-center study. Turk J Haematol. 2015;32:228–33.
16. Naik RP, Streiff MB, Haywood Jr C, Segal JB, Lanzkron S. Venous thromboembolism incidence in the cooperative study of sickle cell disease. J Thromb Haemost. 2014;12:2010–6.
17. Taher A, Isma'eel H, Mehio G, Bignamini D, Kattamis A, Rachmilewitz EA, Cappellini MD. Prevalence of thromboembolic events among 8,860 patients with thalassaemia major and intermedia in the Mediterranean area and Iran. Thromb Haemost. 2006;96:488–91.
18. Branchford BR, Gibson E, Manco-Johnson MJ, Goldenberg NA. Sensitivity of discharge diagnosis ICD-9 codes for pediatric venous thromboembolism is greater than specificity, but still suboptimal for surveillance and clinical research. Thromb Res. 2012;129:662–3.
19. CDC. Determining patient days for summary data collection: observation vs. inpatients. Atlanta, GA: Center for Disease Control and Prevention; 2015.
20. Prevention, Centers for Disease Control. Bloodstream infection event (central line-associated bloodstream infection and non-central line-associated bloodstream infection). 2016. https://www.cdc.gov/nhsn/pdfs/pscmanual/4psc_clabscurrent.pdf.
21. "Federal Plain Language Guidelines." Plain Language.gov Improving Communication from the Federal Government to the Public. 2011. http://www.plainlanguage.gov/howto/guidelines/FederalPLGuidelines/FederalPLGuidelines.pdf.
22. Feifer C, Ornstein SM. Strategies for increasing adherence to clinical guidelines and improving patient outcomes in small primary care practices. Jt Comm J Qual Saf. 2004;30:432–41.
23. Heisler M, Piette JD, Spencer M, Kieffer E, Vijan S. The relationship between knowledge of recent HbA1c values and diabetes care understanding and self-management. Diabetes Care. 2005;28:816–22.
24. Goudie A, Dynan L, Brady PW, Fieldston E, Brilli RJ, Walsh KE. Costs of venous thromboembolism, catheter-associated urinary tract infection, and pressure ulcer. Pediatrics. 2015;136:432–9.
25. Mahajerin A, Branchford BR, Amankwah EK, Raffini L, Chalmers E, van Ommen CH, Goldenberg NA. Hospital-associated venous thromboembolism in pediatrics: a systematic review and meta-analysis of risk factors and risk-assessment models. Haematologica. 2015;100:1045–50.
26. Takemoto CM, Sohi S, Desai K, Bharaj R, Khanna A, McFarland S, Klaus S, Irshad A, Goldenberg NA, Strouse JJ, Streiff MB. Hospital-associated venous thromboembolism in children: incidence and clinical characteristics. J Pediatr. 2014;164:332–8.
27. Athale UH, Siciliano SA, Crowther M, Barr RD, Chan AK. Thromboembolism in children with acute lymphoblastic leukaemia treated on Dana-Farber Cancer Institute protocols: effect of age and risk stratification of disease. Br J Haematol. 2005;129:803–10.
28. van Ommen CH, Heijboer H, Buller HR, Hirasing RA, Heijmans HS, Peters M. Venous thromboembolism in childhood: a prospective two-year registry in The Netherlands. J Pediatr. 2001;139:676–81.

29. Fratino G, Molinari AC, Parodi S, Longo S, Saracco P, Castagnola E, Haupt R. Central venous catheter-related complications in children with oncological/hematological diseases: an observational study of 418 devices. Ann Oncol. 2005;16:648–54.
30. Branchford BR, Mourani P, Bajaj L, Manco-Johnson M, Wang M, Goldenberg NA. Risk factors for in-hospital venous thromboembolism in children: a case-control study employing diagnostic validation. Haematologica. 2012;97:509–15.
31. Meier KA, Clark E, Tarango C, Chima RS, Shaughnessy E. Venous thromboembolism in hospitalized adolescents: an approach to risk assessment and prophylaxis. Hosp Pediatr. 2015;5:44–51.
32. O'Brien SH, Klima J, Termuhlen AM, Kelleher KJ. Venous thromboembolism and adolescent and young adult oncology inpatients in US children's hospitals, 2001 to 2008. J Pediatr. 2011;159:133–7.
33. Tormene D, Simioni P, Prandoni P, Franz F, Zerbinati P, Tognin G, Girolami A. The incidence of venous thromboembolism in thrombophilic children: a prospective cohort study. Blood. 2002;100:2403–5.
34. Halvorson EE, Ervin SE, Russell TB, Skelton JA, Davis S, Spangler J. Association of obesity and pediatric venous thromboembolism. Hosp Pediatr. 2016;6:22–6.
35. Hanson SJ, Punzalan RC, Greenup RA, Liu H, Sato TT, Havens PL. Incidence and risk factors for venous thromboembolism in critically ill children after trauma. J Trauma. 2010;68:52–6.
36. McLean TW, Fisher CJ, Snively BM, Chauvenet AR. Central venous lines in children with lesser risk acute lymphoblastic leukemia: optimal type and timing of placement. J Clin Oncol. 2005;23:3024–9.
37. Revel-Vilk S, Yacobovich J, Tamary H, Goldstein G, Nemet S, Weintraub M, Paltiel O, Kenet G. Risk factors for central venous catheter thrombotic complications in children and adolescents with cancer. Cancer. 2010;116:4197–205.
38. Shah SH, West AN, Sepanski RJ, Hannah D, May WN, Anand KJ. Clinical risk factors for central line-associated venous thrombosis in children. Front Pediatr. 2015;3:35.
39. Male C, Chait P, Andrew M, Hanna K, Julian J, Mitchell L, Parkaa Investigators. Central venous line-related thrombosis in children: association with central venous line location and insertion technique. Blood. 2003;101:4273–8.
40. Journeycake JM, Quinn CT, Miller KL, Zajac JL, Buchanan GR. Catheter-related deep venous thrombosis in children with hemophilia. Blood. 2001;98:1727–31.
41. Mitchell L, Hoogendoorn H, Giles AR, Vegh P, Andrew M. Increased endogenous thrombin generation in children with acute lymphoblastic leukemia: risk of thrombotic complications in L'Asparaginase-induced antithrombin III deficiency. Blood. 1994;83:386–91.
42. Nowak-Gottl U, Junker R, Kreuz W, von Eckardstein A, Kosch A, Nohe N, Schobess R, Ehrenforth S, Group Childhood Thrombophilia Study. Risk of recurrent venous thrombosis in children with combined prothrombotic risk factors. Blood. 2001;97:858–62.
43. Tormene D, Gavasso S, Rossetto V, Simioni P. Thrombosis and thrombophilia in children: a systematic review. Semin Thromb Hemost. 2006;32:724–8.
44. Nowak-Gottl U, Wermes C, Junker R, Koch HG, Schobess R, Fleischhack G, Schwabe D, Ehrenforth S. Prospective evaluation of the thrombotic risk in children with acute lymphoblastic leukemia carrying the MTHFR TT 677 genotype, the prothrombin G20210A variant, and further prothrombotic risk factors. Blood. 1999;93:1595–9.
45. Unal S, Varan A, Yalcin B, Buyukpamukcu M, Gurgey A. Evaluation of thrombotic children with malignancy. Ann Hematol. 2005;84:395–9.
46. Manco-Johnson M, Grabowski EF, Hellgreen M, Kemahli AS, Massicotte MP, Muntean W, Peters M, Mowak-Gottl U. Laboratory testing for thrombophilia in pediatric patients, ISTH. 2002.   https://c.ymcdn.com/sites/www.isth.org/resource/group/13390e81-9b4b-479f-a449-2b66ad574ffd/official_communications/perinatalthrombophilia.pdf.
47. Monagle P, Chan AK, Goldenberg NA, Ichord RN, Journeycake JM, Nowak-Gottl U, Vesely SK, Physicians American College of Chest. Antithrombotic therapy in neonates and children: antithrombotic therapy and prevention of thrombosis, 9th ed: American College of Chest Physicians evidence-based clinical practice guidelines. Chest. 2012;141:e737S–801S.

48. Gerber DE, Segal JB, Levy MY, Kane J, Jones RJ, Streiff MB. The incidence of and risk factors for venous thromboembolism (VTE) and bleeding among 1514 patients undergoing hematopoietic stem cell transplantation: implications for VTE prevention. Blood. 2008;112:504–10.
49. Kansu E. Thrombosis in stem cell transplantation. Hematology. 2012;17(Suppl 1):S159–62.
50. Westerman MP, Green D, Gilman-Sachs A, Beaman K, Freels S, Boggio L, Allen S, Zuckerman L, Schlegel R, Williamson P. Antiphospholipid antibodies, proteins C and S, and coagulation changes in sickle cell disease. J Lab Clin Med. 1999;134:352–62.
51. Khorana AA, Kuderer NM, Culakova E, Lyman GH, Francis CW. Development and validation of a predictive model for chemotherapy-associated thrombosis. Blood. 2008;111:4902–7.
52. Mitchell L, Lambers M, Flege S, Kenet G, Li-Thiao-Te V, Holzhauer S, Bidlingmaier C, Fruhwald MC, Heller C, Schmidt W, Pautard B, Nowak-Gottl U. Validation of a predictive model for identifying an increased risk for thromboembolism in children with acute lymphoblastic leukemia: results of a multicenter cohort study. Blood. 2010;115:4999–5004.
53. Mahajerin A, Webber EC, Morris J, Taylor K, Saysana M. Development and implementation results of a venous thromboembolism prophylaxis guideline in a tertiary care pediatric hospital. Hosp Pediatr. 2015;5:630–6.
54. Raffini L, Trimarchi T, Beliveau J, Davis D. Thromboprophylaxis in a pediatric hospital: a patient-safety and quality-improvement initiative. Pediatrics. 2011;127:e1326–32.
55. Atchison CM, Arlikar S, Amankwah E, Ayala I, Barrett L, Branchford BR, Streiff M, Takemoto C, Goldenberg NA. Development of a new risk score for hospital-associated venous thromboembolism in noncritically ill children: findings from a large single-institutional case-control study. J Pediatr. 2014;165:793–8.
56. Sharathkumar AA, Mahajerin A, Heidt L, Doerfer K, Heiny M, Vik T, Fallon R, Rademaker A. Risk-prediction tool for identifying hospitalized children with a predisposition for development of venous thromboembolism: Peds-Clot clinical Decision Rule. J Thromb Haemost. 2012;10:1326–34.
57. Allenby F, Boardman L, Pflug JJ, Calnan JS. Effects of external pneumatic intermittent compression on fibrinolysis in man. Lancet. 1973;2:1412–4.
58. Cahan MA, Hanna DJ, Wiley LA, Cox DK, Killewich LA. External pneumatic compression and fibrinolysis in abdominal surgery. J Vasc Surg. 2000;32:537–43.
59. Comerota AJ, Chouhan V, Harada RN, Sun L, Hosking J, Veermansunemi R, Comerota Jr AJ, Schlappy D, Rao AK. The fibrinolytic effects of intermittent pneumatic compression: mechanism of enhanced fibrinolysis. Ann Surg. 1997;226:306–13. discussion 13-4
60. Kosir MA, Schmittinger L, Barno-Winarski L, Duddella P, Pone M, Perales A, Lange P, Brish LK, McGee K, Beleski K, Pawlak J, Mammen E, Sajahan NP, Kozol RA. Prospective double-arm study of fibrinolysis in surgical patients. J Surg Res. 1998;74:96–101.
61. Macaulay W, Westrich G, Sharrock N, Sculco TP, Jhon PH, Peterson MG, Salvati EA. Effect of pneumatic compression on fibrinolysis after total hip arthroplasty. Clin Orthop Relat Res. 2002;399:168–76.
62. O'Brien TE, Woodford M, Irving MH. The effect of intermittent compression of the calf on the fibrinolytic responses in the blood during a surgical operation. Surg Gynecol Obstet. 1979;149:380–4.
63. Tarnay TJ, Rohr PR, Davidson AG, Stevenson MM, Byars EF, Hopkins GR. Pneumatic calf compression, fibrinolysis, and the prevention of deep venous thrombosis. Surgery. 1980;88:489–96.
64. Arabi YM, Khedr M, Dara SI, Dhar GS, Bhat SA, Tamim HM, Afesh LY. Use of intermittent pneumatic compression and not graduated compression stockings is associated with lower incident VTE in critically ill patients: a multiple propensity scores adjusted analysis. Chest. 2013;144:152–9.
65. Barrera LM, Perel P, Ker K, Cirocchi R, Farinella E, Morales Uribe CH. Thromboprophylaxis for trauma patients. Cochrane Database Syst Rev. 2013;3:CD008303.
66. Handoll HH, Farrar MJ, McBirnie J, Tytherleigh-Strong G, Milne AA, Gillespie WJ. Heparin, low molecular weight heparin and physical methods for preventing deep vein thrombosis and pulmonary embolism following surgery for hip fractures. Cochrane Database Syst Rev. 2002;4:CD000305.

67. Ho KM, Tan JA. Stratified meta-analysis of intermittent pneumatic compression of the lower limbs to prevent venous thromboembolism in hospitalized patients. Circulation. 2013;128:1003–20.
68. Kakkos SK, Caprini JA, Geroulakos G, Nicolaides AN, Stansby GP, Tsolakis IA, Reddy DJ. Can combined (mechanical and pharmacological) modalities prevent fatal VTE? Int Angiol. 2011;30:115–22.
69. Kahn SR, Lim W, Dunn AS, Cushman M, Dentali F, Akl EA, Cook DJ, Balekian AA, Klein RC, Le H, Schulman S, Murad MH, Physicians American College of Chest. Prevention of VTE in non-surgical patients: antithrombotic therapy and prevention of thrombosis, 9th ed: American College of Chest Physicians evidence-based clinical practice guidelines. Chest. 2012;141:e195S–226S.
70. Massicotte P, Julian JA, Gent M, Shields K, Marzinotto V, Szechtman B, Chan AK, Andrew M, Protekt Study Group. An open-label randomized controlled trial of low molecular weight heparin for the prevention of central venous line-related thrombotic complications in children: the PROTEKT trial. Thromb Res. 2003;109:101–8.
71. Ruud E, Holmstrom H, De Lange C, Hogstad EM, Wesenberg F. Low-dose warfarin for the prevention of central line-associated thromboses in children with malignancies—a randomized, controlled study. Acta Paediatr. 2006;95:1053–9.
72. Schroeder AR, Axelrod DM, Silverman NH, Rubesova E, Merkel E, Roth SJ. A continuous heparin infusion does not prevent catheter-related thrombosis in infants after cardiac surgery. Pediatr Crit Care Med. 2010;11:489–95.
73. Vidal E, Sharathkumar A, Glover J, Faustino EV. Central venous catheter-related thrombosis and thromboprophylaxis in children: a systematic review and meta-analysis. J Thromb Haemost. 2014;12:1096–109.
74. Kabrhel C, Mark Courtney D, Camargo Jr CA, Plewa MC, Nordenholz KE, Moore CL, Richman PB, Smithline HA, Beam DM, Kline JA. Factors associated with positive D-dimer results in patients evaluated for pulmonary embolism. Acad Emerg Med. 2010;17:589–97.
75. Trame MN, Mitchell L, Krumpel A, Male C, Hempel G, Nowak-Gottl U. Population pharmacokinetics of enoxaparin in infants, children and adolescents during secondary thromboembolic prophylaxis: a cohort study. J Thromb Haemost. 2010;8:1950–8.
76. Young G, Yee DL, O'Brien SH, Khanna R, Barbour A, Nugent DJ. FondaKIDS: a prospective pharmacokinetic and safety study of fondaparinux in children between 1 and 18 years of age. Pediatr Blood Cancer. 2011;57:1049–54.
77. Kearon C, Akl EA, Ornelas J, Blaivas A, Jimenez D, Bounameaux H, Huisman M, King CS, Morris TA, Sood N, Stevens SM, Vintch JR, Wells P, Woller SC, Moores L. Antithrombotic therapy for VTE disease: CHEST guideline and expert panel report. Chest. 2016;149:315–52.
78. Kuhle S, Spavor M, Massicotte P, Halton J, Cherrick I, Dix D, Mahoney D, Bauman M, Desai S, Mitchell LG. Prevalence of post-thrombotic syndrome following asymptomatic thrombosis in survivors of acute lymphoblastic leukemia. J Thromb Haemost. 2008;6:589–94.
79. Kahn SR, Galanaud JP, Vedantham S, Ginsberg JS. Guidance for the prevention and treatment of the post-thrombotic syndrome. J Thromb Thrombolysis. 2016;41:144–53.
80. Prandoni P, Lensing AW, Cogo A, Cuppini S, Villalta S, Carta M, Cattelan AM, Polistena P, Bernardi E, Prins MH. The long-term clinical course of acute deep venous thrombosis. Ann Intern Med. 1996;125:1–7.
81. Kuhle S, Koloshuk B, Marzinotto V, Bauman M, Massicotte P, Andrew M, Chan A, Abdolell M, Mitchell L. A cross-sectional study evaluating post-thrombotic syndrome in children. Thromb Res. 2003;111:227–33.
82. Manco-Johnson MJ. Postthrombotic syndrome in children. Acta Haematol. 2006;115:207–13.
83. Bidlingmaier C, Kenet G, Kurnik K, Mathew P, Manner D, Mitchell L, Krumpel A, Nowak-Gottl U. Safety and efficacy of low molecular weight heparins in children: a systematic review of the literature and meta-analysis of single-arm studies. Semin Thromb Hemost. 2011;37:814–25.
84. Stem J, Christensen A, Davis D, Raffini L. Safety of prophylactic anticoagulation at a pediatric hospital. J Pediatr Hematol Oncol. 2013;35:e287–91.

Chapter 13
Blood Product Administration Safety

Jennifer Webb, Rahul Shah, and Naomi Luban

Background

The administration of blood products is a critical component of supportive care for patients with hematologic and oncologic disorders, as well as those undergoing hematopoietic stem cell transplants. Ensuring blood administration safety is a priority for all hospitals due to the potential severity of reactions, extensive regulations regarding these high-risk products, and mandatory reporting of severe adverse events. Furthermore, an error can result in a significant effect on the patient, including death. Blood bank practices are scrutinized as part of hospital accreditation processes. From blood product order to patient samples to administration, patient safety guides transfusion medicine care from blood bank to bedside.

Measurement

Hemovigilance is a set of surveillance procedures that monitor the whole transfusion process, the goal of which is to collect and analyze data to improve transfusion standards, guide policy, and increase safety and quality [1]. It was developed in the 1990s as a safety concept that was applied to all aspects of blood banking and has become an essential branch of transfusion medicine in the United States and abroad. Due to the myriad of steps that span from blood donor to product recipient, data

J. Webb (✉) • R. Shah • N. Luban
Children's National Health System, 111 Michigan Ave NW, Washington, DC, USA
e-mail: jwebb@childrensnational.org; rshah@childrensnational.org; nluban@childrensnational.org

© Springer International Publishing AG 2017   225
C.E. Dandoy et al. (eds.), *Patient Safety and Quality in Pediatric Hematology/Oncology and Stem Cell Transplantation*, DOI 10.1007/978-3-319-53790-0_13

compilation and measurement from multiple sources is necessary to define the spectrum of outcomes and inform the process.

Collection of blood products, including blood donor history and testing, is the initial step in ensuring a safe blood supply, and these practices are integrated at the blood supplier level. These practices fall under the purview of Hemovigilance; however, these are a part of transfusion safety that is outside the focus of this chapter and best covered elsewhere. It is important, however, for hospital-based blood banks to have open communication with their blood supplier to ensure adequate inventory, to procure specialized products when necessary, and to provide continuous feedback regarding product quality and transfusion reactions which may impact future collections from a specific donor or set of donors.

Hemovigilance includes the measurement of frequency, type, and pattern of transfusion reactions suffered by patients. In the United States, the Food and Drug Administration (FDA) mandates notification of all fatal transfusion reactions as soon as possible after the fatality occurs with a complete report of the fatality sent within 7 days (Section 606.170(b) of Title 21, Code of Federal Regulations). Each of these reports is investigated by the FDA and summary data are publically available. Currently, only these most severe of outcomes are subject to mandatory reporting in the United States; however, transfusion safety relies on the accurate measurement of nonfatal transfusion reactions, as well. Indeed, many hospitals have policies in place requiring internal reporting of such events on a periodic basis. Rates are calculated as total number of reactions divided by the number of issued/transfused components. These rates may be further subdivided (intensive care unit vs floor, inpatient vs outpatient, operating room vs floor, indication for transfusion, etc.) to meet the quality control needs of the transfusion service.

In 2010, the US Centers for Disease Control and Prevention (CDC) developed a national recipient Hemovigilance system for voluntary reporting of transfusion reactions. The Hemovigilance Module is part of the National Healthcare Safety Network (NHSN) and provides a framework for defining and quantifying the burden of transfusion reactions on patients, including nonfatal reactions [2]. See Table 13.1 for current transfusion reaction definitions as defined by NHSN. However, it is unclear how applicable these definitions are for pediatric patients, especially those undergoing hematopoietic stem cell transplants (HSCT). Reporting of symptoms may be impossible or delayed in young patients due to lack of language acquisition, so that patient symptoms fail to fit within the Hemovigilance criteria. The use of axillary temperatures in pediatric patients who cannot cooperate with oral temperatures may artificially decrease absolute temperature, thus lowering the patient below the threshold for febrile nonhemolytic transfusion criteria (FNHTR). Strategies to adapt transfusion reaction definition criteria so that there is improved recognition and reporting of transfusion reactions are critical for hospitals caring for pediatric patients.

Currently, participation in the Hemovigilance Module remains voluntary; however, this will likely change in the next few years. Preliminary data reveal that transfusion reaction rates per 100,000 red blood cell (RBC) units reported through the Hemovigilance Module are comparable to rates of transfusion reactions in other

Table 13.1 Definition of transfusion reactions (adapted from National Healthcare Safety Network Biovigilance Component Hemovigilance Module Component Surveillance Protocol v2.3, June 2016)

Type of reaction	Definition
Acute hemolytic transfusion reaction (AHTR)	Occurs during or within 24 h of cessation of transfusion with new onset of any one of the following symptoms: • Back/flank pain • Chills/rigors • Disseminated intravascular coagulation (DIC) • Epistaxis • Fever • Hematuria • Hypotension • Oliguria/anuria • Pain and/or oozing at IV site • Renal failure *And* two or more of the following: • Decreased fibrinogen • Decreased haptoglobin • Elevated bilirubin • Elevated LDH • Hemoglobinemia • Hemoglobinuria • Plasma discoloration consistent with hemolysis • Spherocytes on blood smear And either: • *Immune Mediated:* Positive direct antiglobulin test (DAT) for anti-IgG or anti-C3 and positive elution test • *Non-Immune Mediated:* Serologic testing is negative, and a physical cause (thermal, osmotic, mechanical, etc.) is confirmed
Delayed hemolytic transfusion reaction (DHTR)	Positive direct antiglobulin test (DAT) for antibodies developed between 24 h and 28 days after cessation of transfusion *and* either: • Positive elution with alloantibody present • Newly identified red blood cell alloantibody in recipient serum *And* either: • Inadequate posttransfusion rise in hemoglobin or rapid fall in hemoglobin back to pre-transfusion levels • Unexplained spherocytes on blood smear
Delayed serologic transfusion reaction (DSTR)	Absence of clinical signs of hemolysis and demonstration of new, clinically significant antibodies against red blood cells by either: • Positive direct antiglobulin test (DAT) • Newly identified red blood cell alloantibody in recipient serum
Allergic reaction	Two or more of the following within 4 h of cessation of transfusion: • Conjunctival edema • Edema of the lips, tongue, or uvula • Erythema and edema of the periorbital area • Generalized flushing • Hypotension • Localized angioedema • Maculopapular rash • Pruritus (itching) • Respiratory distress; bronchospasm • Urticaria (hives)

(continued)

Table 13.1 (continued)

Type of reaction	Definition
Febrile nonhemolytic transfusion reaction (FNHTR)	Fever (≥38.0) and a change of at least 1 °C from pre-transfusion value *or* chills and rigors within 4 h of cessation of transfusion
Transfusion-associated circulatory overload (TACO)	New onset of 3 or more within 6 h of cessation of transfusion: • Acute respiratory distress • Elevated brain natriuretic peptide (BNP) • Elevated central venous pressure (CVP) • Evidence of left heart failure • Evidence of positive fluid balance • Radiographic evidence of pulmonary edema
Transfusion-related acute lung injury (TRALI)	*No* evidence of acute lung injury prior to transfusion *and* acute lung injury onset during or within 6 h of transfusion *and* hypoxemia *and* radiographic infiltrates bilaterally *without* elevated left atrial pressure
Transfusion-associated graft versus host disease (TA-GVHD)	A clinical syndrome occurring between 2 days and 6 weeks after cessation of transfusion characterized by: • Characteristic, erythematous, maculopapular rash • Diarrhea • Fever • Hepatomegaly • Liver dysfunction • Bone marrow aplasia • Pancytopenia *And* • Characteristic histological appearance of skin or liver biopsy
Transfusion-transmitted infection (TTI)	Laboratory evidence of a pathogen in the transfusion recipient linked to the donor or the blood component
Posttransfusion purpura (PTP)	Alloantibodies in the patient directed against human platelet antigen (HPA) or other platelet-specific antigen detected at or after development of thrombocytopenia *and* thrombocytopenia (<20% of pre-transfusion count)
Hypotensive transfusion reaction	Hypotension within 1 h of cessation of transfusion *and* other transfusion reactions presenting with hypotension do not apply
Transfusion-associated dyspnea	Acute respiratory distress occurring within 24 h of cessation of transfusion *and* allergic/TACO/TRALI definitions do not apply

countries where reporting is mandatory [3, 4], suggesting that this is a robust collection system with the potential for refinement and expansion.

In other countries, other Hemovigilance reporting systems are in place to measure and monitor transfusion-related outcomes. Some of these systems have been mandatory from inception, while others began as voluntary systems and then, with refinement, became mandatory. They vary as to whether they are active or passive reporting systems, whether they are centralized or decentralized, and in the type of supervising body. They vary as to whether they only collect adverse events or if they also capture near-miss events that never reach the patient [1]. Despite the wide variety of systems in place, national Hemovigilance systems have not only documented areas for process improvement, but they have been able to quantify the success of strategies to improve patient outcomes [1, 5, 6].

Through the use of national Hemovigilance surveillance, the majority of preventable transfusion errors have been identified as due to human or clerical errors [1, 7–10]. This highlights the fact that transfusion safety begins at the hospital level, as soon as the order for transfusion is placed. Hemovigilance modules that include near-miss events identify significantly more near-miss events for every single event that results in patient harm [11, 12]. Root-cause analyses of events emphasize the importance of ensuring the correct blood order is placed for the correct patient, adequate sample collection and labeling, and correct product retrieval from the blood bank [13]. Mislabeled and unacceptable blood specimens have been shown to be 40 times more likely to have a blood grouping discrepancy which carries with it the potential for significant harm [14].

Implementation of Hemovigilance surveillance at the hospital, regional, and national level plays a critical role in identifying and mitigating the risks associated with transfusions. Though some risks are inherent, prospective collection of Hemovigilance data is a powerful tool to measure patient outcomes, identify areas for improvement, and monitor the impact of risk mitigation strategies.

Transfusion practices for pediatric patients vary significantly between institutions. In a survey of blood bank personnel in the United States and Canada, tremendous variation in practice was noted with regard to RBC storage age, irradiation policies, washing policies, and leukoreduction [15]. Thresholds for auditing and benchmarking similarly vary [15]. Some of this may be due to difficulty defining absolute transfusion thresholds in pediatric patients because of physiologic changes that naturally occur. There are also limitations in available evidence, highlighting the need for ongoing research in pediatric transfusion medicine. However, transfusion practices may also be affected by nonclinical factors [16]. Yet for certain populations of patients, modifications to products, such as leukoreduction or irradiation, are critical. For patients receiving significant immunosuppression, such as those undergoing hematopoietic stem cell transplants or receiving high-dose chemotherapy, certain blood products convey a risk of transfusion-associated graft versus host disease (TA-GVHD). TA-GVHD is a rare, but nearly universally fatal transfusion reaction. It can be prevented through irradiation of cellular blood products. Unfortunately, the use of selective irradiation protocols, which require providers to notify the blood bank if a patient is at risk for TA-GVHD, allows for patients to potentially receive nonirradiated products if the notification is not made. Ensuring patients receive appropriately modified products has been identified as an area in need of improvement through Hemovigilance modules [17]. As certain immunodeficiencies also place patients at risk for TA-GVHD, many hospitals have policies in place for irradiation of blood products for patients under a certain age in the hope that a diagnosis will have been made; however, the age threshold for empiric irradiation varies significantly. In a survey of pediatric hospitals, 72% empirically irradiate if patient is less than 4 months of age, 4% if the patient is less than 6 months of age, and 24% if the patient is less than 12 months of age [15]. These variations in practice have not been compared systematically to determine the most cost-effective or safest policy, so hospital blood banks continue to be allowed to determine their own thresholds.

In an effort to improve blood safety, the National Heart, Lung, and Blood Institute (NHLBI) has funded a series of multicenter studies which have made significant contributions to transfusion medicine and blood banking knowledge. The now completed Retroviral Epidemiology and Donor Study (REDS) and REDS-II initially focused on risks of transfusion-transmitted infections including HIV and human T-lymphotropic virus (HTLV) while also capturing data on characterization and motivations of blood donors to ensure blood safety and supply [18]. Key results from REDS and REDS-II have included the evaluation of the performance of a variety of donor screening tests for infectious agents [19–21], the establishment of a rapid response platform for emerging infectious agents [22], an evaluation of the role of incentives on repeat blood donation [23], and a quantification of the efficacy of donor deferral questions in infection prevention [24]. The ongoing REDS-III will further expand upon the research from REDS and REDS-II, while also including data collection on transfusion recipients and transfusion outcomes [25]. As further analyses are published, REDS, REDS-II, and REDS-III will continue to make significant contributions to blood safety.

Strategies for Improvement

Understanding the root cause of transfusion errors or adverse events is the first step in improving transfusion safety. Devising strategies to prevent those events in the future is the critical second step. Though it may seem that the cause of the error is specific to the hospital or transfusion center in which the event occurred, lessons learned in one institution may be applied elsewhere to prevent a similar error. Furthermore, strategies for improvement may include changes to processes or product well before it reaches the hospital blood bank.

Transfusion of the incorrect blood product, defined as a patient receiving blood intended for another recipient, blood products transfused based on phlebotomy errors ("wrong blood in tube"), or blood transfused where there is a laboratory error in selection, testing, or issue of the blood product, is the most commonly reported avoidable adverse event noted in mandatory Hemovigilance modules [10]. As previously noted, human or clerical errors directly contribute to these events [1, 7–10]. In many cases, the final bedside check prior to blood product administration, if done properly, should catch the error highlighting the critical need for correct patient and product identification. Several strategies have been developed to prevent misidentification and incorrect blood administration, including the use of barcoded labeling systems for patient, specimen, and product identification. Barcode identification of patient identification has been shown to simplify patient identification at the time of blood sample collection and at the time of product administration [26]. The use of barcodes also significantly improves rates of correct patient identification including full name and date of birth, as well as increase rates of immediate and correct labeling of specimen tubes with medical record number, name, date of birth, gender, and sample date [27]. It has also been shown to improve accuracy of blood product collection from the blood bank and at time of administration [27]. In one 2-month pilot study, two cases of ABO incompatible transfusions were avoided due to barcoding [28]. However, barcoding systems throughout the transfusion process are not fail-safe. They rely on initial correct patient identification at the time of barcode generation and wristband application, and there are a number of logistic challenges to implementation and use [29]. As with all systems, strict adherence to procedures is critical to ensuring the correct patient receives the correct blood. However, if barcodes simplify and improve the accuracy of those steps, they could significantly improve transfusion safety.

In addition to barcoding, technology has the potential to further improve transfusion safety by eliminating the opportunity for human errors. Electronic crossmatching, which uses software to crossmatch units from blood bank inventory to eligible patients, has been in use since the 1990s and provides another opportunity for hospital blood banks to avoid human error [30, 31]. It has been shown to provide rapid and safe issue of compatible blood while also reducing laboratory work load, blood sample volume requirements, unit expiration, and costs [32]. Blood bank software networking and remote blood refrigeration units allow for electronic remote blood issue (ERBI). ERBI, facilitated by electronic crossmatching, has the potential for rapid issue of crossmatched blood units to sites, such as the hematology/oncology floor, while limiting the potential opportunities for human errors [33]. These systems are fairly new and require further study to provide accurate estimates of quality and safety.

Checklists, which have been shown to improve safety in other high-risk occupations such as the airline industry, are another strategy that has been demonstrated to improve transfusion safety. One study found that implementation of a transfusion checklist and order set improved transfusion safety around prevention of transfusion-associated circulatory overload (TACO) in adults, one of the most common causes of fatal transfusion reactions [34]. The checklist prompted providers to identify specific risk factors for TACO, such as age or history of congestive heart failure, prior to transfusion and then recommended use of IV furosemide following transfusion. Unfortunately, at this time, no published checklists have been adapted for use in pediatric patients; however, if implemented, they have the potential to aid in the elimination of errors. Serious Hazards of Transfusion (SHOT) has published an online checklist that includes steps from ordering to post-transfusion testing freely available to be used for all transfusions [35].

With the increased use of computerized physician order entry (CPOE) in hospitals, there is the potential to embed transfusion criteria and alerting mechanisms at the time of physician blood ordering. Several studies have shown decreased red blood cell usage after the implementation of systems that require physicians to enter a transfusion indication at the time of order placement and/or provide an alert if the patient's hemoglobin does not meet said criteria [36–38]. Despite these promising results, few studies have demonstrated that decreased frequency of transfusion has improved patient outcomes [39]. However, in general, clinical decision supports imbedded in electronic health records and in CPOE systems have been shown to improve indicators of quality in other areas of medicine [40].

Strategies to improve safety may also be implemented at the blood supply level. Currently, in the United States, many blood banks have selective transfusion protocols that require patients to be identified to the blood bank as requiring specific product manipulation, such as irradiation or leukoreduction. Advocates have argued for universal modifications to the blood supply to prevent eligible patients from being missed [41, 42]. Universal irradiation of cellular blood products has been shown to be effective in preventing TA-GVHD in populations at high risk of this disease [43]. However, irradiation of red blood cells may increase potassium leakage into the supernatant which, if infused rapidly, may cause unsafe heart rhythms and potentially death [44–46]. Saline suspension, washing of products, specialized filtration, and the use of additional additives to the supernatant may mitigate these risks; however, these require additional inventory management and come with additional cost [47]. Furthermore, irradiated products have a limited shelf life, which may affect available blood supplies. Though the benefits of leukoreduction of blood products have been well documented, leukoreduction remains elective in the United States, though it has been successfully adopted in other countries as part of universal safety strategies [42]. Universal manipulation of blood products with irradiation or leukoreduction has the potential to protect patients at risk for severe and potentially fatal adverse events by removing the need to identify individuals requiring specialized products. By treating all products, no one will be missed; however, these strategies have the potential to impact blood availability and cost.

Historically, transfusion-transmitted infections have been identified through pathogen-specific donor screening tests, cultures of blood products, or surrogate markers of contamination such as pH testing. Pathogen inactivation systems are being developed and studied with a goal to universally treat blood products and prevent possible infections from a wide variety of known and emerging pathogens. One of the available methods relies on photochemical inactivation through the use of a photosensitizing agent and ultraviolet (UV) light. This causes irreversible cross-linking of nucleotides, preventing the pathogens from replicating [48, 49]. These techniques also inactivate white blood cells and may prevent TA-GVHD, providing a potential alternative to universal irradiation [50]. In mouse models, pathogen reduction methods with UV-C light have been shown to be as effective as irradiation in preventing TA-GVHD [51]. Another method of pathogen inactivation uses solvent/detergent (SD) treatments to kill enveloped viruses [52, 53]. There is some evidence that SD treatments may also inhibit bacterial growth [54]. SD methods have long been in use with factor concentrates and plasma [53]. These methods have the potential to be applied to a wide variety of blood products to proactively protect the blood supply [55, 56]. Currently, only pathogen-reduced plasma and platelets are FDA approved and available in the United States. Despite the promise of sterile blood components, much remains to be learned about the efficacy and safety of these products in pediatric patients, and universal adoption of these systems is not expected in the near future [57].

Transfusion safety strategies may also be educational rather than technological, especially given that the majority of medical schools devote a mere one to 2 h total to transfusion medicine education [58]. The *Choosing Wisely* campaign is an initiative from the American Board of Internal Medicine to reduce the overuse of tests and procedures that are unnecessary and therefore potentially harmful [59]. It provides a framework for engaging patients and physicians in a conversation about care [60]. As blood transfusion is one of the most common procedures performed on a hospitalized patient and overuse of transfusion carries a potential risk of harm, transfusions have become a focus for the *Choosing Wisely* campaign [61]. The American Society of Hematology (ASH) has supported the *Choosing Wisely* campaign by providing specific recommendations for transfusion, such as "Don't transfuse more than the minimum number of RBC units necessary to relieve symptoms of anemia or return a patient to a safe hemoglobin range (7 to 8 g/dL) in stable, non-cardiac in-patients." In pediatric patients, the recommendation is to use specific weight-based dosing calculations [62]. The AABB, an organization devoted to safe transfusion practices, has also supported this endeavor through publication of evidence-based guidelines to help physicians and patients make judicious decisions about blood product transfusion [61]. This guidance is in alignment with the ongoing push for patient blood management (PBM) strategies for all hospitalized patients. The goal of PBM is to appropriately use blood products to optimize patient health and safety and to identify and implement strategies to safely avoid unnecessary transfusion.

AABB and the Joint Commission recently developed a voluntary PBM Certificate which can be earned by hospitals who meet the AABB Standards for a Patient Blood Management Program [63]. Unfortunately, PBM and *Choosing Wisely* are focused on adult patients where guidelines for transfusion are better established. Though there are concepts from both that can be applied to pediatric patients, this highlights the limitations of the evidence for transfusion management in children and neonates. There is a need for ongoing rigorous research and investigation around best practices for transfusion in these patients.

Strategies for Sustainability and Oversight

Successful implementation of safety strategies requires ensuring sustainability of these programs as part of prioritizing a culture of safety. Sustainability requires engagement with key stakeholders throughout the transfusion process. For pediatric hematology/oncology and hematopoietic stem cell transplant patients, that includes engagement of the primary clinical teams, surgical services, intensive care specialists, hospital blood bank, and blood suppliers. With this many providers involved in care, sustainability often falls to one person or group to be the champion for change. Many hospitals have established a new position, a transfusion safety officer (TSO), to be that force for change.

The responsibilities of a TSO often include education of staff on transfusion guidelines or specimen collection, auditing of transfusion orders and blood utilization, transfusion reaction investigation, and implementation of new safety strategies

[64]. TSOs have been widely accepted in other countries where they serve a critical role in national Hemovigilance efforts, supporting nationalized blood supplies [65]. In general, the focus of the TSO is transfusion safety outside of the laboratory. As Hemovigilance, as a concept, grows in the United States, hospitals will likely see the unmistakable need for dedicated TSOs.

Blood utilization committees (BUCs) or transfusion committees may serve a similar role to a TSO or may serve as the body that oversees the TSO. In general, the goal of a BUC is to develop local transfusion policies, educate clinicians, and audit blood use. BUCs are multidisciplinary groups that review blood product usage and compare local results to predefined benchmarks. They report to the medical staff and the board of directors of hospitals. This task is especially challenging in pediatrics as there is limited consensus for transfusion criteria. However, BUCs are a requirement for accreditation from the Joint Commission and the College of American Pathologists which demonstrates the commitment of these governing bodies to safe transfusion practices [66]. Hospitals should empower BUCs to enforce change as a means for ensuring that safety efforts are continuously updated and renewed.

In implementing PBM strategies, adult hospitals have found variable success through establishing transfusion guidelines and providing education in absence of other PBM strategies. The use of single strategies, in isolation, has been shown to be insufficient [67]. However, hospitals that have included proactive auditing and direct feedback regarding transfusion practice have seen not only a reduction in unnecessary transfusions but also significant cost savings [68]. It remains unclear, however, if fewer transfusions improve patient outcomes through avoidance of unnecessary risk, and this is an area of active study. Early adopters of PBM strategies emphasize the need for a multifaceted, interdisciplinary approach to improve safety outcomes [69]. The need for auditing and feedback underscores the absolute necessity of Hemovigilance as part of any safety strategy. It also provides a specific niche where the duties of a TSO align with the goals of PBM.

Processes and policies at all stages of blood administration, from collection to infusion, should be continuously and proactively refined and improved. Strategies for improvement should be shared collaboratively as part of medicine's evolving and iterative culture of safety. Implementation strategies should include strategies for sustainability, such as proactive Hemovigilance and the creation of a TSO position.

References

1. de Vries RR, Faber JC, Strengers PF. Haemovigilance: an effective tool for improving transfusion practice. Vox Sang. 2011;100(1):60–7.
2. Chung KW, Harvey A, Basavaraju SV, Kuehnert MJ. How is national recipient hemovigilance conducted in the United States? Transfusion (Paris). 2015;55(4):703–7.
3. Rogers MA, Rohde JM, Blumberg N. Haemovigilance of reactions associated with red blood cell transfusion: comparison across 17 Countries. Vox Sang. 2015;110(3):266–77.

4. Harvey AR, Basavaraju SV, Chung KW, Kuehnert MJ. Transfusion-related adverse reactions reported to the National Healthcare Safety Network Hemovigilance Module, United States, 2010 to 2012. Transfusion (Paris). 2015;55(4):709–18.
5. Williamson LM, Stainsby D, Jones H, Love E, Chapman CE, Navarrete C, et al. The impact of universal leukodepletion of the blood supply on hemovigilance reports of posttransfusion purpura and transfusion-associated graft-versus-host disease. Transfusion (Paris). 2007;47(8):1455–67.
6. Funk MB, Heiden M, Volkers P, Lohmann A, Keller-Stanislawski B. Evaluation of risk minimisation measures for blood components - based on reporting rates of transfusion-transmitted reactions (1997-2013). Transfus Med Hemother. 2015;42(4):240–6.
7. Bolton-Maggs PH, Cohen H. Serious hazards of transfusion (SHOT) haemovigilance and progress is improving transfusion safety. Br J Haematol. 2013;163(3):303–14.
8. Stainsby D, Williamson L, Jones H, Cohen H. 6 Years of shot reporting—its influence on UK blood safety. Transfus Apher Sci. 2004;31(2):123–31.
9. Stainsby D, Jones H, Asher D, Atterbury C, Boncinelli A, Brant L, et al. Serious hazards of transfusion: a decade of hemovigilance in the UK. Transfus Med Rev. 2006;20(4):273–82.
10. Bolton-Maggs PH. Conference report: the 2015 SHOT symposium and report—what's new? Transfus Med. 2015;25(5):295–8.
11. Kaplan HS. Getting the right blood to the right patient: the contribution of near-miss event reporting and barrier analysis. Transfus Clin Biol. 2005;12(5):380–4.
12. Lundy D, Laspina S, Kaplan H, Rabin Fastman B, Lawlor E. Seven hundred and fifty-nine (759) chances to learn: a 3-year pilot project to analyse transfusion-related near-miss events in the Republic of Ireland. Vox Sang. 2007;92(3):233–41.
13. Callum JL, Kaplan HS, Merkley LL, Pinkerton PH, Rabin Fastman B, Romans RA, et al. Reporting of near-miss events for transfusion medicine: improving transfusion safety. Transfusion (Paris). 2001;41(10):1204–11.
14. Lumadue JA, Boyd JS, Ness PM. Adherence to a strict specimen-labeling policy decreases the incidence of erroneous blood grouping of blood bank specimens. Transfusion (Paris). 1997;37(11–12):1169–72.
15. Spinella PC, Dressler A, Tucci M, Carroll CL, Rosen RS, Hume H, et al. Survey of transfusion policies at US and Canadian children's hospitals in 2008 and 2009. Transfusion (Paris). 2010;50(11):2328–35.
16. Fortin S, Cardona LG, Latreille M, Tucci M, Lacroix J. Blood transfusion in acute and chronic pediatric settings: beliefs and practices. Transfusion (Paris). 2015;56(1):130–8.
17. Bolton-Maggs PH. Bullet points from SHOT: key messages and recommendations from the annual SHOT report 2013. Transfus Med. 2014;24(4):197–203.
18. Kleinman S, King MR, Busch MP, Murphy EL, Glynn SA. The National Heart, Lung, and Blood Institute retrovirus epidemiology donor studies (retrovirus epidemiology donor study and retrovirus epidemiology donor study-II): twenty years of research to advance blood product safety and availability. Transfus Med Rev. 2012;26(4):281–304. e1–2
19. Busch MP, Glynn SA, Wright DJ, Hirschkorn D, Laycock ME, McAuley J, et al. Relative sensitivities of licensed nucleic acid amplification tests for detection of viremia in early human immunodeficiency virus and hepatitis C virus infection. Transfusion (Paris). 2005;45(12):1853–63.
20. Tobler LH, Stramer SL, Lee SR, Baggett D, Wright D, Hirschkorn D, et al. Performance of ORTHO HCV core antigen and trak-C assays for detection of viraemia in pre-seroconversion plasma and whole blood donors. Vox Sang. 2005;89(4):201–7.
21. Tobler LH, Stramer SL, Lee SR, Masecar BL, Peterson JE, Davis EA, et al. Impact of HCV 3.0 EIA relative to HCV 2.0 EIA on blood-donor screening. Transfusion (Paris). 2003;43(10):1452–9.
22. Busch MP, Kleinman SH, Nemo GJ. Current and emerging infectious risks of blood transfusions. JAMA. 2003;289(8):959–62.
23. Sanchez AM, Ameti DI, Schreiber GB, Thomson RA, Lo A, Bethel J, et al. The potential impact of incentives on future blood donation behavior. Transfusion (Paris). 2001;41(2):172–8.

24. Spencer B, Steele W, Custer B, Kleinman S, Cable R, Wilkinson S, et al. Risk for malaria in United States donors deferred for travel to malaria-endemic areas. Transfusion (Paris). 2009;49(11):2335–45.
25. Kleinman S, Busch MP, Murphy EL, Shan H, Ness P, Glynn SA. The National Heart, Lung, and Blood Institute recipient epidemiology and donor evaluation study (REDS-III): a research program striving to improve blood donor and transfusion recipient outcomes. Transfusion (Paris). 2014;54(3 Pt 2):942–55.
26. Turner CL, Casbard AC, Murphy MF. Barcode technology: its role in increasing the safety of blood transfusion. Transfusion (Paris). 2003;43(9):1200–9.
27. Davies A, Staves J, Kay J, Casbard A, Murphy MF. End-to-end electronic control of the hospital transfusion process to increase the safety of blood transfusion: strengths and weaknesses. Transfusion (Paris). 2006;46(3):352–64.
28. Lau FY, Cheng G. To err is human nature. Can transfusion errors due to human factors ever be eliminated? Clin Chim Acta. 2001;313(1–2):59–67.
29. Murphy MF. Application of bar code technology at the bedside: the Oxford experience. Transfusion (Paris). 2007;47(2 Suppl):120S–4S; discussion 30S–31S.
30. Butch SH, Judd WJ, Steiner EA, Stoe M, Oberman HA. Electronic verification of donor-recipient compatibility: the computer crossmatch. Transfusion (Paris). 1994;34(2):105–9.
31. Cheng G. Experiences with "self service" electronic blood banking. Vox Sang. 1998;74(Suppl 2):427–9.
32. Sharma G, Parwani AV, Raval JS, Triulzi DJ, Benjamin RJ, Pantanowitz L. Contemporary issues in transfusion medicine informatics. J Pathol Inform. 2011;2:3.
33. Sellen KM, Jovanovic A, Perrier L, Chignell M. Systematic review of electronic remote blood issue. Vox Sang. 2015;109(1):35–43.
34. Tseng E, Spradbrow J, Cao X, Callum J, Lin Y. An order set and checklist improve physician transfusion ordering practices to mitigate the risk of transfusion-associated circulatory overload. Transfus Med. 2016;26(2):104–10.
35. SHOT. Transfusion Checklist for every transfusion. 2012 [cited 2016 August 29]; http://www. shotuk.org/wp-content/uploads/2010/03/SHOT-Transfusion-Process-Checklist-May-2012.pdf.
36. Smith M, Triulzi DJ, Yazer MH, Rollins-Raval MA, Waters JH, Raval JS. Implementation of a simple electronic transfusion alert system decreases inappropriate ordering of packed red blood cells and plasma in a multi-hospital health care system. Transfus Apher Sci. 2014;51(3):53–8.
37. McWilliams B, Triulzi DJ, Waters JH, Alarcon LH, Reddy V, Yazer MH. Trends in RBC ordering and use after implementing adaptive alerts in the electronic computerized physician order entry system. Am J Clin Pathol. 2014;141(4):534–41.
38. Butler CE, Noel S, Hibbs SP, Miles D, Staves J, Mohaghegh P, et al. Implementation of a clinical decision support system improves compliance with restrictive transfusion policies in hematology patients. Transfusion (Paris). 2015;55(8):1964–71.
39. Hibbs SP, Nielsen ND, Brunskill S, Doree C, Yazer MH, Kaufman RM, et al. The impact of electronic decision support on transfusion practice: a systematic review. Transfus Med Rev. 2015;29(1):14–23.
40. Mishuris RG, Linder JA, Bates DW, Bitton A. Using electronic health record clinical decision support is associated with improved quality of care. Am J Manag Care. 2014;20(10):e445–52.
41. Anderson K. Broadening the spectrum of patient groups at risk for transfusion-associated GVHD: implications for universal irradiation of cellular blood components. Transfusion (Paris). 2003;43(12):1652–4.
42. Bassuni WY, Blajchman MA, Al-Moshary MA. Why implement universal leukoreduction? Hematol Oncol Stem Cell Ther. 2008;1(2):106–23.
43. Uchida S, Tadokoro K, Takahashi M, Yahagi H, Satake M, Juji T. Analysis of 66 patients definitive with transfusion-associated graft-versus-host disease and the effect of universal irradiation of blood. Transfus Med. 2013;23(6):416–22.
44. Hirayama J, Abe H, Azuma H, Ikeda H. Leakage of potassium from red blood cells following gamma ray irradiation in the presence of dipyridamole, trolox, human plasma or mannitol. Biol Pharm Bull. 2005;28(7):1318–20.

45. Winter KM, Johnson L, Kwok M, Reid S, Alarimi Z, Wong JK, et al. Understanding the effects of gamma-irradiation on potassium levels in red cell concentrates stored in SAG-M for neonatal red cell transfusion. Vox Sang. 2015;108(2):141–50.
46. Lee AC, Reduque LL, Luban NL, Ness PM, Anton B, Heitmiller ES. Transfusion-associated hyperkalemic cardiac arrest in pediatric patients receiving massive transfusion. Transfusion (Paris). 2014;54(1):244–54.
47. Vraets A, Lin Y, Callum JL. Transfusion-associated hyperkalemia. Transfus Med Rev. 2011;25(3):184–96.
48. Marschner S, Goodrich R. Pathogen reduction technology treatment of platelets, plasma and whole blood using riboflavin and UV light. Transfus Med Hemother. 2011;38(1):8–18.
49. Henschler R, Seifried E, Mufti N. Development of the S-303 pathogen inactivation technology for red blood cell concentrates. Transfus Med Hemother. 2011;38(1):33–42.
50. Fast LD, Nevola M, Tavares J, Reddy HL, Goodrich RP, Marschner S. Treatment of whole blood with riboflavin plus ultraviolet light, an alternative to gamma irradiation in the prevention of transfusion-associated graft-versus-host disease? Transfusion (Paris). 2013;53(2):373–81.
51. Pohler P, Muller M, Winkler C, Schaudien D, Sewald K, Muller TH, et al. Pathogen reduction by ultraviolet C light effectively inactivates human white blood cells in platelet products. Transfusion (Paris). 2015;55(2):337–47.
52. Horowitz B, Lazo A, Grossberg H, Page G, Lippin A, Swan G. Virus inactivation by solvent/detergent treatment and the manufacture of SD-plasma. Vox Sang. 1998;74(Suppl 1):203–6.
53. Liumbruno GM, Marano G, Grazzini G, Capuzzo E, Franchini M. Solvent/detergent-treated plasma: a tale of 30 years of experience. Expert Rev Hematol. 2015;8(3):367–74.
54. Chou ML, Wu YW, Su CY, Lee LW, Burnouf T. Impact of solvent/detergent treatment of plasma on transfusion-relevant bacteria. Vox Sang. 2012;102(4):277–84.
55. Kleinman S, Stassinopoulos A. Risks associated with red blood cell transfusions: potential benefits from application of pathogen inactivation. Transfusion (Paris). 2015;55(12):2983–3000.
56. Kleinman S. Pathogen inactivation: emerging indications. Curr Opin Hematol. 2015;22(6):547–53.
57. Salunkhe V, van der Meer PF, de Korte D, Seghatchian J, Gutierrez L. Development of blood transfusion product pathogen reduction treatments: a review of methods, current applications and demands. Transfus Apher Sci. 2015;52(1):19–34.
58. Karp JK, Weston CM, King KE. Transfusion medicine in American undergraduate medical education. Transfusion (Paris). 2011;51(11):2470–9.
59. Hurley R. Can doctors reduce harmful medical overuse worldwide? BMJ. 2014;349:g4289.
60. Murphy MF. The choosing wisely campaign to reduce harmful medical overuse: its close association with patient blood management initiatives. Transfus Med. 2015;25(5):287–92.
61. Callum JL, Waters JH, Shaz BH, Sloan SR, Murphy MF. The AABB recommendations for the choosing wisely campaign of the American Board of Internal Medicine. Transfusion (Paris). 2014;54(9):2344–52.
62. ASH. American Society of Hematology: ten things physicians and patients should question. 2013 [cited 2016 August 22, 2016]; http://www.choosingwisely.org/wp-content/uploads/2015/02/ASH-Choosing-Wisely-List.pdf.
63. AABB. Standards for a patient blood managment program. 1st ed. Bethesda: AABB; 2014. p. 33.
64. Dunbar NM, Szczepiorkowski ZM. How do we utilize a transfusion safety officer? Transfusion (Paris). 2015;55(9):2064–8.
65. Dzik WH. Emily Cooley lecture 2002: transfusion safety in the hospital. Transfusion (Paris). 2003;43(9):1190–9.
66. Haynes SL, Torella F. The role of hospital transfusion committees in blood product conservation. Transfus Med Rev. 2004;18(2):93–104.
67. Murphy MF, Casbard AC, Ballard S, Shulman IA, Heddle N, Aubuchon JP, et al. Prevention of bedside errors in transfusion medicine (PROBE-TM) study: a cluster-randomized, matched-paired clinical areas trial of a simple intervention to reduce errors in the pretransfusion bedside check. Transfusion (Paris). 2007;47(5):771–80.

68. Mehra T, Seifert B, Bravo-Reiter S, Wanner G, Dutkowski P, Holubec T, et al. Implementation of a patient blood management monitoring and feedback program significantly reduces trans-fusions and costs. Transfusion (Paris). 2015;55(12):2807–15.
69. LaRocco M, Brient K. Interdisciplinary process improvement for enhancing blood transfusion safety. J Healthc Qual. 2010;32(2):29–34.

Chapter 14
Home Medication Safety and Adherence

Jessica A. Zerillo and Kathleen E. Walsh

Safety

A *medication error* is defined by the Agency for Healthcare Research and Quality (AHRQ) as "any preventable event that may cause or lead to inappropriate medication use or patient harm while the medication is in the control of the health care professional, patient or consumer." [1] Errors occur during drug ordering, dispensing, administering, or monitoring. An *adverse drug event* is an injury resulting from the use of the medication. *Medication adherence* is "the extent to which a person's behavior in taking medications coincides with medical or health advice." [2] In the home setting, nonadherence can be intentional or erroneous. Similarly, medication errors in the home can result in underdosing, overdosing, and missed doses. In children with cancer, any of these possibilities is very serious and can be potentially fatal.

Medication errors can be identified in a variety of ways, including incident reports, medical record reviews, and direct observations (Table 14.1). In the inpatient setting, research on medication errors and adverse events examines all steps in the medication use pathway: ordering, dispensing, administering, and monitoring (see Chap. 10). In the ambulatory setting, medication ordering takes place in a clinic or office, dispensing in an ambulatory or retail pharmacy and administering and monitoring in the clinic or at home (Fig. 14.1).

J.A. Zerillo (✉)
Division of Hematology and Oncology,
Beth Israel Deaconess Medical Center, Boston, MA, USA
e-mail: jzerillo@bidmc.harvard.edu

K.E. Walsh
James M Anderson Center for Health Systems Excellence,
Cincinnati Children's Hospital, Cincinnati, Ohio
e-mail: Kathleen.walsh@cchmc.org

© Springer International Publishing AG 2017
C.E. Dandoy et al. (eds.), *Patient Safety and Quality in Pediatric Hematology/Oncology and Stem Cell Transplantation*, DOI 10.1007/978-3-319-53790-0_14

Table 14.1 Medication error measurement methods

Method	Strengths	Weaknesses
Home visit with direct observation of medication use	Captures the breadth of types of errors which occur	Time and resource intensive Misses some errors with serious harm
Medical record review	Captures errors recorded in chart Efficient	Misses errors parents don't report, doctors don't record Level of detail may not be adequate to ascertain contributing factors
Parent survey	Captures errors parents are aware of and willing to report	Parents may not report or may not know they are making errors
National poison data system	Efficient May capture more serious errors	Level of detail may not be adequate to ascertain contributing factors

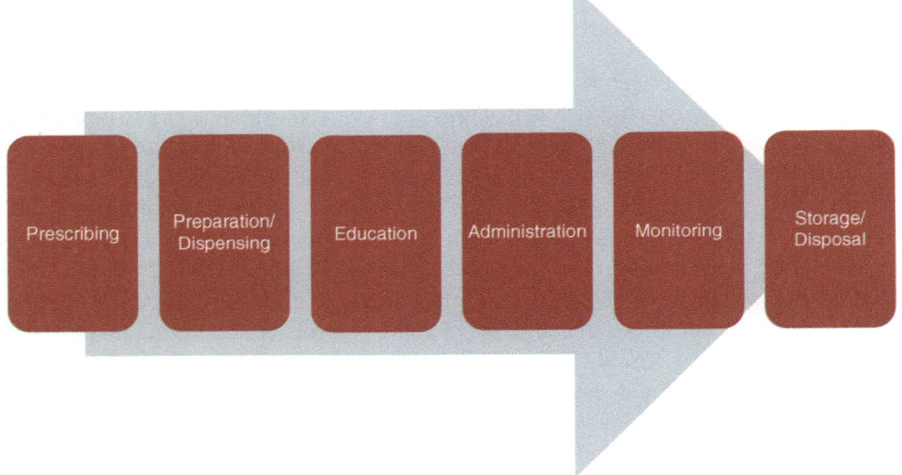

Fig. 14.1 Home medication pathway [3]

Ambulatory pediatric medication use is highly complex due to the use of weight-based dosing, liquid medications [4, 5], the need to cut pills [6], and lack of standardized measurement tools [7, 8]. Published studies on home medication errors employ medical record review (and trigger tools), parent interviews, observed measurements in clinic, home visits, and poison control center data [9–12]. Medical record reviews, sometimes using trigger tools, may detect medication errors at home that the parent or patient reported to the clinical team and that the clinical team recorded in the chart. Parent interviews capture errors parents are aware of and are willing to report; however, parents often are unaware of errors they make [10, 11]. Having parents bring medications to the clinic along with a thorough medication reconciliation process is a good way for clinicians to identify administration errors in their practice, but measurement devices, preparation, and storage of medications will not have been observed. If a parent sprinkles chemotherapy on dinner, for example, that practice will not be detected with this method. Home visits allow direct observation of medication administration in the home, as well as an in-depth understanding of medication storage and support tools used to prevent errors in home medication use. These home visit methods are analogous to direct observation methods used in the hospital, which have been determined to be the most efficient and accurate method to detect nurse administration errors [13–16].

Children are highly vulnerable to dangerous medication errors. Among hospitalized children, the rate of potentially dangerous medication errors is three times that of adults due to the complexity of pediatric medication use [17]. In the ambulatory setting, children take more medication than most people realize: on average, one medication a week [18]. A recent national study of the National Poison Database system indicates that from 2002 to 2012, an average of 63,358 children under 6 years old (one child every 8 min) annually experienced out-of-hospital medication errors [12]. In another study, 3% of pediatric primary care outpatients experienced a preventable adverse event [10].

Caregivers frequently make errors and are not always aware of it. Only half (54%) of parents accurately repeat back the child's medication name and instructions, and half (53%) cannot demonstrate how to measure liquid medications [19, 20]. In calls to poison control centers, the most common medication errors in children were due to giving the same medication twice (presumably due to miscommunication between caregivers), incorrect doses, and confusion about units [9].

Many error-prone processes occur during oral chemotherapy use. These include taking different medications on different days of the week (e.g., trimethoprim/sulfamethoxazole), frequent adjustments in dosing (e.g., 6 mercaptopurine), parent administration [7, 19] use of liquid medicines [8, 21], and cutting or crushing of tablets. In our home visit study, we visited children with cancer who took up to 26 different medications at home; one child took 22.5 oral chemotherapy tablets in a single dose [6–8, 19, 21].

There is little literature on medication errors in the home setting, with only a few studies on oral chemotherapy use among children. Walsh et al. performed a multisite study where she reviewed 117 pediatric and 1262 adult ambulatory medical records for error, using established methods. Children with cancer suffered more than twice as many ambulatory medication errors than adults (18% vs. 7%) [22]. This difference was entirely explained by a very high rate of errors in medications administered at home. Weingart et al. reviewed reports from MedMarx (the medication error reporting program at the United States Pharmacopeia) and from the literature and solicited incident reports from 14 comprehensive cancer centers [23]. The authors identified 99 case reports of injuries due to an oral chemotherapy overdose, including 12 deaths. Taylor et al. asked parents at a single academic health center to bring oral chemotherapy to the clinic and directly observed how parents measured the current doses of their medications [9]. For the 29% of parents who did not bring their medication, the authors provided medication samples to mimic home administration. Of 69 children studied, 19% had at least one medication error, including 10% who were administered the wrong dose, usually due to parents misunderstanding the regimen or measuring incorrectly.

In a multisite study, Walsh et al. directly observed medication use in the home of 92 children with cancer on daily home medications [6]. This study demonstrated very high rates of serious medication error and injuries in the homes of children with cancer. The rate of injuries due to medication error was 3.6%, and 36% of children had serious errors that were not intercepted before reaching the patient.

Walsh et al. also performed a study of home medication use in children with sickle cell disease and epilepsy [24]. The 24 children with sickle cell disease that they visited took 119 medications and experienced 39 errors. The most common errors were missed medication doses (nonadherence) and mistakes administering oral chelation therapy. Errors in the use of non-steroidal anti-inflammatory medications were also common. In this study, parents who used support tools at home for medication use, such as reminders or pill boxes, were significantly less likely to have errors than those who did not. We are aware of no other studies of medication errors in children with sickle cell disease or other hematologic illnesses, such as hemophilia or thalassemia.

In collaboration with parents and clinicians, Walsh et al. developed a home medication support (HoMeS) toolkit to reduce errors in the home care of children with cancer. In a pilot study with 15 parents, the intervention received high marks for usability and acceptability, but the study was underpowered to evaluate its impact on errors [25].

The ordering and dispensing of oral chemotherapy in the ambulatory setting are not subject to the same safety standards as chemotherapy infusions [26, 27]. Standards for oral chemotherapy are written primarily for adult patients, but recent revisions are the first attempts to incorporate pediatrics.

The American Academy of Pediatrics recommends that parents use graduated cups and syringes rather than spoons to measure liquid pediatric medications [28]. In children on liquid medications, color coding and using a marked syringe have been shown to reduce errors. Among 101 parents randomized to determine the dose and measure acetaminophen for their child using a color chart and matching syringe with color lines or a conventional method, there were significantly less errors in the intervention group. In another study of liquid medication use, McMahon et al. found that by demonstrating the dose and providing a syringe with a line marked, the percent of parents who correctly measured the dose improved from 37.5% (verbal instructions only) to 100% [5].

Clinicians use medication calendars to help parents remember which medications and doses are due each day. This is particularly helpful as doses change from day to day. Families also tend to create their own folder containing all the information about their chemotherapy, which some parents referred to as their "medication bible" [29]. Some families used cell phone alerts, excel spreadsheets, pill boxes, and other support tools to prevent errors at home.

In summary, the little available research indicates that medication errors are common in the home care of children with cancer and hematologic conditions, such as sickle cell disease. This is not surprising because children with cancer take many medications at home, with complicated dosing regimens and different forms of medications that must be cut, crushed, or measured in syringes. Children are particularly vulnerable to medication errors due to the complexity of weight-based dosing, stock solutions made for adults, their small size, and other reasons. There is little research testing interventions to prevent errors in home cancer care.

Because of the paucity of literature in this area, there are many opportunities for research and improvement. While it is clear that errors are common and can be dangerous, the types of injuries that occur in home medication use among children with cancer are not well described. The relationship between error and nonadherence has not been well elucidated. This is important because there is a large body of literature both on error prevention in the inpatient setting and on nonadherence in the ambulatory setting. This field could grow upon this work if the relationship between error and nonadherence is elucidated. Finally, interventions need to be developed and systematically tested for the clinic and home setting to prevent errors.

Adherence

The accurate adherence of pediatric hematology/oncology patients to home prescription and nonprescription medications has implications not only for immediate safety but also for long-term outcomes. Underuse or incorrect use can cause recurrence or progression of symptoms or disease. This is most evident with the use of home oral chemotherapy to treat cancer [30].

Epidemiology and the Problem

Pediatric nonadherence is highly prevalent, with long-term oral medication adherence estimated only at 11–83% [31]. A 2002 review found that nonadherence in pediatric patients on oral chemotherapy ranged from 2 to 59% [32], whereas in those with sickle cell disease (SCD), adherence to medications such as antibiotic prophylaxis, iron chelation, and hydroxyurea are 16–89% [33]. There is a long-standing concern for even greater problems with adherence in adolescents [34].

Potential risk factors for pediatric hematology/oncology nonadherence include low-income status [35, 36] and being of older or adolescent age [37, 38]. Conversely, low family stress and satisfaction with the home care regimen are associated with better adherence [39]. In cancer patients, lower adherence is associated with older age, particularly adolescents, time on therapy and number of children in the family [40]. Specifically, in acute lymphoblastic leukemia (ALL), risk factors include being Hispanic, African American, or Asian American, age ≥ 12 years, and being from a single-mother household [41, 42]. Nonadherence in international ALL patients is associated with low socioeconomic and education status, large family size, and high cost for visits [43].

Though nonadherence is prevalent, it is not routinely assessed in a reliable and standardized way. A study of American Society of Pediatric Hematology/Oncology members found that adherence to hydroxyurea in the treatment of SCD was primarily assessed by clinicians using patient and parent interviews (84%) and laboratory levels (70–75%); however, the majority used informal methods [44].

How to Measure Threshold for Adherence and How that Impacts Rates

There is no standardized way to measure adherence nor universal cutoff of what level of adherence is necessary. Depending on the specific disease being treated or prevented, the necessary threshold of adherence to obtain clinical benefit may differ. Additionally, the side effect profile for medications taken at home, from acetaminophen to hydroxyurea, can vary widely, and impact of nonadherence varies depending on the drug used.

There are a variety of methods to measure adherence, along a spectrum from those that rely on patient/family report to those that are more objective, such as direct observation (Table 14.2) [45–47]. While retrospective patient/family report has traditionally been used in clinical practice, there are tools that may improve the accuracy of these self-reports or even adherence itself, including medication diaries [48–51]. Pill and liquid counts allow for providers to assess whether the correct amount of medication has been taken over a given time period. Monitoring through the Medication Event Monitoring System (MEMS) caps has been used in research but is not yet regularly deployed in practice. Other options for adherence assessment include using insurance claims to calculate medication possession ratios and metabolite or drug levels [43, 46, 52–54].

The disadvantage of patient/family report is that it may underestimate nonadherence. The disadvantages of pill counts are that they can be more expensive and do not allow for an assessment of daily adherence to scheduled doses. There are not yet MEMS caps to capture liquid medication use, which make up a large proportion of pediatric home medication drugs. Directly observed therapy (DOT), which has frequently been utilized for tuberculosis and human immunodeficiency virus (HIV) therapies, requires even further resources and is not practical for every patient and every medication. Additionally, DOT alters the environment in which medications are taken and is thus not only a measurement tool but, due to the Hawthorne effect, is itself an intervention. Though considered one of the more objective sources for adherence, metabolite levels may be influenced by biological heterogeneity [55]. As they may be more sensitive in identifying nonadherence, pharmacy prescriptions are also nonspecific and therefore provide an overestimate.

Multiple methods used simultaneously are recommended to understand the true rate of adherence in a population [39]. While different methods may identify

Table 14.2 Adherence measurement methods by reliability

Low reliability	Moderate reliability	High reliability
Medical record note review	Verbal self-report (e.g., Morisky score)	Level and metabolite testing
Clinician prescription review	Written self-report (e.g., diary)	Video-observed therapy
	Pharmacy fill data	Directly observed therapy
	Insurance claims data	
	Pill or liquid count	
	Microelectronic monitoring systems	
	Treatment response	

different rates of adherence and thus may not give a "true" value of adherence, each may be useful for benchmarking and monitoring for change in adherence overtime within and across populations. It is controversial whether the best current tool to stand alone as a measurement of adherence is serum and urine testing or the MEMS cap. For those drugs without serum and urine testing available, the widespread use of the MEMS cap is currently limited by cost [56, 57]. Such devices are increasingly allowing now only for monitoring but also for reminding and alerting functionality.

Studies have applied the described methods of measurement to assess baseline adherence in hematology/oncology pediatric patients with SCD, hemophilia, iron deficiency anemia, and ALL. Notably, many of these studies have occurred outside of the United States. Using MEMS caps and metabolite levels in patients with hematologic malignancies, mostly with acute ALL, adherence has been variable, between 7 and 98% [38, 42, 53]. There is less information about pediatric patients with other forms of cancer, with the only study not using self-report by Tebbi et al., citing adherence as 60.5% [40]. For patients with hemophilia and SCD, studies have found adherence of 34% [58] and 49–85% [59, 60] respectively. Similar efforts are needed to fill gaps in understanding adherence in other populations including bone marrow transplant, solid tumor and other heme-malignancy cancer patients, as well as those with other benign hematologic disorders.

The adherence measurement tools are likely complementary to one another, and multiple methods of assessment should be used in each adherence study. A study of 39 patients on maintenance therapy for ALL identified nonadherence through interviews with parents, a medical record chart review, and drug metabolite levels. Thirteen of the 21 nonadherent patients were identified through only one of these methods and only two through all three [35]. In another study, self-report and metabolite noncompliance was only 66.7% concordant [37].

Unfortunately, available studies have applied various measurement tools and cut-offs for adherence. There is a need for research to standardize what adherence methods are most reliable and effective. If serum or urine testing is used, clearly defined levels with sensitivity and specificity for optional adherence to achieve a desired clinical endpoint need to be determined.

Summary of Findings

Though adherence is not routinely assessed in a reliable and standardized way, the available literature suggests a need for adherence improvement in pediatric hematology/oncology patients. This literature also emphasizes the need to examine effects of adherence on patient outcomes. Adherence of patients with SCD has been associated with better health-related quality of life [60], whereas other studies have not shown a difference in hospitalizations with antibiotic prophylaxis for these patients [51]. And while one adherence study of patients with hemophilia did not show an impact on major bleeding events or hospitalizations [58], it was associated with less chronic pain in another [61]. In the most recent convincing evidence for outcomes influenced by adherence, Bhatia et al. identified a 3.9 times greater risk of recurrence with adherence of less than 90% for patients with ALL [42].

Interventions and Improvement Strategies

Interventions to improve adherence in pediatric hematology/oncology are desperately needed; however, few have been done and only rarely have they been evaluated with vigorous methodology.

Despite the fact that ALL is the most common pediatric malignancy, with convincing data on the importance of high adherence levels, interventions have not been targeted to this population. Most interventions have been in SCD and anemia, with only one vigorous study as a randomized control trial in patients with malignancy.

Published interventions, particularly in anemia, have generally been in low-resource settings and when they used people, utilized non-clinicians, such as trained volunteers. Similar work was done using social workers providing information sessions explaining the pathogenesis and complications from SCD as well as conducting weekly phone calls and providing a calendar to patients on penicillin [51]. Other interventions included a combination of education; reminder devices, such as text messaging; incentives; and modified treatment schedules. One study of patients with SCD used text-messaging reminders [52]. In the case of patients with malignancy, a video game was used to try to improve adherence for pediatric patients on oral chemotherapy and antibiotics [62].

As drug delivery (oral versus injectable) and side effect profiles may alter adherence for the pediatric hematology/oncology population, changing drug delivery has also been used to attempt to improve adherence [63]. The creative design of drug delivery, to meet patients existing needs and align with their home and school processes, may help to improve adherence. One example is overnight disposable pumps for desferrioxamine to meet the needs of teenage thalassemia patients requiring chelation therapy [64]. Some studies have demonstrated improved adherence and outcomes with flexible scheduling. This may be appropriate for some conditions and drugs, such as the use of iron in iron deficiency anemia [65] or adolescents being treated with prophylaxis for hemophilia [66].

The ambulatory use of medications and the need to ensure adherence are long-standing problems in other populations. Within pediatrics, this has been a problem faced by those in infectious disease, particularly in regard to care for patients with HIV disease. Ensuring adherence has been an issue in adults, specifically for medications related to chronic diseases such as diabetes and hypertension and anticoagulation management. Within the general adult adherence literature, interventions have been multidimensional, and none has stood out as a clear best practice [67]. Oral chemotherapy for adult cancer patients is a growing need for which the intervention research is not yet clear, and practices are also still struggling to even measure adherence [68].

Summary and Next Steps

There is a paucity of data on adherence interventions in pediatric hematology/oncology, particularly for those with cancer. Understanding the mechanisms that drive nonadherence is of primary importance before the development of interventions to promote adherence. To understand the drivers of nonadherence, it is necessary to understand the patient and family perspective. These perspectives and their associated interventions will vary depending on the age and developmental status of the child and adolescent.

Even reverting back to parenteral therapy in the controlled clinical environment may be necessary to treat those select patient populations requiring more urgent therapy or with high nonadherence risk [69]. This may be necessary until there are more robust systems to support adherence of home medications in pediatric hematology/oncology. Such systems may require the creative integration and engagement of home care services and community programs to support patients and their caregivers.

Opportunities for Research and Improvement

While there has been a growing literature on pediatric hematology/oncology adherence, there are still many populations where we are without an understanding of baseline adherence rates, unanswered questions about ideal adherence, and, most importantly, a need for further work to identify the interventions that are most successful. The changing location of care from inpatient and the clinic to the home and the changing providers of this care from clinical teams to families leave these patients vulnerable. New systems are needed to meet this need and ensure standardization of adherence programs.

A better understanding of patient, parent, and caregiver needs to improve adherence to home medications in hematology/oncology is needed. It is necessary to understand the patient perspective, particularly for adolescents, in order to design interventions and processes that promote adherence. Additional research to identify risk factors and causes for nonadherence for adolescents and then interventions targeting those at highest risk for severe nonadherence are particularly needed.

We need to identify the causes and treatments of nonadherence beyond the traditional research setting in order to implement changes that are effective and practical in the real world. Observational studies and modeling that describe risks and reasons for nonadherence, as well as descriptions of situations when adherence is high, could be used to design interventions that facilitate adherence through embedding successful processes in patients' and families' usual workflow [70]. For example, as one study in ALL found that patients were more adherent with evening than morning doses [71], evening could be explored as the time to encourage medication scheduling. Implementation science researches and system engineers may be particularly valuable collaborators as these new home medication systems are designed.

It is both a challenge and an opportunity that there are a multitude of stakeholders involved in home medication adherence. Thinking creatively how to integrate specialty pharmacies, visiting nurses, caretakers, and schools as well as how to reintegrate nursing into patient care may help to spread the burden of resources needed for interventions to be scalable and sustainable. Outside of research, national professional and patient organizations should lead in developing standards and guidelines and allow for sharing of best practices across organizations. Quality improvement efforts at the institutional and practice level may then be used to address local needs.

With the growth of home medications to treat pediatric hematology/oncology patients, ensuring adherence is a problem that will only grow. By helping to design interventions and processes within the home and ambulatory setting, the traditional clinical care team can assist the growing care team of patients and families in improving adherence.

Conclusions

There is little research on medication adherence in the homes of children with hematologic/oncologic conditions and less on errors in home medication use. There is a need for rigorous evaluations of interventions to support home care. The relationship between errors and nonadherence in children is unclear. It is possible that some nonadherence is unintentional and due to error. Similarly, some patients who experience errors may also be nonadherent. Improvement in medication adherence when patients do not understand how to use their medications may paradoxically increase rates of errors. The relationship between these two types of problems needs to be elucidated. In addition, since errors and nonadherence likely coexist in the same patient population, in the same clinical setting, interventions that address both errors and nonadherence should be developed and tested.

Sidebar: A 13-Year-Old with Leukemia [72]

A 13-year-old male child was diagnosed with acute lymphoblastic leukemia. The patient attended private and group educational sessions with his mother about his diagnosis and treatment. He was treated with vincristine and prednisone and maintenance therapy with daily 6-mercaptopurine, weekly methotrexate, and prednisone daily for 28 days every fourth of the month. The patient was distressed by the side effects he experienced—hair loss, weight gain, and facial puffiness.

Approximately 2 years later, the child experienced a relapse. In a meeting with his parents and doctors, the patient described that he had only taken his medications intermittently during the recent months. The 15-year-old was then treated as an outpatient with vincristine and prednisone and, after his bone marrow continued to show disease, was admitted for inpatient therapy, at which point he achieved remission.

A urine test for prednisone compliance showed that the adolescent was not adherent to the regimen during the maintenance phase or the initial reinduction attempt. Were there any demographic, disease, or treatment characteristics that could have alerted this patient's providers that he was at high risk of nonadherence? If he was at high risk, are there any proven interventions available to reduce the risk of nonadherence? Was there any way to pick up this nonadherence sooner and intervene on it? These are all questions that need answers.

Sidebar: Nursing Verification of Pediatric Oral Chemotherapy [73]

At the Dana-Farber/Boston Children's Cancer and Blood Disorders Clinic, a program was initiated in 2015 to incorporate verification of oral chemotherapy prescription orders as well as a standardized nursing education [74]. The mean time required for verification was 12.4 min (SD 10.1) per nurse. In over 110 prescription verifications, there were three good catches identified by nurses—an 80% underdose of everolimus, an incorrect pill number and dose of everolimus, and a 22 mL instead of a 2.2 mL dose of cyclophosphamide. The program was expanded in 2016 to include standardized nursing teaching for new oral chemotherapy starts [74].

References

1. Department of Health and Human Services. Advancing Patient Safety Implementation through Safety Medication Use Research (R18). http://grants.nih.gov/grants/guide/pa-files/PA-14-002.html.
2. Hasford J. Compliance and the benefit/risk relationship of antihypertensive treatment. J Cardiovasc Pharmacol. 1992;20 Suppl 6:S30–4.
3. Zerillo JA, Goldenberg BA, Kotecha RR, Tewari A, Kryzanowska MK, Jacobson JO. Interventions to improve oral chemotherapy safety and quality: a systematic and grey literature review. J Clin Oncol. 2017;35(suppl 8S): Abstract 97.
4. Yin HS, Dreyer BP, Foltin G, van Schaick L, Mendelsohn AL. Association of low caregiver health literacy with reported use of nonstandardized dosing instruments and lack of knowledge of weight-based dosing. Ambul Pediatr. 2007;7(4):292–8.
5. Frush KS, Luo X, Hutchinson P, Higgins JN. Evaluation of a method to reduce over-the-counter medication dosing error. Arch Pediatr Adolesc Med. 2004;158(7):620–4.
6. Walsh KE, Roblin DW, Weingart SN, Houlahan KE, Degar B, Billett A, et al. Medication errors in the home: a multisite study of children with cancer. Pediatrics. 2013;131(5):e1405–14.
7. Yin HS, Mendelsohn AL, Wolf MS, Parker RM, Fierman A, van Schaick L, et al. Parents' medication administration errors: role of dosing instruments and health literacy. Arch Pediatr Adolesc Med. 2010;164(2):181–6.
8. Yin HS, Wolf MS, Dreyer BP, Sanders LM, Parker RM. Evaluation of consistency in dosing directions and measuring devices for pediatric nonprescription liquid medications. JAMA. 2010;304(23):2595–602.
9. Taylor JA, Winter L, Geyer LJ, Hawkins DS. Oral outpatient chemotherapy medication errors in children with acute lymphoblastic leukemia. Cancer. 2006;107(6):1400–6.

10. Kaushal R, Goldmann DA, Keohane CA, Christino M, Honour M, Hale AS, et al. Adverse drug events in pediatric outpatients. Ambul Pediatr. 2007;7(5):383–9.
11. Weingart SN, Spencer J, Buia S, Duncombe D, Singh P, Gadkari M, et al. Medication safety of five oral chemotherapies: a proactive risk assessment. Journal of oncology practice/American Society of Clinical Oncology. 2011;7(1):2–6.
12. Smith MD, Spiller HA, Casavant MJ, Chounthirath T, Brophy TJ, Xiang H. Out-of-hospital medication errors among young children in the United States, 2002-2012. Pediatrics. 2014;134(5):867–76.
13. Flynn EA, Barker KN, Pepper GA, Bates DW, Mikeal RL. Comparison of methods for detecting medication errors in 36 hospitals and skilled-nursing facilities. Am J Health Syst Pharm. 2002;59(5):436–46.
14. Landrigan CP, Rothschild JM, Cronin JW, Kaushal R, Burdick E, Katz JT, et al. Effect of reducing interns' work hours on serious medical errors in intensive care units. N Engl J Med. 2004;351(18):1838–48.
15. Buckley MS, Erstad BL, Kopp BJ, Theodorou AA, Priestley G. Direct observation approach for detecting medication errors and adverse drug events in a pediatric intensive care unit. Pediatr Crit Care Med. 2007;8(2):145–52.
16. Walsh KE, Stille CJ, Mazor KM, Gurwitz JH. Using home visits to understand medication errors in children. In: Henriksen K, Battles JB, Keyes MA, Grady ML, editors. Advances in patient safety: new directions and alternative approaches (Vol 4: Technology and medication safety). Rockville: Advances in Patient Safety; 2008.
17. Kaushal R, Bates DW, Landrigan C, McKenna KJ, Clapp MD, Federico F, et al. Medication errors and adverse drug events in pediatric inpatients. JAMA. 2001;285(16):2114–20.
18. Vernacchio L, Kelly JP, Kaufman DW, Mitchell AA. Medication use among children <12 years of age in the United States: results from the Slone survey. Pediatrics. 2009;124(2):446–54.
19. McMahon SR, Rimsza ME, Bay RC. Parents can dose liquid medication accurately. Pediatrics. 1997;100(3 Pt 1):330–3.
20. Moon RY, Cheng TL, Patel KM, Baumhaft K, Scheidt PC. Parental literacy level and understanding of medical information. Pediatrics. 1998;102(2):e25.
21. Li SF, Lathcer B, Crain EF. Acetaminophen and ibuprofen dosing by parents. Pediatr Emerg Care. 2000;16:394–7.
22. Walsh KE, Dodd KS, Seetharaman K, Roblin DW, Herrinton LJ, Von Worley A, et al. Medication errors among adults and children with cancer in the outpatient setting. Journal of clinical oncology : official journal of the American Society of Clinical Oncology. 2009;27(6):891–6.
23. Weingart SN, Toro J, Spencer J, Duncombe D, Gross A, Bartel S, et al. Medication errors involving oral chemotherapy. Cancer. 2010;116(10):2455–64.
24. Walsh KE, Mazor KM, Stille CJ, Torres I, Wagner JL, Moretti J, et al. Medication errors in the homes of children with chronic conditions. Arch Dis Child. 2011;96(6):581–6.
25. Walsh KE, Biggins C, Blasko D, Christiansen SM, Fischer SH, Keuker C, et al. Home medication support for childhood cancer: family-centered design and testing. Journal of oncology practice / American Society of Clinical Oncology. 2014;10(6):373–6.
26. Weingart SN, Brown E, Bach PB, Eng K, Johnson SA, Kuzel TM, et al. NCCN task force report: oral chemotherapy. Journal of the National Comprehensive Cancer Network : JNCCN. 2008;6(Suppl 3):S1–14.
27. Weingart SN, Flug J, Brouillard D, Morway L, Partridge A, Bartel S, et al. Oral chemotherapy safety practices at US cancer centres: questionnaire survey. BMJ. 2007;334(7590):407.
28. American Academy of Pediatrics. Don't use household spoons for liquid medicines. http://www.aappublications.org/content/36/4/26.5. Published: 3/30/2015, Accessed: 6 Dec 2016.
29. Walsh KE, Mazor KM, Roblin D, Biggins C, Wagner JL, Houlahan K, et al. Multisite parent-centered risk assessment to reduce pediatric oral chemotherapy errors. Journal of oncology practice / American Society of Clinical Oncology. 2013;9(1):e1–7.
30. Lilleyman JS, Lennard L. Non-compliance with oral chemotherapy in childhood leukaemia. BMJ. 1996;313(7067):1219–20.
31. Davies HA, Lilleyman JS. Compliance with oral chemotherapy in childhood lymphoblastic leukaemia. Cancer Treat Rev. 1995;21(2):93–103.

32. Partridge AH, Avorn J, Wang PS, Winer EP. Adherence to therapy with oral antineoplastic agents. J Natl Cancer Inst. 2002;94(9):652–61.
33. Walsh KE, Cutrona SL, Kavanagh PL, Crosby LE, Malone C, Lobner K, et al. Medication adherence among pediatric patients with sickle cell disease: a systematic review. Pediatrics. 2014;134(6):1175–83.
34. Ruddy K, Mayer E, Partridge A. Patient adherence and persistence with oral anticancer treatment. CA Cancer J Clin. 2009;59(1):56–66.
35. de Oliveira BM, Viana MB, Zani CL, Romanha AJ. Clinical and laboratory evaluation of compliance in acute lymphoblastic leukaemia. Arch Dis Child. 2004;89(8):785–8.
36. Lee WS, Toh TH, Chai PF, Soo TL. Self-reported level of and factors influencing the compliance to desferrioxamine therapy in multitransfused thalassaemias. J Paediatr Child Health. 2011;47(8):535–40.
37. Hawwa AF, Millership JS, Collier PS, McCarthy A, Dempsey S, Cairns C, et al. The development of an objective methodology to measure medication adherence to oral thiopurines in paediatric patients with acute lymphoblastic leukaemia--an exploratory study. Eur J Clin Pharmacol. 2009;65(11):1105–12.
38. Smith SD, Rosen D, Trueworthy RC, Lowman JT. A reliable method for evaluating drug compliance in children with cancer. Cancer. 1979;43(1):169–73.
39. Treadwell MJ, Law AW, Sung J, Hackney-Stephens E, Quirolo K, Murray E, et al. Barriers to adherence of deferoxamine usage in sickle cell disease. Pediatr Blood Cancer. 2005;44(5):500–7.
40. Tebbi CK, Cummings KM, Zevon MA, Smith L, Richards M, Mallon J. Compliance of pediatric and adolescent cancer patients. Cancer. 1986;58(5):1179–84.
41. Bhatia S, Landier W, Shangguan M, Hageman L, Schaible AN, Carter AR, et al. Nonadherence to oral mercaptopurine and risk of relapse in Hispanic and non-Hispanic white children with acute lymphoblastic leukemia: a report from the children's oncology group. Journal of clinical oncology : official journal of the American Society of Clinical Oncology. 2012;30(17):2094–101.
42. Bhatia S, Landier W, Hageman L, Kim H, Chen Y, Crews KR, et al. 6MP adherence in a multiracial cohort of children with acute lymphoblastic leukemia: a Children's oncology group study. Blood. 2014;124(15):2345–53.
43. Khalek ER, Sherif LM, Kamal NM, Gharib AF, Shawky HM. Acute lymphoblastic leukemia: are Egyptian children adherent to maintenance therapy? J Cancer Res Ther. 2015;11(1):54–8.
44. Brandow AM, Panepinto JA. Monitoring toxicity, impact, and adherence of hydroxyurea in children with sickle cell disease. Am J Hematol. 2011;86(9):804–6.
45. Kruske SG, Ruben AR, Brewster DR. An iron treatment trial in an aboriginal community: improving non-adherence. J Paediatr Child Health. 1999;35(2):153–8.
46. Creary SE, Gladwin MT, Byrne M, Hildesheim M, Krishnamurti L. A pilot study of electronic directly observed therapy to improve hydroxyurea adherence in pediatric patients with sickle-cell disease. Pediatr Blood Cancer. 2014;61(6):1068–73.
47. Bharti S. Feasibility of "directly observed home-based twice-daily iron therapy" (DOHBIT) for management of anemia in rural patients: a pilot study. Indian J Med Sci. 2004;58(10):431–8.
48. De Moerloose P, Urbancik W, Van Den Berg HM, Richards M. A survey of adherence to haemophilia therapy in six European countries: results and recommendations. Haemophilia. 2008;14(5):931–8.
49. Thornburg CD, Pipe SW. Adherence to prophylactic infusions of factor VIII or factor IX for haemophilia. Haemophilia. 2006;12(2):198–9.
50. Alvarez O, Rodriguez-Cortes H, Robinson N, Lewis N, Pow Sang CD, Lopez-Mitnik G, et al. Adherence to deferasirox in children and adolescents with sickle cell disease during 1-year of therapy. J Pediatr Hematol Oncol. 2009;31(10):739–44.
51. Berkovitch M, Papadouris D, Shaw D, Onuaha N, Dias C, Olivieri NF. Trying to improve compliance with prophylactic penicillin therapy in children with sickle cell disease. Br J Clin Pharmacol. 1998;45(6):605–7.
52. Estepp JH, Winter B, Johnson M, Smeltzer MP, Howard SC, Hankins JS. Improved hydroxyurea effect with the use of text messaging in children with sickle cell anemia. Pediatr Blood Cancer. 2014;61(11):2031–6.
53. Lancaster D, Lennard L, Lilleyman JS. Profile of non-compliance in lymphoblastic leukaemia. Arch Dis Child. 1997;76(4):365–6.

54. Al-Kloub MI, MA AB, Al Khawaldeh OA, Al Tawarah YM, Froelicher ES. Predictors of non-adherence to follow-up visits and deferasirox chelation therapy among jordanian adolescents with thalassemia major. Pediatr Hematol Oncol. 2014;31(7):624–37.
55. Gaynon PS. Treatment adherence and 6-mercaptopurine metabolites. Pediatr Blood Cancer. 2006;46(2):120–1.
56. Rohan JM, Drotar D, Alderfer M, Donewar CW, Ewing L, Katz ER, et al. Electronic monitoring of medication adherence in early maintenance phase treatment for pediatric leukemia and lymphoma: identifying patterns of nonadherence. J Pediatr Psychol. 2015;40(1):75–84.
57. Martin S, Elliott-DeSorbo DK, Calabrese S, Wolters PL, Roby G, Brennan T, et al. A comparison of adherence assessment methods utilized in the United States: perspectives of researchers, HIV-infected children, and their caregivers. AIDS Patient Care STDs. 2009;23(8):593–601.
58. Armstrong EP, Malone DC, Krishnan S, Wessler MJ. Adherence to clotting factors among persons with hemophilia a or B. Hematology. 2015;20(3):148–53.
59. Thornburg CD, Calatroni A, Telen M, Kemper AR. Adherence to hydroxyurea therapy in children with sickle cell anemia. J Pediatr. 2010;156(3):415–9.
60. Al Jaouni SK, Al Muhayawi MS, Halawa TF, Al Mehayawi MS. Treatment adherence and quality of life outcomes in patients with sickle cell disease. Saudi Med J. 2013;34(3):261–5.
61. McLaughlin JM, Witkop ML, Lambing A, Anderson TL, Munn J, Tortella B. Better adherence to prescribed treatment regimen is related to less chronic pain among adolescents and young adults with moderate or severe haemophilia. Haemophilia. 2014;20(4):506–12.
62. Kato PM, Cole SW, Bradlyn AS, Pollock BH. A video game improves behavioral outcomes in adolescents and young adults with cancer: a randomized trial. Pediatrics. 2008;122(2):e305–17.
63. Afzal M, Qureshi SM, Lutafullah M, Iqbal M, Sultan M, Khan SA. Comparative study of efficacy, tolerability and compliance of oral iron preparations (iron edetae, iron polymatose complex) and intramuscular iron sorbitol in iron deficiency anaemia in children. J Pak Med Assoc. 2009;59(11):764–8.
64. Lombardo T, Frontini V, Ferro G, Sergi P, Guidice A, Lombardo G. Laboratory evaluation of a new delivery system to improve patient compliance with chelation therapy. Clin Lab Haematol. 1996;18(1):13–7.
65. Ip H, Hyder SM, Haseen F, Rahman M, Zlotkin SH. Improved adherence and anaemia cure rates with flexible administration of micronutrient sprinkles: a new public health approach to anaemia control. Eur J Clin Nutr. 2009;63(2):165–72.
66. Khair K, Gibson F, Meerabeau L. The benefits of prophylaxis: views of adolescents with severe haemophilia. Haemophilia. 2012;18(3):e286–9.
67. Nieuwlaat R, Wilczynski N, Navarro T, Hobson N, Jeffery R, Keepanasseril A, et al. Interventions for enhancing medication adherence. Cochrane Database Syst Rev. 2014;11:CD000011.
68. Zerillo JA, Pham TH, Kadlubek P, Severson JA, Mackler E, Jacobson JO, et al. Administration of oral chemotherapy: results from three rounds of the quality oncology practice initiative. Journal of oncology practice / American Society of Clinical Oncology. 2015;11(2):e255–62.
69. Wali YA, Taqi A, Deghaidi A. Study of intermittent intravenous deferrioxamine high-dose therapy in heavily iron-loaded children with beta-thalassemia major poorly compliant to subcutaneous injections. Pediatr Hematol Oncol. 2004;21(5):453–60.
70. Valdez RS, Holden RJ, Novak LL, Veinot TC. Transforming consumer health informatics through a patient work framework: connecting patients to context. J Am Med Inform Assoc. 2015;22(1):2–10.
71. Lau RC, Matsui D, Greenberg M, Koren G. Electronic measurement of compliance with mercaptopurine in pediatric patients with acute lymphoblastic leukemia. Med Pediatr Oncol. 1998;30(2):85–90.
72. Smith SD, Cairns NU, Sturgeon JK, Lansky SB. Poor drug compliance in an adolescent with leukemia. Am J Pediatr Hematol Oncol. 1981;3(3):297–300.
73. Zerillo JA, Santacroce E, Zimmerman MA, Freeman M, Lau Greenberg T, Nguyen P, Chi SN, Bandopadhayay P, Lane S, Szabatura A, Houlahan K, Billett A. Building a new process: nursing verification of pediatric oral chemotherapy. J Clin Oncol 2016;34 (suppl 7S; abstr 199).
74. Santacroce E. Standardizing nursing education for ambulatory pediatric oncology patients. 48th Congress of the International Society of Paediatric Oncology, October 19-22, 2016. Dublin, Ireland.

Chapter 15
Implementation of Evidence-Based Care in Pediatric Hematology/Oncology Practice

Eric J. Werner and Dana E. Ramirez

Timely Antibiotic Administration in Febrile Immunocompromised Patients

Febrile illnesses are a common part of a child's life and, in the vast majority of instances, do not represent life-threatening illness. Within the pediatric hematology/oncology community, however, there are several populations who have an increased risk for life-threatening infection, in particular, those with neutropenia, functional or anatomic asplenia, and central venous catheters. When such patients present with fever, it is often to facilities that manage large numbers of febrile children, only a small proportion of which have these risk factors, so processes need to be implemented, monitored, and improved to achieve rapid patient evaluation and treatment for this population.

E.J. Werner, MD, MMM (✉)
Chief Medical Quality Officer and Member, Division of Pediatric Hematology/Oncology, Children's Specialty Group, Norfolk, VA, USA

Co-Chief Medical Information Officer, Children's Hospital of The King's Daughters, Norfolk, VA, USA

Professor of Pediatrics, Eastern Virginia Medical School, Norfolk, VA, USA
e-mail: Eric.werner@chkd.org

D.E. Ramirez, MD
Director, Pediatric Residency, Associate Professor of Pediatrics, Eastern Virginia Medical School, Norfolk, VA, USA

Associate Medical Director for Quality and Patient Safety, Children's Hospital of The King's Daughters, Norfolk, VA, USA

Member, Division of Pediatric Emergency Medicine, Children's Specialty Group, Norfolk, VA, USA
e-mail: dana.ramirez@chkd.org

© Springer International Publishing AG 2017
C.E. Dandoy et al. (eds.), *Patient Safety and Quality in Pediatric Hematology/Oncology and Stem Cell Transplantation*, DOI 10.1007/978-3-319-53790-0_15

Time to Antibiotics in Pediatric Cancer Patients with Febrile Neutropenia

Populations and Locations of QI Projects

Factors other than the absolute neutrophil count alone contribute to a patient's risk for bacteremia. While a risk stratification tool has become standard for adult patients with fever and neutropenia, it has several components that make it not applicable for a pediatric population [1]. There have been many stratification tools aimed at the pediatric population validated and reported, but none has yet been found to have reliability across a broad range of clinical environments [2]. Hence, most of the quality improvement projects to date have not separated "high-risk" from "low-risk" febrile neutropenia patients.

There are three locations where time to antibiotic administration can be analyzed; the emergency department, the ambulatory oncology clinic, and inpatient areas. Time from initial fever, which is usually in the home, until antibiotic administration would be a worthwhile target for reduction. Some issues affecting this time have been described [3]. However, other than patient/family education, most of these are currently out of control of the health system. Therefore, majority of the literature thus far available on time to antibiotics (TTA) in pediatric hematology/oncology patients has been from quality improvement projects within emergency departments, inpatient units, and/or ambulatory clinics.

Goals and Outcomes of QI Projects

Based on adult guidelines, a goal of less than 1 h for administration of antibiotics in febrile, immunocompromised pediatric patients is widely cited [4]. Some recent pediatric data supports this goal time frame. Using a composite adverse event outcome measure (in-hospital mortality, PICU admission, and/or fluid resuscitation), Fletcher et al. found that febrile neutropenic cancer patients who had a time to antibiotics (TTA) of 61–120 min had an increased odds ratio of this adverse outcome when compared to those who received antibiotics in ≤60 min [5]. Looking at a similar population treated in an ambulatory pediatric oncology clinic, Salstrom et al. analyzed the outcomes of 143 patients who had a TTA <60 min to 77 patients with a TTA over 60 min and found a 20% decrease in ICU admissions [6]. They also found one death in the shorter TTA group compared with three in the longer group.

The comparative TTA in reported febrile neutropenia quality improvement studies is shown in Table 15.1 [6–17]. There was an 53% decrease in the average TTA reported in these studies. Seven of the projects achieved the goal of ≤60 min, and three additional institutions were within 10 min of this goal. The majority of quality improvement interventional studies were performed in the emergency department. While the inclusion criteria, such as the definition of neutropenia, vary within these reports, many share quality improvement methods (Table 15.2). For instance, these include standardized processes such as algorithms and/or clinical pathways, multidisciplinary involvement in design, standardized patient/parent/caregiver and staff education, and sharing of data with key stakeholders. Iterative process improvement trials using the plan-do-study-act approach have been utilized [8]. Common factors delaying TTA included failure to rapidly identify and triage at-risk patients; time for laboratory

Table 15.1 Time to antibiotics (TTA) in pediatric cancer patients with febrile neutropenia

Author	Year	Location	TTA before QI process (Min)	TTA after QI process (Min)	Percent decrease
Amado [7]	2011	PICU	164	55	66%
Pakakasam [14]	2011	ED	180	75	58%
Burry [10]	2012	ED	216	Not stated	–
Volpe [8]	2012	ED	99	49	51%
Dobrasz [13]	2013	ED1	103	44	57%
Dobrasz [13]	2013	ED2	141	61	57%
Cash [11]	2014	ED	154	95	38%
Vedi [15]	2014	ED1	148	76	49%
Vedi [15]	2014	ED2	221	65	71%
Cohen [12]	2015	ED	97	64	34%
Salstrom [6]	2015	Hem/Onc Clinic	134	54	60%
Jobson [9]	2015	ED	65	30	54%
Dandoy [17]	2016	ED	137	<50	>63%
Green [16]	2016	Inpatient	99	50	49%

Table 15.2 Quality improvement techniques to reduce time to antibiotics in febrile neutropenic pediatric cancer patients	
	Clinical practice guidelines or management algorithm
	Multidisciplinary involvement in process design
	Data sharing with key stakeholders
	Staff and patient/parent/caregiver education
	Process improvement methodology such as Lean
	"Sign and hold" orders
	Release of auto-diff results without manual confirmation
	Rapid identification and triage of at-risk patients
	Availability of antibiotics near the patient treatment areas
	Patient/parent/caregiver application of topical anesthetic cream prior to arrival in clinic
	Documentation and discussion of an inpatient patient-specific fever plan

results, primarily absolute neutrophil counts, to complete; delays in obtaining antibiotic orders; and/or availability of the antibiotic for infusion [6, 8, 9]. Examples of process improvements used to overcome such obstacles include tools to rapidly identify at-risk patients [8, 13, 17], having parents apply topical anesthetic cream prior to ED arrival [6], not waiting for blood count results to start antibiotics in selected patient groups [12], and maintaining a stock of antibiotics in the treatment area [9].

Time to Antibiotics in Other Pediatric Hematology/Oncology Populations

The incidence of bacteremia in febrile children with sickle cell disease has been reported to be as high as 3–5% [18]. The rate may be lower now due to vaccination against *Streptococcus pneumoniae* and *Haemophilus influenzae* and the use of prophylactic penicillin in young children with sickle cell disease. Still, bacteremia is still a major concern in this population [18, 19]. While to our knowledge, there are no studies that look at time to antibiotic versus clinical outcome in febrile sickle cell disease patients, administration of parenteral broad spectrum antibiotics in less than 60 min to febrile sickle cell disease patients has been identified as a quality indicator of high importance for this disorder [20]. Quality improvement studies for time to antibiotics are lacking in this population but have been done for time to pain medication [21, 22].

Using a series of interventions in a population of febrile pediatric patients with central venous catheters in a pediatric academic emergency department, Jobson et al. increased the percentage who had a TTA <60 min from 66 to 99%, sustained for over 2 years, and decreased the mean TTA from a mean of 65 to 30 min. Of note, a baseline racial disparity in the TTA disappeared after these interventions. Key components identified included standardized processes, patient identification cards, and communication of the data with providers and staff [9].

Sepsis in the Hematology/Oncology Patient

Defining Sepsis

As mentioned previously, there is a population of hematology/oncology patients, specifically those with neutropenia, functional or anatomic asplenia, or central venous catheters who are at increased risk of life-threatening infections. Before addressing how to identify and treat these patients, there must first be an understanding of the definitions associated with life-threating infection. At the 2005 International Pediatric Sepsis Consensus Conference, definitions [23] (see Fig. 15.1) were created for systemic inflammatory response syndrome (SIRS), sepsis, severe sepsis, and septic shock in the pediatric population. SIRS requires the presence of at least two of the following: fever/hypothermia, tachypnea/respiratory failure, leukopenia/bandemia, and tachycardia/bradycardia. Sepsis is defined as the presence of a suspected or confirmed infection combined with SIRS. Severe sepsis includes sepsis with either cardiovascular dysfunction, respiratory distress syndrome, or dysfunction of at least two other organ systems. Figure 15.2 describes the definition of organ dysfunction in the pediatric population [23]. Finally, septic shock is defined as persistent hypotension despite fluid resuscitation or evidence of tissue hypoperfusion (e.g., altered mental status, decreased urinary output) [23] (Fig. 15.1).

Early Goal-Directed Therapy

Early goal-directed therapy (EGDT) has been of primary focus from the Surviving Sepsis Campaign, an international collaborative that created guidelines for management of severe sepsis and septic shock revised in 2012 and again in 2016. Principles of EGDT include providing oxygen, aggressive fluid resuscitation, early antibiotic administration, inotropic support for fluid-resistant shock, and steroid administration for inotropic resistant shock [24]. The newest guidelines used large validated adult data to change the guidelines emphasizing infection and dysfunction of two organ

SIRS[a]

The presence of at least two of the following four criteria, **one of which must be abnormal temperature or leukocyte count:**

- Core[b] temperature of > 38.5°C or < 36°C.
- Tachycardia, defined as a mean heart rate > 2 SD above normal for age in the absence of external stimulus, chronic drugs, or painful stimuli; or otherwise unexplained persistent elevation over a 0.5- to 4-h time period **OR for children < 1 year old: bradycardia, defined as a mean heart rate <10th percentile for age in the absence of external vagal stimulus, β-blocker drugs, or congenital heart disease; or otherwise unexplained persistent depression over a 0.5-h time period.**
- Mean respiratory rate > 2 SD above normal for age or mechanical ventilation for an acute process not related to underlying neuromuscular disease or the receipt of general anesthesia.
- Leukocyte count elevated or depressed for age (not secondary to chemotherapy-induced leukopenia) or > 10% immature neutrophils.

Infection

A suspected or proven (by positive culture, tissue stain, or polymerase chain reaction test) infection caused by any pathogen OR a clinical syndrome associated with a high probability of infection. Evidence of infection includes positive findings on clinical exam, imaging, or laboratory tests (e.g., white blood cells in a normally sterile body fluid, perforated viscus, chest radiograph consistent with pneumonia, petechial or purpuric rash, or purpura fulminans)

Sepsis

SIRS in the presence of or as a result of suspected or proven infection.

Severe sepsis

Sepsis plus one of the following: cardiovascular organ dysfunction OR acute respiratory distress syndrome OR two or more other organ dysfunctions. Organ dysfunctions are defined in Table 15.4.

Septic shock

Sepsis and cardiovascular organ dysfunction as defined in Table 15.4.

Modifications from the adult definitions are highl ighted in boldface.
[a]See Table 15.3 for age-specific ranges for physiologic and laboratory variables; [b]core temperature must be measured by rectal, bladder, oral, or central catheter robe.

Fig. 15.1 Definitions of systemic inflammatory response syndrome (SIRS), infection, sepsis, severe sepsis, and septic shock. Reprinted with permission from [23]

Cardiovascular dysfunction

- Despite administration of isotonic intravenous fluid bolus ≥40 mL/kg in 1 h
  - Decrease in BP (hypotension) < 5th percentile for age or systolic BP <2 so below normal for age[a]

    OR
  - Need for vasoactive drug to maintain BP in normal range (dopamine >5 µg/kg/min or dobutamine, epinephrine, or norepinephrine at any dose)

    OR
  - Two of the following
    Unexplained metabolic acidosis: base deficit >5.0 mEq/L
    Increased arterial lactate >2 times upper limit of normal
    Oliguria: urine output < 0.5 mL/kg/hr
    Prolonged capillary refill: >5 s
    Core to peripheral temperature gap > 3°C

Respiratory[b]

- PaO_2/FIO_2 <300 in absence of cyanotic heart disease or preexisting lung disease

  OR
- $PaCO_2$ > 65 torr or 20 mm Hg over baseline $Paco_2$

  OR
- Proven need[c] or > 50% FIO_2 to maintain saturation ≥92%

  OR
- Need for nonelective invasive or noninvasive mechanical ventilation[d]

Neurologic

- Glasgow Coma Score ≤11 (57)

  OR
- Acute change in mental status with a decrease in Glasgow Coma Score ≥3 points from abnormal baseline

Hematologic

- Platelet count <80,000/mm³ or a decline of 50% in platelet count from highest value recorded over the past 3 days (for chronic hematology/oncology patients)

  OR
- International normalized ratio >2

Renal

- Serum creatinine ≥2 times upper limit of normal for age or twofold increase in baseline creatinine

Hepatic

- Total bilirubin ≥4 mg/dL (not applicable for newborn)

  OR
- ALT 2 times upper limit of normal for age

BP, blood pressure; ALT, alanine transaminase.

[a]See Table 15.2; [b]acute respiratory distress syndrome must include a Pao_2/FIO_2 ratio :S200 mm Hg, bilateral infiltrates, acute onset, and no evidence of left heart failure (Refs. 58 and 59). Acute lung injury is defined identically except the Pao_2/FIO_2 ratio must be ≤300 mm Hg; [c]proven need assumes oxygen requirement was tested by decreasing flow with subsequent increase in flow if required; [d]in postoperative patients, this requirement can be met if the patient has developed an acute inflammatory infectious process in the lungs that prevents him or her from bein extubated.

Fig. 15.2 Organ dysfunction criteria. Reprinted with permission from [23]

Table 15.3 Surviving sepsis campaign bundles

To be completed within 3 h:
(1) Measure lactate level
(2) Obtain blood cultures prior to administration of antibiotics
(3) Administer broad spectrum antibiotics
(4) Administer 30 mL/kg crystalloid for hypotension or lactate 4 mmol/L
To be completed within 6 h:
(5) Apply vasopressors (for hypotension that does not respond to initial fluid resuscitation) to maintain a mean arterial pressure (MAP) ≤ 65 mm Hg
(6) In the event of persistent arterial hypotension despite volume resuscitation (septic shock) or initial lactate 4 mmol/L (36 mg/dL):   - Measure central venous pressure (CVP)[a]   - Measure central venous oxygen saturation (ScvO2)[a]
(7) Remeasure lactate if initial lactate was elevated[a]

[a]Targets for quantitative resuscitation included in the guidelines are CVP of ≥8 mm Hg, ScvO2 of ≥70%, and normalization of lactate

Modified from [33]

Table 15.4 Pediatric advanced life support septic shock (SS) guidelines

Timely recognition of septic shock	Initiation of interventions/frequent reassessment
Placement of PIV	Within 5 min of recognition
20 cc/kg isotonic crystalloid fluid	Within 5 min of recognition then reassess
Antibiotic administration	Within 60 min of recognition
Vasoactive agent administration	Within 60 min of recognition

Modified from [26–28]

systems as the best indicators of sepsis [25]. While the Surviving Sepsis Campaign guidelines have been used as a gold standard for sepsis evaluation and treatment, the definitions are not pediatric specific, and the Goldstein criteria [23] remain the most frequently cited pediatric sepsis definitions. In 2010, the addition of pediatric recommendations were released by the American Heart Association as part of Pediatric Advanced Life Support [26] and further revised in 2015 [27, 28] (see Table 15.4).

When focusing on pediatric specific literature, studies have reported a noteworthy increase over the past decade in the number of sepsis cases identified in pediatric hospitals [29]. Yet, the rate of sepsis in the pediatric population differs from study to study likely due to a myriad of factors including different patient populations, study design, reporting bias, detection bias, differing sets of diagnostic criteria, and differing sources of data [30].

Early identification of the febrile patient who is likely neutropenic, functionally or anatomically asplenic, has an indwelling central venous line, or is immunosuppressed is critical to assess for SIRS, sepsis and septic shock in the hematology/oncology population. Once suspicion of sepsis is identified, initial management should include EGDT with concentration on frequent assessment [26–28]. Intravenous access must be quickly established followed by a 20 mL/kg bolus with isotonic fluid and timely reassessment for tissue hypoperfusion [28]. Additional fluid boluses should be considered based on these frequent assessments [27].

Compared with adults, children can remain in compensated shock with persistent tachycardia. They may also present later with hypotension as a sign of irreversible cardiovascular collapse [26]. The pediatric consensus guidelines are designed to identify patients with compensated septic shock allowing for early intervention to prevent cases of profound decompensation [23].

During fluid resuscitation, the clinician should also remain aware of the patient's respiratory status. The Fluid Expansion as Supportive Therapy [31] trial looked at treatment of children with a febrile illness complicated by impaired consciousness, respiratory distress or both, and impaired perfusion. The trial concluded that early fluid therapy increased mortality [31]. However, further review of subsequent literature analyzing the FEAST trial was included in the Pediatric Advanced Life Support: 2015 International Consensus on Cardiopulmonary Resuscitation which does not recommend limiting resuscitation fluids for children in septic shock but does recommend utilizing caution if the resuscitation occurs in a place with extremely limited critical care resources [27, 28].

The other principles of EGDT: providing oxygen, early antibiotic administration, and inotropic support for fluid-resistant shock [24], also should each be addressed as soon as signs of SIRS/sepsis/septic shock are recognized. As oxygen delivery is dependent on cardiac output and the oxygen-carrying capacity of blood, oxygen delivery can be increased by first providing 100% inspired oxygen and additionally by volume expansion with rapid infusion of isotonic fluid or packed red blood cells when indicated by hemoglobin and hematocrit results. The administration of intravenous antibiotics must be administered within the first hour of suspected sepsis or septic shock [32].

Performance Improvement

Poor patient outcomes from sepsis can be mitigated with early identification of sepsis and subsequent timely initiation of proven therapies [33]. The Surviving Sepsis Campaign 2012 recommendations include the utilization of performance improvement methods to improve patient outcomes [32]. The original campaign implemented a set of goals in the form of a bundle in multiple hospital settings and demonstrated not only improved quality of treatment of sepsis but additionally decreased mortality [33] (see Table 15.3).

Implementation of standardized sepsis protocols in pediatrics foster improved recognition of septic patients [34, 35] and more timely delivery of critical interventions [34, 36] in both inpatient and emergency department settings. Early identification of patients who may require EGDT for possible sepsis can be achieved by training staff on age-appropriate vital signs and abnormal variation in vital signs based on temperature elevation [34–36]. Additional training must focus on compliance with current treatment guidelines. Paul et al. were able to increase compliance with PALS sepsis guidelines with the use of QI methodology [36]. As pediatric institutions continue to undertake development of plans for adapting and sustaining sepsis protocols, collaboration and continued quality improvement will remain vital to reaching the goal of enhancing outcomes. In addition to institutional quality improvement efforts, national and international efforts may offer the opportunity for more rapid learning through shared quality improvement collaboration as done in the past by the Surviving Sepsis Campaign [32] and currently by the Children's Hospital Association Improving Sepsis Outcomes Collaborative [37].

Safe Handoffs in Pediatric Hematology/Oncology

All care providers must transition the care of their patients to an oncoming provider at the end of a clinical shift. Hematology/oncology patients frequently have complicated conditions; thus, it is important for providers to be competent in patient handovers.

A successful handoff is defined by The Joint Commission's Center for Transforming Healthcare as "a transfer and acceptance of responsibility for patient care that is achieved through effective communication. It is a real time process of passing patient-specific information from one caregiver to another or from one team of caregivers to another to ensure the continuity and safety of that patient's care [38]. In 2006, The Joint Commission identified handoffs as a major risk to patient safety. In response one of its national patient safety goals was for hospitals "to implement a standardized approach to "hand off" communications, including an opportunity to ask and respond to questions." [39, 40] When a provider relinquishes the care of a hematology/oncology patient to another provider, the effective transfer of information becomes critical to patient safety, and the loss of critical information can lead to medical error and adverse events [41].

Increased attention to handoffs occurred when the American Council for Graduate Medical Education (ACGME) restricted resident work hours to 80 h per week in 2003 and then added additional restrictions in 2011 [42, 43]. This resulted in a significant increase in the number of patient transitions of care. The increased number of patient handoffs subsequently led to delayed care [44], delayed disposition [45], redundancy in work [46], and uncertainty regarding future care [47].

Currently, the ACGME requires residents to be competent at handing over patients [48]. Yet, initial exploration of resident ability to transition patients demonstrated that interns often overestimate the effectiveness of their handoffs. Additionally, in one study residents reported that a patient was harmed 50% of the time on their previous rotation due to a handoff error [49]. To achieve handoff consistency among residents in an academic institution, it has been suggested that standardization of handoffs and a content checklist are crucial to appropriate communication [50].

As research progressed in the field of handoffs, communication was noted to be an essential part of an effective handoff (1, Joint Commission 2007). Poor communication has been cited by The Joint Commission as the root cause of up to two-thirds of sentinel events [51]. In addition, it has been estimated that up to one quarter

Fig. 15.3 Elements of the
I-pass handoff tool.
Reprinted from [54] with
permission from the
I-PASS Study Group

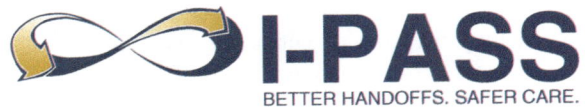

I	Illness Severity	• Stable, "watcher," unstable
P	Patient Summary	• Summary statement • Evens leading up to admission • Hospital course • Ongoing assessment • Plan
A	Action List	• To do list • Time line and ownership
S	Situation Awareness and Contingency Planning	• Know what's going on • Plan for what might happen
S	Synthesis by Receiver	• Receiver summarizes what was heard • Asks questions • Restates key action/to do Items

of all malpractice claims are a direct result of communication errors [52]. To improve communication, one suggested strategy is the utilization of mnemonics which can provide structure and act as a memory aid [53]. In pediatrics, the I-Pass mnemonic [54] (Fig. 15.3) and the use of checklists [50] have established improvement in handoffs. The I-Pass mnemonic, when implemented as part of a handoff bundle to include standardized communication, training, as well as efforts to minimize distraction, ultimately revealed decreased rates of medical errors [41]. Measurement of improvement in communication can be done using a Likert scale to score elements of communication such as confidence, organization, and included/excluded content [50] (Fig. 15.4). Additionally, for improved handoff communication, one should strive to communicate face to face which has proven to be the superior method of communication when compared with phone, email, and paper communication [55].

Two additional factors that can weaken handoff quality are lack of formal training [39] and lack of standardized tools to assess handoffs [53, 56] Thus, whether a health system ultimately chooses to utilize a checklist or a mnemonic for care transition, it is imperative that all providers receive standardized training on the tool.

Transfer of Care Global Evaluation Scale

Evaluator: _____   Date _____

Evaluates _____   □ intern □ resident □ student □ other _____

Situation: □ End of shift □ Transfer between services   □ Admission

Type: □ face-to-face □ phone □ Notes

Organization

1	2	3	4	5
Information followed a logical order for the patient.		The learner seemed to follow a series of topics; however, there were some items/topics out of order.		The learner provided information that was disjointed and unorganized.

Economy

1	2	3	4	5
The learner provided the ideal amount of information.		The learner included a fair amount of extraneous information		The learner provided far too much extraneous information.

Confidence

1	2	3	4	5
The learner spoke without hesitation.		The learner was occasionally hesitant.		The learner was frequently hesitant.

Presentation Order
Presents sickest patients first

1	2	3	4	5
Always	Usually	Sometimes	Rarely	Never

Seeks Comprehension
Ensures that recipient understands information and concerns/plans for next shift

1	2	3	4	5
Always	Usually	Sometimes	Rarely	Never

Professionalism
Appropriate comments re: patient, family, staff, etc

1	2	3	4	5
Always	Usually	Sometimes	Rarely	Never

Overall Rating: _____

Fig. 15.4 Reprinted with permission from [50]

By providing standardization, providers obtain structure so that the "rules" of inter-action (e.g., content and order) do not need to be negotiated; if no information is given, it implies there was nothing that required mention, and information is con-veyed more efficiently and reliably [56]. One must also develop an assessment tool for ongoing evaluation and improvement [53]. For example, a global assessment tool (Fig. 15.4) encourages evaluation by direct observation [50].

Once the health system has determined the tool, education, and assessment that will be implemented, there are some general strategies that will be undertaken to make handoffs as successful as possible. These include being clear, concise, and organized and asking the receiver if they have any questions after each patient; being certain to impart critical data including pertinent positives and negatives about the patient; allowing the appropriate amount of time to relay information; and doing it where interruptions are minimized. For instance, implement a page-free zone or a designated quiet space in which to handover patients. Identify and present the most critical patients first when the receivers' attention is at its best. Finally, the receiver should be empowered to not accept a poor patient handoff and to ask clarifying questions.

Influenza Vaccination in Pediatric Hematology/ Oncology Practices

Influenza, a common upper respiratory tract infection, can cause major complications, especially in the immune compromised host [57, 58]. Complications include respiratory failure, secondary pneumonia and bacteremia, and prolonged viral shedding. Cancer treatment delays are common [59]. Therefore, preventing this infection in children with sickle cell disease or cancer is of high importance. The percentage of patients in each of these groups who did receive the appropriate influenza vaccine in the recommended time frame for each year is a good process measure for influenza prevention.

Influenza Vaccination in Pediatric Cancer Patients

Pediatric cancer patients are at increased risk for severe influenza-related illness. Two studies in the recent era assessed influenza complications in hospitalized pediatric oncology patients. In a 5-year period with 27 clinical encounters due to influenza, 63% of which were treated with antiviral medication, Tasian et al. [59] found that 15% required mechanical ventilation, 22% required oxygen support, 15% developed bacteremia, and 11% had hospitalizations in excess of 30 day. The influenza vaccination status of these patients was not reported. In a similar 5-year period, Kersun et al. [60] describe 39 patients, 46% of which had received immunization. Of these, 20% had respiratory complications, 10% intensive care admissions, and 5% died.

Treatment with antiviral agents such as oseltamivir or zanamivir for specific strains of influenza and in appropriately aged patients can decrease the severity of infection and complication rate for pediatric cancer patients infected with influenza [58]. However, because complications exist even in treated patients, the potential for cancer treatment interruption, and possible exposure of other at-risk patients to the illness, prevention is a better strategy. As infection of patients can occur from healthcare personnel, universal vaccination of pediatric hematology/oncology providers and staff should be performed [58].

Influenza Vaccination Safety and Efficacy in Pediatric Cancer Patients

Overall, patients receiving chemotherapy have a decreased serologic response to influenza vaccine when compared to healthy children. Patients with AML or within 1 year of stem-cell transplant have lower response rates [58]. Mavinkurve-Groothuis et al. [61] found that 92% of patients with a normal absolute lymphocyte count for age had a protective immune response to H1N1 vaccine as opposed to 33% with a low absolute lymphocyte count. They did not find a difference between hematologic malignancy (mostly ALL) and solid tumor patients in response to H1N1 vaccine. None of their patients with an absolute T-cell count below 200 per microliter achieved protective levels. Older age or perhaps the larger dose administered to older children may predict a higher vaccine response rate in children with ALL [62, 63]. It is not clear that the serologic titer associated with a protective effect in healthy individuals is applicable to pediatric oncology patients [58, 63]. Children who have completed therapy for cancer, with the exception of stem-cell transplant patients, have a better response to immunization [63].

The adverse reaction rate to inactivated influenza vaccine is not higher in pediatric cancer patients than in the general population [58, 63]. Thus, despite lower serologic response rates for children on chemotherapy compared to the general pediatric population, that a significant proportion of on-therapy patients do respond, that off-therapy patients respond well, the low adverse reaction rate and the significant morbidity of influenza in this population give strong support to the recommendation that this population be vaccinated against this infection with the inactivated form of the vaccine.

Influenza Vaccination Rates in Pediatric Oncology Patients

Despite the above reasons for vaccinating pediatric cancer patients against influenza, vaccination rates in this population have been disappointing [58, 60]. Some of the stated barriers to adequate vaccination are noted in Table 15.5. Adult survivors of childhood cancer who are also at high risk for influenza-related complications due to late effects of their cancer treatments also have a low rate of vaccination [64].

Freedman et al. [65] used five interventions to increase influenza vaccination rates in their pediatric oncology program: (a) parent/family education, (b) use of the electronic health record to identify vaccine-eligible patients, (c) brightly-colored identification bracelets attached to vaccine-eligible patients in the ambulatory environment, (d) inclusion of influenza vaccine in the discharge order set, and (e) provider education. As a result, when compared to the prior year's population, there was a significant increase in the percentage of fully immunized patients (64.5% vs. 44.4%, $p = 0.001$) and a proportionate decrease in unimmunized patients (45.2% vs. 22.5%, $p = 0.001$). The percentage of patients who were partially immunized did not change significantly (13.0% vs. 10.4%, $p = 0.19$). They demonstrate, as with most

Table 15.5 Barriers to influenza vaccination in pediatric cancer patients	
	Parental concern about vaccine side effects
	Parental fear that vaccination will cause influenza illness
	Provider belief that vaccination is ineffective
	System failure to identify unimmunized children
	System failure to administer vaccine to eligible children

quality improvement projects to improve adherence in pediatrics, multidisciplinary and patient/parent/family education, and systemic factors need to be addressed.

Influenza Vaccination in Pediatric Sickle Cell Disease

Sickle cell disease (SCD) patients are also at increased risk for adverse outcomes from influenza infection [57]. The hospitalization rate for influenza illness in children with sickle cell disease is 56 times that of children without SCD and even higher for children identified as having homozygous HbSS disease [66]. Influenza can cause acute chest syndrome [67].

Influenza vaccine is both safe and effective in SCD. Unlike pediatric cancer patients, the large majority of children with SCD achieve protective antibody titers in response to inactivated influenza vaccine [68–71]. Purohit et al. [68] did report a decreased response to inactivated H1N1 in SCD patients on chronic transfusion. Hydroxyurea use and splenectomy did not appear to impact response [68, 69]. The vaccine is well tolerated in this population [69–71]. The inactivated trivalent influenza vaccine does not appear to increase the rate of hospitalization for vaso-occlusive crisis within 2 weeks of administration [72]. Because of the morbidity of influenza in SCD patients and the proven efficacy and safety of the inactivated vaccine, the CDC, AAP, and WHO all recommend influenza vaccination for sickle cell disease [57]. An annual influenza vaccine is a recommended quality measure for sickle cell disease [20].

Despite this recommendation, adherence with influenza vaccination in children remains poor [73]. An analysis of a Wisconsin Medicaid database showed that over a 5-year period, only 30% of children with SCD received 80% of their influenza vaccines annually, while 46% received less than 50% [74]. Barriers likely are quite similar to those described for pediatric cancer patients, although concern of poor response should not be a factor. Additional factors include that the seasonal availability of the vaccine may not coincide with the patient's clinic visit and primary care or specialty provider's assumptions that the other will manage this aspect of the patient's care [75].

Improvement in Influenza Immunization in Pediatric Sickle Cell Disease Patients

Quality improvement methods have been used in increase influenza immunization in other high-risk pediatric populations [65, 76]. Repeated contact with a hematologist was shown to increase the likelihood of influenza immunization in sickle cell disease patients, suggesting that information provided from this source is valued [77]. Zimmerman et al. [78]. identified tools to facilitate three major approaches to increasing influenza vaccination rates among high-risk pediatric populations including

Table 15.6 Strategies to increase influenza vaccination in children and adolescents with sickle cell disease [79]

Patient/parent and provider education
Enhanced electronic health record
Establishment of patient registry
Use of care coordinators

sickle cell disease in a low-income urban environment. These tools included parent information devices (e.g., flyers, posters, letters, etc.), increased access to immunizations (walk-in and Saturday clinics), and systems-based interventions including electronic provider reminders, staff education, and standing orders. While these interventions nearly doubled the immunization rate, going from 10.4 to 18.7%, it remained quite poor. Recently, Sobota et al. [79] used four strategies (Table 15.6) to increase both the rate of influenza immunization and the timing of this vaccination in their SCD patients treated in an urban pediatric hematology ambulatory environment. Implemented and refined over a 2-year period, these approaches dramatically increased the influenza vaccination rate from 45 to 90%. The immunization rate exceeded 80% even for patients 18–21 years of age. An additional secondary goal was to have patients receive their immunization early in the season. Seventy-one percent were immunized by mid-November of the last year reported.

Despite data demonstrating safety and utility, albeit the latter perhaps less well demonstrated for pediatric cancer than SCD patients, there appears to be significant opportunity for improvement. Two recent publications, one for each population, have demonstrated that dedicated teams adequately resourced and using systems-based approaches can achieve high influenza immunization rates. Implementation of such practices and use of evolving tools such as interoperable vaccine registry databases to identify unimmunized patients, secure provider-to-provider electronic communication to facilitate care coordination between practices, and electronic patient portals to send education and reminders to patients may soon help achieve similar vaccination rates across all pediatric hematology/oncology practices.

Iron Overload and Its Management

Iron homeostasis is a complex process that tightly regulates iron absorption and iron excretion, with relatively small quantities of this element moving in either direction on a daily basis [80]. In the average adult, iron balance is achieved by the absorption of 1–2 mg/day of iron from the gut and the loss of 1–2 mg/day of iron, primary from shedding of GI mucosal cells and blood loss [81]. As there are no physiologic pathways to increase iron excretion, the main control mechanism is to limit iron absorption from the diet through a complex series of interacting regulating proteins, principally hepcidin and ferroportin [82, 83]. Causes of iron overload are shown in Table 15.7. As each unit of red blood cells transfused contains 200–250 mg of iron, [84] a 60-kg individual transfused 2 units/month receives roughly 7–8 mg/day of iron. More than one mechanism may be present in any given patient. For example, patients with the more severe thalassemic disorders, especially β-thalassemia major,

Table 15.7 Causes of iron overload

1. Defects in iron metabolism regulatory proteins. Example hereditary hemochromatosis
2. Excessive iron intake. Example transfusional iron overload
3. Ineffective erythropoiesis. Example thalassemia intermedia

4. Combination of factors. Examples:
  a. Thalassemia with transfusional therapy
  b. Long-term therapeutic doses of iron in patients with hereditary hemochromatosis
    or thalassemia

have both ineffective erythropoiesis and frequent transfusions [85]. Ineffective erythropoiesis causes suppression of hepcidin synthesis leading to increased GI iron absorption and iron overload, even without or with only limited red blood cell transfusion. When the amount of iron in the plasma exceeds the transferrin binding capacity, labile plasma iron can induce free radicals which cause oxidative intracellular damage, in particular, in the liver, heart, pancreas, and endocrine organs [86].

Determination of iron overload is made by measurement of iron levels in various organs. Serum ferritin can reflect iron overload but correlates poorly with hepatic and most importantly cardiac iron deposition. Liver iron concentration by liver biopsy has long been the gold standard but is invasive. Recently, MRI techniques ($R2^*$) have been shown to correlate well with hepatic liver iron concentration as determined by liver biopsy [81]. Cardiac iron as determined by $T2^*$ has also been shown to be predictive of cardiac dysfunction [81, 84] It is very important that the MRI unit and technique have appropriate validation and calibration [81]. Symptomatic cardiac overload can occur even without major hepatic disease, especially if there is ineffective erythropoiesis or the patient has undergone chelation with desferrioxamine that preferentially removes hepatic iron [84].

Management of Iron Overload

Non-pharmacologic techniques include ingesting tea, which can inhibit iron absorption [87], dietary restriction of iron-containing foods, and carefully counseling patients to avoid iron supplements. In most instances, such interventions will not be adequate to prevent iron overload. Use of exchange transfusions rather than simple transfusions to remove aging erythrocytes has been shown to be effective in reducing iron overload for patients on chronic transfusion regimens but requires adequate venous access and increases the donor exposures [88].

Three iron chelators are currently licensed in the United States. Desferrioxamine has been available for decades. It is typically administered as a 12-h subcutaneous infusion 4–5 times/week. Higher-dose, intravenous infusions may also be used for selected patients [89]. Desferrioxamine has been associated with several significant toxicities including retinal damage, hearing loss, bone changes, local reactions at the infusion site, poor growth, Yersinia infections, and allergic reactions [84, 86]. High doses can cause neurologic and pulmonary toxicity [84]. While effective for hepatic iron overload, desferrioxamine is not always effective at limited cardiac iron overload, and patients have developed fatal cardiac disease while on the medication [84]. Not surprisingly, poor adherence to desferrioxamine regimens has long been recognized [86, 90].

Deferiprone (DFP) is an oral iron chelator approved by the FDA in 2011 [86]. Due to a short half-life of 4 h, it is typically taken three times daily. DFP may have advantages over DFO for management of cardiac iron overload [84, 91]. Toxicities include nausea and vomiting, arthropathy, zinc deficiency, and elevated liver enzymes. The most serious toxicity is neutropenia or agranulocytosis that occurs in approximately 1% of drug recipients and requires close monitoring of blood counts throughout treatment [84].

Deferasirox (DFX), approved by the FDA in 2005, has a longer experience in the United States but not in Europe. DFX promotes fecal iron excretion. Its half-life permits once-daily dosing. DFX has been shown to be effective in reducing hepatic and cardiac iron in pediatric and adult patients with transfusion-iron overload [84]. Common toxicities include gastrointestinal symptoms (nausea, vomiting, diarrhea, abdominal pain), rash, hearing loss, and cytopenias. Significant hepatic and renal toxicity has been noted, and a "Black Box" warning exists for renal and hepatic failure, with frequent laboratory testing recommended. A Black Box warning also exists for GI hemorrhage but this problem is noted more frequently in the elderly.

Alternating or combined chelator trials have been performed, albeit generally in small numbers of patients, and further trials are needed to determine the optimal approach for management of iron overload in children [84, 92, 93].

Medication Adherence with Chelation Therapy

To date, several studies have focused on medication adherence. There are some studies noted below that also measured clinical outcome measures such as hepatic iron concentration or hospitalization rates.

Not surprisingly for a medication with a requirement for long-term painful sub-cutaneous infusions, early on nonadherence to desferrioxamine regimens was identified as a barrier to its effectiveness [90]. A series of large studies put the estimated adherence with DFO at 59–78% [94]. Nonadherence is associated with an increased incidence of poor outcomes including death [94, 95]. Based on survey responses in a multinational study, Ward et al. found that outside of India and Iran where access to medication was the most frequent reason for missing doses, the patient's beliefs and feelings about the medication and medication side effects were the most common reasons. Additionally, age was also correlated with nonadherence with children under 10 years having the highest rate of adherence, while patients over 18 years of age had the lowest rate [96]. Adherence has been shown to be better for deferiprone than desferrioxamine [97].

An Iranian study reported increase patient self-reported adherence to DSX as compared with DFO [98]. As part of a larger study of adherence to chelation in thalassemia patients, Trachtenberg et al. found that adherence did increase for a subset who changed from DFO to DSX. Predictors of poor adherence included side effects, smoking, age, and difficulties with DFO [99]. Using a medication possession ratio and analysis of Medicaid claims from three states, Jordan et al. found a higher adherence rate and decreasing hospitalization rate for sickle cell disease patients on DSX compared with DFO [100]. Compliance with chelation therapy had a more significant role in prevention of iron-induced cardiac disease than choice of chelation agent in transfused adults with beta thalassemia major [101].

Improvement Trials in Chelation Adherence

While nonadherence is well documented in patients with transfusional iron overload, and several contributing factors have been identified, there are relatively few studies of effective interventions. Pakbaz et al. used a Numerical Likert Scale adherence assessment tool and then discussion of hepatic iron content results, education regarding chelation, and barrier to adherence solutions to improve adherence and decrease hepatic iron in a subgroup of 15 patients who had serial measurements over 15 months [102].

Iron overload remains a major problem for many populations with impact on quality and quantity of life, particularly for those patients on chronic transfusion therapy. Medication non-adherence contributes significantly to adverse patient outcome. Factors associated with decreased adherence to chelation regimens are similar to other disorders including patient beliefs, side effects, decreased access to medication, and regimens that are difficult to understand or complete. Access to oral iron chelation agents appears to increase medication adherence, but concerns about toxicity have prevented consensus that these should be the front line agents for all such patients [93]. Few studies have been performed in this population to increase adherence, and these are limited to small patient numbers and short term interventions.

Conclusion

Efficacy of evidence-based care is dependent upon its reliable delivery. Many of the quality improvement activities cited in this chapter used common tools in the quality improvement toolbox including identified measurable targets for improvement, multidisciplinary team approaches to design and implementation, standardized processes, patient/parent/caregiver engagement, and iterative cycles of improvement activity. More in-depth discussion of quality improvement science and some of its potential applications in pediatric hematology/oncology is found elsewhere in this book. However, many opportunities remain for future development and implementation of improvement methods for these and many other areas within our specialty.

References

1. Sung L, Phillips R, Lehrnbecher T. Time for paediatric febrile neutropenia guidelines—children are not little adults. Eur J Cancer. 2011;47:811–3.
2. Phillips RS, Lehrnbecher T, Alexander S, Sung L. Updated systematic review and meta-analysis of the performance of risk prediction rules in children and young people with febrile neutropenia. PLoS One. 2012;7:e38300.
3. Gavidia R, Fuentes SL, Vasquez R, et al. Low socioeconomic status is associated with prolonged times to assessment and treatment, sepsis and infectious death in pediatric fever in El Salvador. PLoS One. 2012;7:e43639.
4. McCavit TL, Winick N. Time-to-antibiotic administration as a quality of care measure in children with febrile neutropenia: a survey of pediatric oncology centers. Pediatr Blood Cancer. 2012;58:303–5.
5. Fletcher M, Hodgkiss H, Zhang S, et al. Prompt administration of antibiotics is associated with improved outcomes in febrile neutropenia in children with cancer. Pediatr Blood Cancer. 2013;60:1299–306.
6. Salstrom JL, Coughlin RL, Pool K, et al. Pediatric patients who receive antibiotics for fever and neutropenia in less than 60 min have decreased intensive care needs. Pediatr Blood Cancer. 2015;62:807–15.
7. Amado VM, Vilela GP, Queiroz A Jr, Amaral AC. Effect of a quality improvement intervention to decrease delays in antibiotic delivery in pediatric febrile neutropenia: a pilot study. J Crit Care. 2011;26:103. e9–12
8. Volpe D, Harrison S, Damian F, et al. Improving timeliness of antibiotic delivery for patients with fever and suspected neutropenia in a pediatric emergency department. Pediatrics. 2012;130:e201–10.
9. Jobson M, Sandrof M, Valeriote T, Liberty AL, Walsh-Kelly C, Jackson C. Decreasing time to antibiotics in febrile patients with central lines in the emergency department. Pediatrics. 2015;135:e187–95.
10. Burry E, Punnett A, Mehta A, Thull-Freedman J, Robinson L, Gupta S. Identification of educational and infrastructural barriers to prompt antibiotic delivery in febrile neutropenia: a quality improvement initiative. Pediatr Blood Cancer. 2012;59:431–5.
11. Cash T, Deloach T, Graham J, Shirm S, Mian A. Standardized process used in the emergency department for pediatric oncology patients with fever and neutropenia improves time to the first dose of antibiotics. Pediatr Emerg Care. 2014;30:91–3.
12. Cohen C, King A, Lin CP, Friedman GK, Monroe K, Kutny M. Protocol for reducing time to antibiotics in pediatric patients presenting to an emergency department with fever and neutropenia: efficacy and barriers. Pediatr Emerg Care. 2016;32(11):739–45.
13. Dobrasz G, Hatfield M, Jones LM, Berdis JJ, Miller EE, Entrekin MS. Nurse-driven protocols for febrile pediatric oncology patients. J Emerg Nurs. 2013;39:289–95.
14. Pakakasama S, Surayuthpreecha K, Pandee U, et al. Clinical practice guidelines for children with cancer presenting with fever to the emergency room. Pediatr Int. 2011;53:902–5.
15. Vedi A, Pennington V, O'Meara M, et al. Management of fever and neutropenia in children with cancer. Support Care Cancer. 2015;23:2079–87.
16. Green AL, Yi J, Bezler N, et al. A prospective cohort quality improvement study to reduce the time to antibiotics for new fever in neutropenic pediatric oncology inpatients. Pediatr Blood Cancer. 2016;63:112–7.
17. Dandoy CE, Hariharan S, Weiss B, et al. Sustained reductions in time to antibiotic delivery in febrile immunocompromised children: results of a quality improvement collaborative. BMJ Qual Saf. 2016;25:100–9.
18. Baskin MN, Goh XL, Heeney MM, Harper MB. Bacteremia risk and outpatient management of febrile patients with sickle cell disease. Pediatrics. 2013;131:1035–41.
19. Buchanan GR, Ballas SK, Afenyi-Annan AN, et al. Evidence-based management of sickle cell disease. U.S. Department of Health and Human Services: Washington; 2014.

20. Wang CJ, Kavanagh PL, Little AA, Holliman JB, Sprinz PG. Quality-of-care indicators for children with sickle cell disease. Pediatrics. 2011;128:484–93.
21. Kavanagh PL, Sprinz PG, Wolfgang TL, et al. Improving the management of vaso-occlusive episodes in the pediatric emergency department. Pediatrics. 2015;136:e1016–25.
22. Treadwell MJ, Bell M, Leibovich SA, et al. A quality improvement initiative to improve emergency department care for pediatric patients with sickle cell disease. J Clin Outcomes Manag. 2014;21:62–70.
23. Goldstein B, Giroir B, Randolph A, International Consensus Conference on Pediatric S. International pediatric sepsis consensus conference: definitions for sepsis and organ dysfunction in pediatrics. Pediatr Crit Care Med. 2005;6:2–8.
24. Silverman AM. Septic shock: recognizing and managing this life-threatening condition in pediatric patients. Pediatr Emerg Med Pract. 2015;12:1–25. quiz 6–7
25. Jacob JA. New sepsis diagnostic guidelines shift focus to organ dysfunction. JAMA. 2016;315:739–40.
26. Kleinman ME, Chameides L, Schexnayder SM, et al. Pediatric advanced life support: 2010 American Heart Association Guidelines for Cardiopulmonary Resuscitation and Emergency Cardiovascular Care. Pediatrics. 2010;126:e1361–99.
27. de Caen AR, Maconochie IK, Aickin R, et al. Part 6: Pediatric basic life support and pediatric advanced life support: 2015 International Consensus on Cardiopulmonary Resuscitation and Emergency Cardiovascular Care Science With Treatment Recommendations. Circulation. 2015;132:S177–203.
28. American Heart Association. Web-based integrated guidelines for cardiopulmonary resuscitation and emergency cardiovascular care—part 12: Pediatric advanced life support. 2015. https://eccguidelines.heart.org/index.php/circulation/cpr-ecc-guidelines-2/part-12-pediatric-advanced-life-support/?strue=1&id=3-3n. Accessed April, 2016.
29. Balamuth F, Weiss SL, Neuman MI, et al. Pediatric severe sepsis in U.S. children's hospitals. Pediatr Crit Care Med. 2014;15:798–805.
30. Fontela P, Lacroix J. Sepsis or SEPSIS: does it make a difference? Pediatr Crit Care Med. 2014;15:893–4.
31. Maitland K, Kiguli S, Opoka RO, et al. Mortality after fluid bolus in African children with severe infection. N Engl J Med. 2011;364:2483–95.
32. Dellinger RP, Levy MM, Rhodes A, et al. Surviving sepsis campaign: international guidelines for management of severe sepsis and septic shock: 2012. Crit Care Med. 2013;41:580–637.
33. Levy MM, Dellinger RP, Townsend SR, et al. The surviving sepsis campaign: results of an international guideline-based performance improvement program targeting severe sepsis. Crit Care Med. 2010;38:367–74.
34. Cruz AT, Perry AM, Williams EA, Graf JM, Wuestner ER, Patel B. Implementation of goal-directed therapy for children with suspected sepsis in the emergency department. Pediatrics. 2011;127:e758–66.
35. Bradshaw C, Goodman I, Rosenberg R, Bandera C, Fierman A, Rudy B. Implementation of an Inpatient Pediatric Sepsis Identification Pathway. Pediatrics. 2016;137:1–8.
36. Paul R, Melendez E, Stack A, Capraro A, Monuteaux M, Neuman MI. Improving adherence to PALS septic shock guidelines. Pediatrics. 2014;133:e1358–66.
37. Children's Hospital Association. Join the fight against pediatric sepsis with new collaborative. 2016.
38. Healthcare JCCfT. Facts about the hand-off communications project. The Joint Commission; 2016.
39. Arora V, Johnson J. A model for building a standardized hand-off protocol. Jt Comm J Qual Patient Saf. 2006;32:646–55.
40. The Joint Commission. Handoff Communications: Toolkit for Implementing the National Patient Safety Goal. Oakbrook Terrace, IL. Joint Commission Resources, 2008.
41. Starmer AJ, Sectish TC, Simon DW, et al. Rates of medical errors and preventable adverse events among hospitalized children following implementation of a resident handoff bundle. JAMA. 2013;310:2262–70.

42. Philibbert I, Taradejna C. A brief history of duty hours and resident education. In: The ACGME 2011 Duty Hour Standards: Enhancing quality of care, supervision and resident professional development. Chicago, IL: Accreditation Counciel for Graduate Medical Education; 2011.
43. Accreditation Council for Graduate Medical Education. Common program requirements. Chicago: Accreditation Council for Graduate Medical Education; 2016.
44. Smith D, Burris JW, Mahmoud G, Guldner G. Residents' self-perceived errors in transitions of care in the emergency department. J Grad Med Educ. 2011;3:37–40.
45. Greenberg CC, Regenbogen SE, Studdert DM, et al. Patterns of communication breakdowns resulting in injury to surgical patients. J Am Coll Surg. 2007;204:533–40.
46. Horwitz LI, Krumholz HM, Green ML, Huot SJ. Transfers of patient care between house staff on internal medicine wards: a national survey. Arch Intern Med. 2006;166:1173–7.
47. Arora V, Johnson J, Lovinger D, Humphrey HJ, Meltzer DO. Communication failures in patient sign-out and suggestions for improvement: a critical incident analysis. Qual Saf Health Care. 2005;14:401–7.
48. Nasca TJ, Day SH, Amis Jr ES, Force ADHT. The new recommendations on duty hours from the ACGME Task Force. N Engl J Med. 2010;363:e3.
49. Chang VY, Arora VM, Lev-Ari S, D'Arcy M, Keysar B. Interns overestimate the effectiveness of their hand-off communication. Pediatrics. 2010;125:491–6.
50. Britt RC, Ramirez DE, Anderson-Montoya BL, Scerbo MW. Resident handoff training: initial evaluation of a novel method. J Healthc Qual. 2015;37:75–80.
51. The Joint Commission Sentinel event data root causes by event type 2004–2013. 2013.
52. Riesenberg LA, Berg K, Berg D, et al. Resident and attending physician perception of maladaptive response to stress in residents. Med Educ Online. 2014;19:25041.
53. Abraham J, Kannampallil T, Patel VL. A systematic review of the literature on the evaluation of handoff tools: implications for research and practice. J Am Med Inform Assoc. 2014;21:154–62.
54. Starmer AJ, Spector ND, Srivastava R, et al. I-pass, a mnemonic to standardize verbal handoffs. Pediatrics. 2012;129:201–4.
55. Cockburn A. Communicating, cooperating teams. Humans and Technology; 2013.
56. Patterson ES, Wears RL. Patient handoffs: standardized and reliable measurement tools remain elusive. Jt Comm J Qual Patient Saf. 2010;36:52–61.
57. Gill PJ, Ashdown HF, Wang K, et al. Identification of children at risk of influenza-related complications in primary and ambulatory care: a systematic review and meta-analysis. Lancet Respir Med. 2015;3:139–49.
58. Kersun LS, Reilly AF, Coffin SE, Sullivan KE. Protecting pediatric oncology patients from influenza. Oncologist. 2013;18:204–11.
59. Tasian SK, Park JR, Martin ET, Englund JA. Influenza-associated morbidity in children with cancer. Pediatr Blood Cancer. 2008;50:983–7.
60. Kersun LS, Coffin SE, Leckerman KH, Ingram M, Reilly AF. Community acquired influenza requiring hospitalization: vaccine status is unrelated to morbidity in children with cancer. Pediatr Blood Cancer. 2010;54:79–82.
61. Mavinkurve-Groothuis AM, van der Flier M, Stelma F, van Leer-Buter C, Preijers FW, Hoogerbrugge PM. Absolute lymphocyte count predicts the response to new influenza virus H1N1 vaccination in pediatric cancer patients. Clin Vaccine Immunol. 2013;20:118–21.
62. Leahy TR, Smith OP, Bacon CL, et al. Does vaccine dose predict response to the monovalent pandemic H1N1 influenza a vaccine in children with acute lymphoblastic leukemia? A single-centre study. Pediatr Blood Cancer. 2013;60:1656–61.
63. Chisholm JC, Devine T, Charlett A, Pinkerton CR, Zambon M. Response to influenza immunisation during treatment for cancer. Arch Dis Child. 2001;84:496–500.
64. Ojha RP, Offutt-Powell TN, Gurney JG. Influenza vaccination coverage among adult survivors of pediatric cancer. Am J Prev Med. 2014;46:552–8.
65. Freedman JL, Reilly AF, Powell SC, Bailey LC. Quality improvement initiative to increase influenza vaccination in pediatric cancer patients. Pediatrics. 2015;135:e540–6.

66. Bundy DG, Strouse JJ, Casella JF, Miller MR. Burden of influenza-related hospitalizations among children with sickle cell disease. Pediatrics. 2010;125:234–43.
67. Strouse JJ, Reller ME, Bundy DG, et al. Severe pandemic H1N1 and seasonal influenza in children and young adults with sickle cell disease. Blood. 2010;116:3431–4.
68. Purohit S, Alvarez O, O'Brien R, Andreansky S. Durable immune response to inactivated H1N1 vaccine is less likely in children with sickle cell anemia receiving chronic transfusions. Pediatr Blood Cancer. 2012;59:1280–3.
69. Long CB, Ramos I, Rastogi D, et al. Humoral and cell-mediated immune responses to monovalent 2009 influenza A/H1N1 and seasonal trivalent influenza vaccines in high-risk children. J Pediatr. 2012;160:74–81.
70. Hakim H, Allison KJ, Van De Velde LA, Li Y, Flynn PM, McCullers JA. Immunogenicity and safety of inactivated monovalent 2009 H1N1 influenza A vaccine in immunocompromised children and young adults. Vaccine. 2012;30:879–85.
71. Souza AR, Braga JA, de Paiva TM, Loggetto SR, Azevedo RS, Weckx LY. Immunogenicity and tolerability of a virosome influenza vaccine compared to split influenza vaccine in patients with sickle cell anemia. Vaccine. 2010;28:1117–20.
72. Hambidge SJ, Ross C, Glanz J, et al. Trivalent inactivated influenza vaccine is not associated with sickle cell crises in children. Pediatrics. 2012;129:e54–9.
73. Howard-Jones M, Randall L, Bailey-Squire B, Clayton J, Jackson N. An audit of immunisation status of sickle cell patients in Coventry, UK. J Clin Pathol. 2009;62:42–5.
74. Beverung LM, Brousseau D, Hoffmann RG, Yan K, Panepinto JA. Ambulatory quality indicators to prevent infection in sickle cell disease. Am J Hematol. 2014;89:256–60.
75. Rickert D, Santoli J, Shefer A, Myrick A, Yusuf H. Influenza vaccination of high-risk children: what the providers say. Am J Prev Med. 2006;30:111–8.
76. Ledwich LJ, Harrington TM, Ayoub WT, Sartorius JA, Newman ED. Improved influenza and pneumococcal vaccination in rheumatology patients taking immunosuppressants using an electronic health record best practice alert. Arthritis Rheum. 2009;61:1505–10.
77. Bundy DG, Muschelli J, Clemens GD, et al. Preventive care delivery to young children with sickle cell disease. J Pediatr Hematol Oncol. 2016;38(4):294–300.
78. Zimmerman RK, Hoberman A, Nowalk MP, et al. Improving influenza vaccination rates of high-risk inner-city children over 2 intervention years. Ann Fam Med. 2006;4:534–40.
79. Sobota AE, Kavanagh PL, Adams WG, McClure E, Farrell D, Sprinz PG. Improvement in influenza vaccination rates in a pediatric sickle cell disease clinic. Pediatr Blood Cancer. 2015;62:654–7.
80. Kim A, Nemeth E. New insights into iron regulation and erythropoiesis. Curr Opin Hematol. 2015;22:199–205.
81. Quinn CT, St Pierre TG. MRI measurements of iron load in transfusion-dependent patients: implementation, challenges, and pitfalls. Pediatr Blood Cancer. 2016;63:773–80.
82. Ganz T. Systemic iron homeostasis. Physiol Rev. 2013;93:1721–41.
83. Heeney MM. Iron clad: iron homeostasis and the diagnosis of hereditary iron overload. Hematology Am Soc Hematol Educ Program. 2014;2014:202–9.
84. Hoffbrand AV, Taher A, Cappellini MD. How I treat transfusional iron overload. Blood. 2012;120:3657–69.
85. Amid A, Saliba AN, Taher AT, Klaassen RJ. Thalassaemia in children: from quality of care to quality of life. Arch Dis Child. 2015;100:1051–7.
86. Marsella M, Borgna-Pignatti C. Transfusional iron overload and iron chelation therapy in thalassemia major and sickle cell disease. Hematol Oncol Clin North Am. 2014;28:703–27. vi
87. de Alarcon PA, Donovan ME, Forbes GB, Landaw SA, Stockman JA 3rd. Iron absorption in the thalassemia syndromes and its inhibition by tea. N Engl J Med. 1979;300:5–8.
88. Fasano RM, Leong T, Kaushal M, Sagiv E, Luban NL, Meier ER. Effectiveness of red blood cell exchange, partial manual exchange, and simple transfusion concurrently with iron chelation therapy in reducing iron overload in chronically transfused sickle cell anemia patients. Transfusion. 2016;56(7):1707–15.

89. Nelson SC, Hennessy JM, McDonough EA, Guck KL. Weekend very high-dose intravenous deferoxamine in children with transfusional iron overload. J Pediatr Hematol Oncol. 2006;28:182–5.
90. Olivieri NF. Adherence to deferoxamine therapy: heeding Hippocrates and Osler. Am J Hematol. 2004;76:415–6.
91. Pennell DJ, Berdoukas V, Karagiorga M, et al. Randomized controlled trial of deferiprone or deferoxamine in beta-thalassemia major patients with asymptomatic myocardial siderosis. Blood. 2006;107:3738–44.
92. Fisher SA, Brunskill SJ, Doree C, Chowdhury O, Gooding S, Roberts DJ. Oral deferiprone for iron chelation in people with thalassaemia. Cochrane Database Syst Rev. 2013;8:CD004839.
93. Fisher SA, Brunskill SJ, Doree C, Gooding S, Chowdhury O, Roberts DJ. Desferrioxamine mesylate for managing transfusional iron overload in people with transfusion-dependent thalassaemia. Cochrane Database Syst Rev. 2013;8:CD004450.
94. Delea TE, Edelsberg J, Sofrygin O, et al. Consequences and costs of noncompliance with iron chelation therapy in patients with transfusion-dependent thalassemia: a literature review. Transfusion. 2007;47:1919–29.
95. Brittenham GM, Griffith PM, Nienhuis AW, et al. Efficacy of deferoxamine in preventing complications of iron overload in patients with thalassemia major. N Engl J Med. 1994;331:567–73.
96. Ward A, Caro JJ, Green TC, et al. An international survey of patients with thalassemia major and their views about sustaining life-long desferrioxamine use. BMC Clin Pharmacol. 2002;2:3.
97. Hoffbrand AV, Cohen A, Hershko C. Role of deferiprone in chelation therapy for transfusional iron overload. Blood. 2003;102:17–24.
98. Haghpanah S, Zarei T, Zahedi Z, Karimi M. Compliance and satisfaction with deferasirox (Exjade(R)) compared with deferoxamine in patients with transfusion-dependent beta-thalassemia. Hematology (Amsterdam, Netherlands). 2014;19:187–91.
99. Trachtenberg FL, Gerstenberger E, Xu Y, et al. Relationship among chelator adherence, change in chelators, and quality of life in thalassemia. Qual Life Res. 2014;23:2277–88.
100. Jordan LB, Vekeman F, Sengupta A, Corral M, Guo A, Duh MS. Persistence and compliance of deferoxamine versus deferasirox in Medicaid patients with sickle-cell disease. J Clin Pharm Ther. 2012;37:173–81.
101. Origa R, Danjou F, Cossa S, et al. Impact of heart magnetic resonance imaging on chelation choices, compliance with treatment and risk of heart disease in patients with thalassaemia major. Br J Haematol. 2013;163:400–3.
102. Pakbaz Z, Fischer R, Treadwell M, et al. A simple model to assess and improve adherence to iron chelation therapy with deferoxamine in patients with thalassemia. Ann N Y Acad Sci. 2005;1054:486–91.

Chapter 16
Implementation of Evidence-Based Care in the Sickle Cell and Hemophilia Patient Population

Karen A. Kalinyak, Christopher E. Dandoy, and Rachelle Nuss

Introduction

Sickle cell disease (SCD) is an inherited disorder caused by mutations of the beta hemoglobin chain and is hallmarked by vaso-occlusive crisis (VOC) manifest as intense pain in bones and associated with progressive multi-organ damage that has a major detrimental impact on health, life expectancy, and quality of life (QOL) [1–3]. Approximately 100,000 people in the United States are affected with an estimated annual cost of 1.1 billion dollars in 2009 [4].

Worldwide it is estimated that 300,000 affected babies are born each year; the vast majority is unidentified and die in early childhood. Universal newborn screening, antibiotic prophylaxis, supplemental immunizations, and the timely treatment of febrile events result in a significant reduction of early mortality [5–11]. Despite marked improvement in outcomes, morbidity and early mortality exists as life expectancy is limited in patients with SCD [2, 4, 12, 13].

Quality and safety improvement interventions are clearly indicated to improve the outcome for people with SCD. In the United States, a hemoglobinopathy learning collaborative was formed between centers funded for the Sickle Cell Disease Treatment Program, the National Initiative for Children's Health Care Quality,

K.A. Kalinyak (✉)
Division of Hematology, Cancer and Blood Disease Institute, Cincinnati Children's Hospital Medical Center, 3333 Burnet Ave, Cincinnati, OH, USA
e-mail: Karen.Kalinyak@cchmc.org

C.E. Dandoy
Division of Bone Marrow Transplantation and Immune Deficiency, Cancer and Blood Disease Institute, Cincinnati Children's Hospital Medical Center,
3333 Burnet Ave, Cincinnati, OH, USA

R. Nuss
Department of Pediatric Hematology, Children's Hospital Colorado,
13123 East 16th Ave, Aurora, CO, USA

© Springer International Publishing AG 2017
C.E. Dandoy et al. (eds.), *Patient Safety and Quality in Pediatric Hematology/Oncology and Stem Cell Transplantation*, DOI 10.1007/978-3-319-53790-0_16

Boston Medical Center, and the Sickle Cell Disease Association of America. The goal of the collaborative was to address quality of care through the development and implementation of evidence-based guidelines and measurements of healthcare quality through ongoing quality improvement initiatives. Many of the initiatives described below were performed through the learning collaborative.

Timely Pain Management

Severe pain secondary to VOC is the hallmark of SCD and is the number one indication for patients to seek care in the emergency department (ED) as well as require hospitalization [14–17]. Frequent episodes of VOC affect QOL, are associated with anxiety and depression, and lead to an increase in urgent healthcare utilization, thereby escalating healthcare costs [2, 13, 18].

Pain Management in the Outpatient Setting

When a child with SCD develops VOC, the family is expected to attempt to manage the pain at home. In an attempt to maximize home management, Crosby et al. utilized quality improvement methodology to develop individualized home pain management plans (HPMP) that included both pharmacologic as well as non-pharmacologic strategies for children with SCD ages 5 years and older [19] (Fig. 16.1). The plans were successfully integrated into the daily workflow of their busy outpatient clinic. The

---

Individualized home Pain Management Plan Example

Problem Detail

Noted: 12/9/2012
  Overview Signed 12/9/2012   3:33 PM by Provider

  Mild pain: Rest, increased fluids, and heat. Also take Ibuprofen 600 mg every 6–8 h as needed for mild pain. While for the medication to start working, practice relaxation skills (belly breathing or relaxing muscles).

  Moderate pain: Continue rest, increased fluids, heat, Ibuprofen and relaxation skills (belly breathing, relaxing muscles, thinking about relaxing places). Oxycodone 5 mg every 4 h as needed for moderate pain with zofran 8 mg every 8 h because it upsets stomach. Also start Miralax 17g by mouth once daily.

  Severe pain: Continue rest, increased fluids, heat, Ibuprofen, Miralax, relaxation skills and Oxycodone. Start taking OxyContin 10 mg every 12 h. If pain continues or worsens, call and come to clinic/ED for further pain management.

  Example homework recommendations provided by psychology provider:
  Practice diaphragmatic (belly) breathing for 5 min each day and track practice on the calender provided. Belly breathing includes:
  - Breathing in through nose and out through mouth
  - Taking slow, deep breaths
  - Having belly rise and fall and chest remain still

Fig. 16.1 Individualized home pain management plan example

implementation process was monitored and tracked using 2 weekly run charts: one that displayed the percentage of eligible SCD patients who needed a HPMP each week compared to the number who actually received one and another that showed the overall number of eligible children with a HPMP. The outcome was evaluated by analyzing a monthly control chart showing the percentage of SCD patients seen in the ED. With a HPMP the number of ED visits for uncomplicated VOC was reduced from 6.9 to 1.1%. With ongoing monitoring and HPMP updates every 6 months, the reduction in ED visits has been sustained (unpublished data).

Pain Management in the Acute Care Setting (Day Hospital and ED)

Guidelines from the National Heart, Lung, and Blood Institute (NHLBI) as well as from the American Pain Society for VOC refractory to home therapy recommend rapid evaluation and treatment with parenteral analgesia in an acute care setting followed by timely follow-up pain assessments and administration of repeat analgesia doses as needed [20–22]. The NHLBI guidelines indicate a parenteral analgesic should be administered within 60 min of check-in or 30 min of triage, and the American Pain Society guidelines indicate administration of a parenteral analgesic within 30 min of assessment. Timely and appropriate administration of analgesics relieves the acute pain and may also prevent the development of a chronic pain syndrome necessitating frequent subsequent ED visits and hospitalizations [23]. However, despite detailed guidelines and quality indicators for the management of acute VOC, both pediatric and adult SCD patients generally experience marked delays to treatment in the ED [18, 24] and accusations of drug seeking which result in poor patient satisfaction and increased healthcare costs [4].

Day Hospital

A successful quality improvement initiative is the establishment of a "day" hospital as alternative to the ED. Day hospitals are generally infusion centers capable of managing uncomplicated VOC for children as well as adults. The Texas Children's Sickle Cell Center developed a pediatric day hospital program in 2000. A day hospital admission was defined as a minimum of two consecutive days during which children received aggressive pain management, including parenteral hydration and analgesics, supported by home treatment in the evening and overnight with oral medications. Seventy-one percent of the children admitted to the day hospital avoided inpatient hospitalization, and only 7% returned for further acute care within 48 h of discharge compared with a national average of 23% readmission after inpatient hospitalization for VOC [25]. The day hospital, when compared with inpatient hospitalization, provided efficient and timely management of VOC with a reduced length of stay [25]. Similarly, adults with VOC managed in a day hospital are significantly less likely to need inpatient admission (8.3%) compared to those seen in the ED (42.7%). The cost savings for the hospital was estimated to be approximately $1.7 million [26]. The association between day hospital and decreased inpatient admission rates and lower hospital costs has been validated [27].

A quality improvement project at Johns Hopkins sought to determine variables affecting the ability to achieve timely parenteral opiate administration in the infusion center/day hospital. The authors determined that to improve time to first dose of parenteral analgesic, the primary target for improvement was to reduce the nurse-to-patient ratio [28].

Emergency Department

Misconceptions about the treatment, including timely administration of appropriate doses of pain medication and variation of care amongst providers, have been addressed by the development of care guidelines for VOC by the NIH expert panel and the American Pain Society. However, there are many barriers to appropriate treatment of VOC in the ED. The primary barriers include, but are not limited to: (a) delays in patient assessment, (b) misconceptions about the treatment including appropriate pain medication dosing, (c) variation of care among providers, and (d) infrequent pain reassessments [20]. Quality improvement interventions are evaluating how to overcome the barriers.

In response to the barriers found in the ED, Tanabe et al. developed the adult emergency department sickle cell assessment of needs and strengths (ED-SCANS), a research-based decision support and quality improvement tool. It includes decision algorithms including (a) triage, (b) analgesic management, (c) diagnostic evaluation, (d) identification of the high risk (severe disease) or high user, (e) disposition, (f) need for an analgesic prescription (if discharged home), and (g) needs for referrals, physicians, or psychosocial services (if discharged home) [29]. Subsequently, the authors developed a family-centered pediatric ED-SCANS [30]. The ED-SCANS suggest that if the Emergency Severity Index (ESI) Version 4 triage system is utilized, patients presenting with VOC should be triaged as ESI level 2 (very high priority) [31] and seen promptly. However, this triage system is in place in only about one-half of the United States. ED-SCANS, or similar support tools, can serve as the base for quality improvement interventions.

Givens et al. studied the impact of an ED pain management guideline in concert with clinical case management on ED utilization, clinic visits, and hospital admissions comparing the year prior to 3 years after implementing the quality improvement project. They found that ED visits decreased significantly over the 4-year time period and clinic visits steadily increased. In addition, there was a significant reduction in repeat ED visits within 30 days. Although total hospitalizations did not change, there was a reduction from 43% to 29% of those being seen in the ED being admitted to the hospital [32].

Fig. 16.2 Interventions to
improve timely analgesia
delivery in VOC [31–34]

- Individual prescribing and monitoring protocol
- Proper triage of patients presenting with VOC
- Standardized timing of reassessment
- Standardized time-specific VOE protocol
- Intranasal fentanyl as the first parenteral pain medication
- Pain medication calculator
- Provider and patient/family education
- Clinical practice guidelines

Treadwell et al. showed through their quality improvement initiative that they were able to decrease time to first assessments and administration of pain medication as well as improve the percentage of patients reassessed within 30 min of initial analgesic therapy [33]. Using QI methodology, Kavanagh et al. decreased the mean time to first analgesia from 56 to 23 min, a result that has been sustained for 4 years [34]. The improvement group developed standardized ED-based protocols or algorithms to reduce provider variability. Furthermore, they added the use of intranasal fentanyl as part of the initial pain management strategy, thus significantly decreasing the time to first dose of pain medications, and developed a pain medication calculator and held training sessions for ED providers. They found that the number of repeat ED visits and the length of stay for patients who were sent home decreased [34].

Ender et al. used a clinical pathway in an attempt to improve quality of care for children seen in the ED with VOC. They found the time to first parenteral opioid could be improved from 94 to 46 min ($p = 0.013$). Others have similarly shown that implementation of clinical practice guidelines significantly improves the ability to deliver timely and effective analgesia [35]. The various interventions used to improve timely analgesia delivery are outlined in Fig. 16.2.

Inpatient Management of VOC

Acute VOC episodes are the most frequent cause of hospitalization for patients with SCD. [36] Several randomized control trials as well as observational studies support the use of around-the-clock analgesics versus intermittent analgesic administration in treating SCD patients with VOC [37–42]. The development and implementation of pain guidelines or algorithms have been shown to be effective in improving pain assessment and management in both pediatric and adult populations [43–48]. Treadwell et al. reported their use of quality improvement strategies to enhance pediatric pain assessment which improved pain management practices and resulted in increased patient and staff satisfaction [33]. Inpatient care pathways have been used successfully and have led to less variability among providers, decreased length of inpatient stay by 1.44 days, and increased use of patient-controlled analgesia [49].

Timely, appropriate management of VOC is an effective mechanism to reduce duration of symptoms, improve quality of life, and reduce resource utilization. It is important for healthcare professions to actively engage in QI efforts to improve timely appropriate analgesia for VOC.

Hydroxyurea

Hydroxycarbamide (hydroxyurea) is an oral medication that inhibits ribonucleotide reductase which leads to decreased production of red cells containing sickle hemoglobin and increased production of fetal hemoglobin. In addition, hydroxyurea decreases white blood cell and platelet production [50]. It is also a nitric oxide donor, acting as a vasodilator. Over the past 30 years, hydroxyurea has emerged as a beneficial disease-modifying therapy for adults and children with SCD [51, 52].

Administration of oral hydroxyurea is associated with a decreased incidence of VOC, acute chest, stroke, transfusion requirement, and hospitalizations [20, 53–57]. Importantly, the use of hydroxyurea is associated with improved survival in both adults and children with SCD [58–60]. Hydroxyurea is a well-tolerated medication with very little toxicity. Accordingly, the NHLBI's evidence-based clinical guideline for the management of patients with sickle cell disease recommends that all children with homozygous sickle cell anemia or sickle β^0 thalassemia should be offered hydroxyurea therapy beginning at 9 months of age, regardless of clinical severity [20].

Despite the evidence supporting its benefits, there are two primary barriers: practice implementation and home medication adherence. In 2005, Zumberg et al. surveyed physicians in Florida and North Carolina and found that the barriers to wider use of HU included physician concerns about carcinogenic potential, doubts about HU effectiveness, perceived patient apprehension about adverse effects, concern about lack of contraceptive use, and patient adherence [61]. Other barriers to implementation include parental acceptance, differences in practice management, and perhaps most importantly, barriers to access of care with physician familiar with SCD and use of hydroxyurea [62].

As to practice implementation, Stettler et al. showed that three out of four patients who would benefit from hydroxyurea were not receiving it [63]. In New York, there are statistically significant differences between centers regarding the percentage of patients treated with hydroxyurea and overall compliance with therapy. Practice differences between treatment centers and inadequate compliance is limiting the full disease-modifying effects of hydroxyurea [62].

As to adherence, poor medication adherence is common in chronic disease and is generally defined as intake below 80% of daily prescribed medication use. Among children with chronic medical conditions, adolescents have especially high rates of poor adherence [64, 65]. Children with sickle cell disease who stop taking hydroxyurea indicate they do not want to take daily medication, they think it makes them feel badly, and do not believe it will improve their symptoms. [66] Daily hydroxyurea adherence is particularly challenging because benefits may not be apparent until 3–6 months after starting therapy, and treatment requires frequent blood monitoring [67].

In a small quality improvement initiative with 19 subjects, Inoue et al. found that the two most common barriers to hydroxyurea adherence were lack of daily reminders to take it and difficulty with obtaining hydroxyurea from the pharmacy [68].

These findings were similar to those reported by Thornburg et al. [67] A quality improvement initiative that has been successful in improving hydroxyurea adherence is incorporating a pharmacist into clinic visits. When a clinical pharmacist met with the families, the rate of hydroxyurea dose escalation (a sign of adherence and compliance) was improved [69].

Promoting hydroxyurea adherence requires a multifaceted approach, consisting of multidisciplinary teams integrating medication adherence-related assessments, education, and anticipatory guidance into standard clinical care [70, 71].

Reducing the Incidence of Stroke

The incidence of overt stroke in a child with SCD as determined by The Cooperative Study of Sickle Cell Disease was 1.02 per 100 patient-years with the highest incidence in children 2–5 years of age [72]. Historically, 11% of children would suffer an overt stroke by the age of 20 years.

Fortunately, transcranial Doppler ultrasonography (TCD), a noninvasive test, has been shown to identify children at high risk for stroke. The Stroke Prevention Trial in Sickle Cell Anemia enrolled children with the highest risk for stroke, those with homozygous sickle cell anemia, or sickle β^0 thalassemia. The trial found a greater than 90% reduction in overt stroke for those identified as high risk by TCD who then received prophylactic transfusion therapy [73–78]. A recent review of national databases demonstrates a decrease in the mean annual incidence rate of hospitalizations secondary to overt stroke from 0.51 per 100 patient years in 1993–1998 to 0.28 per 100 patient years in 1999–2009 following the publication of the trial [79].

Based upon the findings, the American Academy of Pediatrics and National Institute of Health evidence-based guidelines recommend screening all children with homozygous sickle cell anemia or sickle β^0 thalassemia, with TCD screening beginning at 2 years and continuing yearly until 16 years of age [20, 74, 80, 81]. A recent study has demonstrated the two-step approach is a cost-effective strategy [82]. However, implementation of the guidelines has been difficult. One sickle cell program reported that only 45% of at risk patients were undergoing yearly TCD screening [83].

Both provider and patient adherence to TCD/transfusion guidelines contribute to the low screening rate. Barriers cited include low patient uptake and/or increased distance from a center skilled at doing the studies [76, 83, 84]. Patient/family fear of chronic transfusions, distrust of the healthcare team, and financial barriers such as large deductibles, copayments, or inadequate insurance coverage have also been suggested by physicians as obstacles [76]. There is a lack of understanding about the importance, purpose, technique, and frequency of TCD screening and hesitation that monthly transfusions would be recommended if the screen was abnormal. [85] A practical barrier to successfully completing a TCD study, especially on a very young child, has been getting the cooperation of the child during the exam as he must be awake and lay still [86].

In order for an efficacious intervention, such as TCD screening and prophylactic transfusion to be clinically effective and achieve the intended outcome, several criteria must be met: (i) the intervention must be easily accessible to all patients, (ii) the appropriate patients needing the intervention need to be identified, (iii) the recommendations need to be accepted and implemented by providers, and (iv) the recommendations must be accepted and adhered to by the patients and caregivers [87].

A failure analysis for TCD at the Cincinnati Comprehensive Sickle Cell Center revealed numerous barriers including variability in processes related to identifying eligible children, educating of caregivers, scheduling the TCD, tracking TCD completion, and acting on the results. In response, the multidisciplinary quality assurance team developed a reliable process for TCD screening which is consistent with the national recommendations. Through this work the successful screening rate for all eligible young children ages 24–27 months improved from 25 to 75%. Changes to the process included the development of a TCD care algorithm used by all providers, standardization of the process for implementation, standardized family education, and caregiver/patient preparation, including pre-visit planning, to allow for successful completion of TCD screening. To identify the patients eligible for TCD screening, a self-generating electronic medical record (EMR) report was created to identify and alert the team of children approaching the age for their first TCD. To assist the provider and family, the TCD is scheduled prior to the physician visit, and the imaging results are given to the provider prior to the visit so the results can be discussed and plan developed prior to the family leaving the clinic visit [88] (Fig. 16.3).

In contrast with the large-scale quality improvement project reported above, Munta et al. evaluated a low-cost quality improvement intervention to increase screening for stroke risk with TCD. They found that when families received personalized reminder letters, information on screening, and a refrigerator magnet imprinted with the recommended date for TCD screening, they were able to improve screening from 54 to 79% [90].

The evidence is overwhelming that screening with TCD identifies those patients at highest risk of stroke, and almost all strokes can be prevented with initiation of a prophylactic transfusion program. Quality improvement initiatives can be used to identify barriers and develop a standardized process that is reliable to deliver coordinated, high-quality care that ensures all patients have the opportunity to be screened and treated to reduce the risk for stroke.

- Completing TCD during the clinic appointment
- Hiring and/or training a nurse to be able to do TCD exams in the clinic
- Development of standardized and reliable process
- family education
- Caregiver/patient preparation to allow for successful completion of TCD
- Reliable process to identify eligible patients
- Completion of the TCD prior to the clinic visit

Fig. 16.3 Interventions to improve transcranial Doppler (*TCD*) screening compliance [86, 88, 89]

Immunizations

As a consequence of functional hyposplenism, which can develop as early as at 4 months of age, infants and young children with SCD are at high risk of serious infection with encapsulated organisms. In addition, they are at risk for respiratory symptoms secondary to influenza. Bundy et al. analyzed hospitalizations during two influenza seasons from the healthcare cost and utilization project state inpatient databases. They found children with SCD were hospitalized with influenza at 56 times the rate of children without SCD [91].

Therefore, in addition to routine vaccinations indicated for all children, children with SCD must receive supplemental vaccines including immunizations against pneumococcus, meningococcus, and influenza. Immunization against pneumococcus has been shown to decrease the rate of invasive pneumococcal disease by 90.8 and 93.45% in children under 2 years and 5 years of age, respectively [92]. The rate is also decreased from 161 cases to 99 cases per 100,000 in children 5 years or greater.

Two quality initiatives have shown that immunization rates in children with sickle cell disease can be improved. Sobota et al. used quality improvement methods to improve influenza vaccination rates in a population of children with SCD. They increased provider and parent education about the importance of the vaccine. To identify children, the team enhanced their electronic health record and used a patient registry. Prior to the clinic visit, a reminder call was completed by a patient navigator. Through their efforts, they were able to improve the vaccination rate to 90% of their patients [93].

Han et al. had a clinical pharmacist meet with families during a child's SCD outpatient visit to provide education and support. By doing so, the immunization rate for the 23-valent pneumococcal polysaccharide vaccine, the 13 valent-pneumococcal conjugate vaccine, and influenza vaccine increased to 66%, 47%, and 62%, respectively. The number of pharmacist encounters correlated with improved immunization completion rates [69].

Quality improvement can be achieved for immunization uptake by families with SCD.

Hemophilia

Hemophilia is primarily due to an X-linked recessive bleeding disorder caused by deficiency or dysfunction of a clotting protein, most often factor VIII (hemophilia A) or factor IX (hemophilia B), and is associated with a substantially increased risk for excessive hemorrhage into any organ although most often into joints and muscles precipitating chronic arthropathy [94, 95].

There are approximately 20,000 people with hemophilia in the United States, most with either factor VIII deficiency (hemophilia A) or factor IX deficiency (hemophilia B), and worldwide there are about 400,000 affected individuals [94–96].

Worldwide, intravenous replacement therapy with the missing or dysfunctional clotting protein episodically and on demand (when the hemorrhage occurs) has been the mainstay of treatment where accessible [97]. In the United States, the annual estimated mean healthcare costs for patients with hemophilia is upward of $140,000 per year in the absence of inhibitors, with the majority of expenditures going toward factor concentrate [98, 99]. Even with on-demand administration of factor concentrate, hemophilia patients develop joint destruction, reduced mobility, chronic pain, and poor quality of life.

In 2012, the National Hemophilia Program Coordinating Center (NHPCC) was funded in the United States by the Human Research Services Agency (HRSA) to coordinate and collaborate with regional hemophilia networks to establish standardized national efforts to identify national priorities for improvement in hemophilia care and collect national metrics. Beginning in 2017, HRSA grants will require regions to implement QI projects at their hemophilia treatment centers.

The current World Federation of Hemophilia Treatment Guidelines are shown in Fig. 16.4. The WHF recommends "The wide ranging needs of people with hemophilia and their families are best met through the coordinated delivery of comprehensive care by a multidisciplinary team of healthcare professionals, in accordance with accepted protocols that are practical and national treatment guidelines, if available." [97] Potential process and outcome measures are shown.

Acute bleeds should be treated as quickly as possible, preferably within 2 h	• Percentage of patients who receive factor within 120 min of acute bleed o (number of patients receiving treatment within 120 min / number of patients with acute bleeds) • Median time from acute bleed to factor administration
Children should be seen by all core team members of a comprehensive multidisciplinary team every 6 months	• Percentage of hemophilia patients receiving comprehensive 6-month evaluation o (patients receiving comprehensive care / total hemophilia patients)
Prophylaxis prevents bleeding and joint destruction and should be the goal of therapy to preserve normal musculoskeletal function	• Percentage of patients receiving >95% of recommended o (number of patients receiving > 95% of scheduled factor doses / total number of patients receiving prophylaxis)

Fig. 16.4 Selected practice statements from the World Federation of Hemophilia Treatment Guidelines Working Group [97] and associated process/outcome measurement

Urgent Care

Patients with hemophilia with active bleeding who seek care in the ED should be triaged as either ESI 1 or 2, depending upon whether or not the hemorrhage is immediately life threatening. A standardized process similar to the ED-SPRANS will need to be developed to rapidly identify, triage, gain venous access, and administer factor concentrate and could serve as the template for quality improvement [100]. Additionally, The World Federation of Hemophilia Treatment Guidelines Working Group recommendation states "To facilitate appropriate management in emergency situations, all patients should carry easily accessible identification, indicating the diagnosis, severity of the bleeding disorder, inhibitor status, type of treatment product used, initial dosage for treatment of severe, moderate, and mild bleeding, and contact information of the treating physician/clinic." [97] Incorporating an identification card into the template is recommended.

Unlike sickle cell, where analgesics and fluids are readily available and prescribed in the ED, due to the rare nature of hemophilia, the majority of urgent care physicians are not knowledgeable about hemophilia therapy, and factor concentrates are not routinely available except in tertiary hospitals due to their low utilization, exorbitant cost, and outdating. Even where available, administration may be delayed due to pharmacy and nursing lack of knowledge about reconstitution and administration of the products. Suggested process measures to improve the time to factor concentrate should include standardized pre-arrival notification, rapid identification of eligible patients, standardized post-arrival process, faculty and staff knowledge of urgency, family engagement, and timely vascular access [101–103].

Tagliaferri et al. integrated a web-based algorithm among 44 emergency departments in Italy which included extensive treatment information corresponding with patients' electronic clinical records including the first dose of concentrate for each type and severity of bleed or trauma in the ED. The intervention reduced triage-assessment and triage-treatment times by approximately 25% [104].

Compliance with Prophylaxis

Home administration of prophylactic, parenteral factor concentrate is the standard therapy for patients with severe hemophilia. Prophylactic therapy prevents morbidity due to hemophilic arthropathy and mortality due to lethal hemorrhage [105, 106]. Long-term adherence to prophylactic therapy requires life-long dedication of the patient and caregiver [107].

For children with severe hemophilia, lack of adherence to prophylactic infusion of factor concentrate will be associated with hemorrhage, potentially life threatening, but more likely joint hemorrhage precipitating joint destruction and necessitating replacement. There is no gold standard for adherence; patient report is accepted. Quality initiatives to measure adherence are by checking frequency of pharmacy ordering records as the majority of infusions are done at home, familial questioning, and clinical outcomes, i.e., number of joint hemorrhages [108] are targets to better assess adherence.

A quality improvement strategy that may prove beneficial for children is to have a family member do the factor infusion rather than relying on the child to do it himself. Higher adherence to prophylaxis has been reported if a child is infused by a family member rather than reliant on self-infusion [109].

Similar to hydroxyurea for SCD patients, adolescents and young adults have poor adherence to prophylactic factor replacement, so targeting process measures to address this population is critical. The reported most important motivators for adherence are a good relationship with the healthcare provider and belief that the treatment is important [107].

Process improvement strategies to promote adherence include team motivation, ensuring a sense of normality, encouraging a positive attitude toward the disease and treatment, developing mechanisms to increase energy and will-power, and minimization of the impact of the disease. In a systematic review of barriers and motivators for home prophylactic adherence, Schriever et al. identified absence of or infrequency of symptoms and increasing age as the largest barriers to prophylactic adherence. Witkop et al. developed a validated hemophilia regimen treatment adherence scale which was administered to 73 males receiving prophylactic infusions. Final logistic regression modeling suggested that 18–25-year-olds were 6.2 times more likely to be nonadherent as compares with 13–17-year-olds [110].

As personalized care is embraced, quality initiatives to assess whether or not individualized pharmacokinetic dosing regimens improve the quality of joint outcome will be indicated [111, 112]. In addition, factor concentrates with prolonged half-lives are becoming available, and quality initiatives should be conducted to assess their impact on reducing joint hemorrhage and damage as well as quality of life [113].

Sufficient Factor Supplies

Since factor concentrate is given generally at home parenterally to those with severe hemophilia, in addition to the factor concentrate, supplies such as tourniquets, needles, tubing, alcohol wipes, band aids, and gauze must be supplied. Even for those patients with mild and moderate hemophilia, at least one if not two doses and supplies are often delivered to the home to be taken to the ED when needed, since not all urgent care centers stock factor concentrate.

Process improvement interventions could include determining the optimal number of each supply to be delivered with each dose of the factor concentrate so families are always well prepared. A process in the pharmacy whereby the pharmacy is notified when home factor concentrate is administered should trigger replacement with adequate supplies.

Transition to Adult Care

Transitions from inpatient and outpatient care and pediatric to adult care are associated with increased mortality. Patients with sickle cell disease and hemophilia share many difficulties in the transition from pediatric to adult care [114]. These include taking over responsibility for their care from parents, generally their mothers, learning to order their medications, communicating their needs, asking questions, coordinating multi-specialty care, asserting independence, understanding their insurance, establishing trust in the new setting for the adult care world, and advocating for themselves. Learning to integrate geographic moves and maintain chronic care is problematic. School and work absence complicates the ability to receive necessary care. In addition, patients with sickle cell disease deal with accusations of narcotic seeking [115].

Porter et al. from St. Jude Children's Research Hospital used quality improvement methodology to implement an assessment tool for readiness to transition. Seventy two adolescents with SCD participated in the program. The team concluded the tool was informative and could be helpful for planning and preparation for transition [116].

Frost et al. conducted a quality improvement project collecting information from focus groups and key informant interviews to identify gaps and opportunities for a health information technology tool as a means to improve care transition for patients with sickle cell disease. Patients, caregivers, and adult and pediatric providers of children with SCD supported the development of a health information technology tool as a means to convey "clinician-endorsed plans" in the hope it could "lessen the opportunity for racial bias," thereby overcoming some barriers and enabling delivery of quality care [117].

As for patients with hemophilia, the NHPCC conducted a patient needs assessment and staff technical assistance survey with hemophilia HRSA grantees. Both surveys identified transition as problematic. Because of those results and the annual expectation that HRSA hemophilia grantees demonstrate improvement in transition of care to meet the Healthy People 2020 measure to " increase the proportion of youth with special health care needs whose provider has discussed transition planning from pediatric to adult health care," NHPCC targeted transition for quality improvement projects. The Dartmouth Institute Microsystem Academy (TIDMA) is a consultant for the projects. Each HRSA grantee is expected to perform a quality initiative on transition.

Conclusion

Process improvement has improved care for patients with SCD and is predicted to do so for those with hemophilia as well. However, for SCD as well as hemophilia, there is much work to be done. Although there is extensive literature on the science of hemophilia and sickle cell disease and many guidelines, data evaluating barriers and interventions to improve delivery of care and adherence with proven interventions are needed to further improve outcomes. Processes and policies at all stages of care delivery should be continuously and proactively refined and improved, and strategies for improvement should be shared.

References

1. Platt OS, Thorington BD, Brambilla DJ, et al. Pain in sickle cell disease. Rates and risk factors. N Engl J Med. 1991;325(1):11–6.
2. Panepinto JA, O'Mahar KM, DeBaun MR, Loberiza FR, Scott JP. Health-related quality of life in children with sickle cell disease: child and parent perception. Br J Haematol. 2005;130(3):437–44.
3. Rees DC, Williams TN, Gladwin MT. Sickle-cell disease. Lancet. 2010;376(9757):2018–31.
4. Kauf TL, Coates TD, Huazhi L, Mody-Patel N, Hartzema AG. The cost of health care for children and adults with sickle cell disease. Am J Hematol. 2009;84(6):323–7.
5. Gaston MH, Verter JI, Woods G, et al. Prophylaxis with oral penicillin in children with sickle cell anemia. A randomized trial. N Engl J Med. 1986;314(25):1593–9.
6. Vichinsky E, Hurst D, Earles A, Kleman K, Lubin B. Newborn screening for sickle cell disease: effect on mortality. Pediatrics. 1988;81(6):749–55.
7. Tsevat J, Wong JB, Pauker SG, Steinberg MH. Neonatal screening for sickle cell disease: a cost-effectiveness analysis. J Pediatr. 1991;118(4 Pt 1):546–54.
8. Shafer FE, Lorey F, Cunningham GC, Klumpp C, Vichinsky E, Lubin B. Newborn screening for sickle cell disease: 4 years of experience from California's newborn screening program. J Pediatr Hematol Oncol. 1996;18(1):36–41.
9. Chesney PJ, Wilimas JA, Presbury G, et al. Penicillin- and cephalosporin-resistant strains of Streptococcus pneumoniae causing sepsis and meningitis in children with sickle cell disease. J Pediatr. 1995;127(4):526–32.
10. O'Brien KL, Swift AJ, Winkelstein JA, et al. Safety and immunogenicity of heptavalent pneumococcal vaccine conjugated to CRM(197) among infants with sickle cell disease. Pneumococcal Conjugate Vaccine Study Group. Pediatrics. 2000;106(5):965–72.
11. Ammann AJ, Addiego J, Wara DW, Lubin B, Smith WB, Mentzer WC. Polyvalent pneumococcal-polysaccharide immunization of patients with sickle-cell anemia and patients with splenectomy. N Engl J Med. 1977;297(17):897–900.
12. Platt OS, Brambilla DJ, Rosse WF, et al. Mortality in sickle cell disease. Life expectancy and risk factors for early death. N Engl J Med. 1994;330(23):1639–44.
13. McClish DK, Penberthy LT, Bovbjerg VE, et al. Health related quality of life in sickle cell patients: the PiSCES project. Health Qual Life Outcomes. 2005;3:50.
14. Mvundura M, Amendah D, Kavanagh PL, Sprinz PG, Grosse SD. Health care utilization and expenditures for privately and publicly insured children with sickle cell disease in the United States. Pediatr Blood Cancer. 2009;53(4):642–6.
15. Smith WR, Penberthy LT, Bovbjerg VE, et al. Daily assessment of pain in adults with sickle cell disease. Ann Intern Med. 2008;148(2):94–101.
16. Yusuf HR, Atrash HK, Grosse SD, Parker CS, Grant AM. Emergency department visits made by patients with sickle cell disease: a descriptive study, 1999-2007. Am J Prev Med. 2010;38(4 Suppl):S536–41.
17. Brousseau DC, Owens PL, Mosso AL, Panepinto JA, Steiner CA. Acute care utilization and rehospitalizations for sickle cell disease. JAMA. 2010;303(13):1288–94.
18. Wang CJ, Kavanagh PL, Little AA, Holliman JB, Sprinz PG. Quality-of-care indicators for children with sickle cell disease. Pediatrics. 2011;128(3):484–93.

19. Crosby LE, Simmons K, Kaiser P, et al. Using quality improvement methods to implement an electronic medical record (EMR) supported individualized home pain management plan for children with sickle cell disease. J Clin Outcomes Manag. 2014;21(5):210–7.
20. Yawn BP, Buchanan GR, Afenyi-Annan AN, et al. Management of sickle cell disease: summary of the 2014 evidence-based report by expert panel members. JAMA. 2014;312(10):1033–48.
21. Jacob E. Pain management in sickle cell disease. Pain Manag Nurs. 2001;2(4):121–31.
22. Benjamin L. Pain management in sickle cell disease: palliative care begins at birth? Hematol Am Soc Hematol Educ Program. 2008:466–74
23. Ballas SK. Pain management of sickle cell disease. Hematol Oncol Clin North Am. 2005;19(5):785–802. v
24. Todd KH, Green C, Bonham Jr VL, Haywood Jr C, Ivy E. Sickle cell disease related pain: crisis and conflict. J Pain. 2006;7(7):453–8.
25. Raphael JL, Kamdar A, Wang T, Liu H, Mahoney DH, Mueller BU. Day hospital versus inpatient management of uncomplicated vaso-occlusive crises in children with sickle cell disease. Pediatr Blood Cancer. 2008;51(3):398–401.
26. Benjamin LJ, Swinson GI, Nagel RL. Sickle cell anemia day hospital: an approach for the management of uncomplicated painful crises. Blood. 2000;95(4):1130–6.
27. Adewoye AH, Nolan V, McMahon L, Ma Q, Steinberg MH. Effectiveness of a dedicated day hospital for management of acute sickle cell pain. Haematologica. 2007;92(6):854–5.
28. Whiteman LN, Lanzkron S, Stewart RW, Haywood C, Strouse JJ, Feldman L. Quality improvement process in a sickle cell infusion center. Am J Med. 2015;128(5):541–4.
29. Tanabe P, Thornton VL, Martinovich Z, Todd KH, Wun T, Lyons JS. The emergency department sickle cell assessment of needs and strengths (ED-SCANS): reliability and validity. Adv Emerg Nurs J. 2013;35(2):143–53.
30. Tanabe P, Dias N, Gorman L. Care of children with sickle cell disease in the emergency department: parent and provider perspectives inform quality improvement efforts. J Pediatr Oncol Nurs. 2013;30(4):205–17.
31. Gilboy N, Tanabe P, Travers DA. The emergency severity index version 4: changes to ESI level 1 and pediatric fever criteria. J Emerg Nurs. 2005;31(4):357–62.
32. Givens M, Rutherford C, Joshi G, Delaney K. Impact of an emergency department pain management protocol on the pattern of visits by patients with sickle cell disease. J Emerg Med. 2007;32(3):239–43.
33. Treadwell MJ, Bell M, Leibovich SA, et al. A quality improvement initiative to improve emergency Department Care for Pediatric Patients with sickle cell disease. J Clin Outcomes Manag. 2014;21(2):62–70.
34. Kavanagh PL, Sprinz PG, Wolfgang TL, et al. Improving the Management of Vaso-Occlusive Episodes in the pediatric emergency department. Pediatrics. 2015;136(4):e1016–25.
35. Morrissey LK, Shea JO, Kalish LA, Weiner DL, Branowicki P, Heeney MM. Clinical practice guideline improves the treatment of sickle cell disease vasoocclusive pain. Pediatr Blood Cancer. 2009;52(3):369–72.
36. Olney RS. Preventing morbidity and mortality from sickle cell disease. A public health perspective. Am J Prev Med. 1999;16(2):116–21.
37. Udezue E, Herrera E. Pain management in adult acute sickle cell pain crisis: a viewpoint. West Afr J Med. 2007;26(3):179–82.
38. Gonzalez ER, Bahal N, Hansen LA, et al. Intermittent injection vs patient-controlled analgesia for sickle cell crisis pain. Comparison in patients in the emergency department. Arch Intern Med. 1991;151(7):1373–8.
39. McPherson E, Perlin E, Finke H, Castro O, Pittman J. Patient-controlled analgesia in patients with sickle cell vaso-occlusive crisis. Am J Med Sci. 1990;299(1):10–2.
40. van Beers EJ, van Tuijn CF, Nieuwkerk PT, Friederich PW, Vranken JH, Biemond BJ. Patient-controlled analgesia versus continuous infusion of morphine during vaso-occlusive crisis in sickle cell disease, a randomized controlled trial. Am J Hematol. 2007;82(11):955–60.
41. Cole TB, Sprinkle RH, Smith SJ, Buchanan GR. Intravenous narcotic therapy for children with severe sickle cell pain crisis. Am J Dis Child. 1986;140(12):1255–59.

42. Holbrook CT. Patient-controlled analgesia pain management for children with sickle cell disease. J Assoc Acad Minor Phys. 1990;1(3):93–6.

43. Alexander M, Richtsmeier AJ, Broome ME, Barkin R. A multidisciplinary approach to pediatric pain: an empirical analysis. Child Health Care. 1993;22(2):81–91.

44. Dalton JA, Blau W, Lindley C, Carlson J, Youngblood R, Greer SM. Changing acute pain management to improve patient outcomes: an educational approach. J Pain Symptom Manag. 1999;17(4):277–87.

45. Miaskowski C, Nichols R, Brody R, Synold T. Assessment of patient satisfaction utilizing the American pain Society's quality assurance standards on acute and cancer-related pain. J Pain Symptom Manag. 1994;9(1):5–11.

46. Ward SE, Gordon D. Application of the American pain society quality assurance standards. Pain. 1994;56(3):299–306.

47. Bookbinder M, Coyle N, Kiss M, et al. Implementing national standards for cancer pain management: program model and evaluation. J Pain Symptom Manag. 1996;12(6):334–47. discussion 331-333

48. Francke AL, Luiken JB, de Schepper AM, Abu-Saad HH, Grypdonck M. Effects of a continuing education program on nurses' pain assessment practices. J Pain Symptom Manag. 1997;13(2):90–7.

49. Allen Liles E, Kirsch J, Gilchrist M, Adem M. Hospitalist management of vaso-occlusive pain crisis in patients with sickle cell disease using a pathway of care. Hosp Pract (1995). 2014;42(2):70–76.

50. Platt OS. Hydroxyurea for the treatment of sickle cell anemia. N Engl J Med. 2008;358(13):1362–9.

51. Platt OS, Orkin SH, Dover G, Beardsley GP, Miller B, Nathan DG. Hydroxyurea enhances fetal hemoglobin production in sickle cell anemia. J Clin Invest. 1984;74(2):652–6.

52. McGann PT, Ware RE. Hydroxyurea therapy for sickle cell anemia. Expert Opin Drug Saf. 2015;14(11):1749–58.

53. Ware RE, Davis BR, Schultz WH, et al. Hydroxycarbamide versus chronic transfusion for maintenance of transcranial doppler flow velocities in children with sickle cell anaemia-TCD with transfusions changing to hydroxyurea (TWiTCH): a multicentre, open-label, phase 3, non-inferiority trial. Lancet. 2016;387(10019):661–70.

54. Wang WC, Ware RE, Miller ST, et al. Hydroxycarbamide in very young children with sickle-cell anaemia: a multicentre, randomised, controlled trial (BABY HUG). Lancet. 2011;377(9778):1663–72.

55. Charache S, Terrin ML, Moore RD, et al. Effect of hydroxyurea on the frequency of painful crises in sickle cell anemia. Investigators of the multicenter study of hydroxyurea in sickle cell anemia. N Engl J Med. 1995;332(20):1317–22.

56. Charache S, Barton FB, Moore RD, et al. Hydroxyurea and sickle cell anemia. Clinical utility of a myelosuppressive "switching" agent. The multicenter study of hydroxyurea in sickle cell anemia. Medicine (Baltimore) 1996;75(6):300–326.

57. Hankins JS, Ware RE, Rogers ZR, et al. Long-term hydroxyurea therapy for infants with sickle cell anemia: the HUSOFT extension study. Blood. 2005;106(7):2269–75.

58. Steinberg MH, McCarthy WF, Castro O, et al. The risks and benefits of long-term use of hydroxyurea in sickle cell anemia: a 17.5 year follow-up. Am J Hematol. 2010;85(6):403–8.

59. Voskaridou E, Christoulas D, Bilalis A, et al. The effect of prolonged administration of hydroxyurea on morbidity and mortality in adult patients with sickle cell syndromes: results of a 17-year, single-center trial (LaSHS). Blood. 2010;115(12):2354–63.

60. Lobo CL, Pinto JF, Nascimento EM, Moura PG, Cardoso GP, Hankins JS. The effect of hydroxcarbamide therapy on survival of children with sickle cell disease. Br J Haematol. 2013;161(6):852–60.

61. Zumberg MS, Reddy S, Boyette RL, Schwartz RJ, Konrad TR, Lottenberg R. Hydroxyurea therapy for sickle cell disease in community-based practices: a survey of Florida and North Carolina hematologists/oncologists. Am J Hematol. 2005;79(2):107–13.

62. Anders DG, Tang F, Ledneva T, et al. Hydroxyurea use in young children with sickle cell anemia in New York state. Am J Prev Med. 2016;51(1 Suppl 1):S31–8.
63. Stettler N, McKiernan CM, Melin CQ, Adejoro OO, Walczak NB. Proportion of adults with sickle cell anemia and pain crises receiving hydroxyurea. JAMA. 2015;313(16):1671–2.
64. Taddeo D, Egedy M, Frappier JY. Adherence to treatment in adolescents. Paediatr Child Health. 2008;13(1):19–24.
65. Green NS, Manwani D, Qureshi M, Ireland K, Sinha A, Smaldone AM. Decreased fetal hemoglobin over time among youth with sickle cell disease on hydroxyurea is associated with higher urgent hospital use. Pediatr Blood Cancer. 2016;63(12):2146–53.
66. Haywood C, Beach MC, Bediako S, et al. Examining the characteristics and beliefs of hydroxyurea users and nonusers among adults with sickle cell disease. Am J Hematol. 2011;86(1):85–7.
67. Thornburg CD, Calatroni A, Telen M, Kemper AR. Adherence to hydroxyurea therapy in children with sickle cell anemia. J Pediatr. 2010;156(3):415–9.
68. Inoue S, Kodjebacheva G, Scherrer T, et al. Adherence to hydroxyurea medication by children with sickle cell disease (SCD) using an electronic device: a feasibility study. Int J Hematol. 2016;104(2):200–7.
69. Han J, Bhat S, Gowhari M, Gordeuk VR, Saraf SL. Impact of a clinical pharmacy service on the management of patients in a sickle cell disease outpatient center. Pharmacotherapy. 2016;36(11):1166–72.
70. Pai AL, McGrady ME. Assessing medication adherence as a standard of Care in Pediatric Oncology. Pediatr Blood Cancer. 2015;62(Suppl 5):S818–28.
71. McGrady ME, Ryan JL, Gutiérrez-Colina AM, Fredericks EM, Towner EK, Pai AL. The impact of effective paediatric adherence promotion interventions: systematic review and meta-analysis. Child Care Health Dev. 2015;41(6):789–802.
72. Ohene-Frempong K, Weiner SJ, Sleeper LA, et al. Cerebrovascular accidents in sickle cell disease: rates and risk factors. Blood. 1998;91(1):288–94.
73. Lee MT, Piomelli S, Granger S, et al. Stroke prevention trial in sickle cell anemia (STOP): extended follow-up and final results. Blood. 2006;108(3):847–52.
74. Adams RJ, McKie VC, Hsu L, et al. Prevention of a first stroke by transfusions in children with sickle cell anemia and abnormal results on transcranial Doppler ultrasonography. N Engl J Med. 1998;339(1):5–11.
75. Fullerton HJ, Adams RJ, Zhao S, Johnston SC. Declining stroke rates in Californian children with sickle cell disease. Blood. 2004;104(2):336–9.
76. Armstrong-Wells J, Grimes B, Sidney S, et al. Utilization of TCD screening for primary stroke prevention in children with sickle cell disease. Neurology. 2009;72(15):1316–21.
77. Enninful-Eghan H, Moore RH, Ichord R, Smith-Whitley K, Kwiatkowski JL. Transcranial Doppler ultrasonography and prophylactic transfusion program is effective in preventing overt stroke in children with sickle cell disease. J Pediatr. 2010;157(3):479–84.
78. Lehman LL, Fullerton HJ. Changing ethnic disparity in ischemic stroke mortality in US children after the STOP trial. JAMA Pediatr. 2013;167(8):754–8.
79. McCavit TL, Xuan L, Zhang S, Flores G, Quinn CT. National trends in incidence rates of hospitalization for stroke in children with sickle cell disease. Pediatr Blood Cancer. 2013;60(5):823–7.
80. Genetics SoHOCo, Pediatrics AAo. Health supervision for children with sickle cell disease. Pediatrics. 2002;109(3):526–35.
81. Claster S, Vichinsky EP. Managing sickle cell disease. BMJ. 2003;327(7424):1151–5.
82. Cherry MG, Greenhalgh J, Osipenko L, et al. The clinical effectiveness and cost-effectiveness of primary stroke prevention in children with sickle cell disease: a systematic review and economic evaluation. Health Technol Assess. 2012;16(43):1–129.
83. Raphael JL, Shetty PB, Liu H, Mahoney DH, Mueller BU. A critical assessment of transcranial doppler screening rates in a large pediatric sickle cell center: opportunities to improve healthcare quality. Pediatr Blood Cancer. 2008;51(5):647–51.

84. Fullerton HJ, Gardner M, Adams RJ, Lo LC, Johnston SC. Obstacles to primary stroke prevention in children with sickle cell disease. Neurology. 2006;67(6):1098–9.
85. Bollinger LM, Nire KG, Rhodes MM, Chisolm DJ, O'Brien SH. Caregivers' perspectives on barriers to transcranial Doppler screening in children with sickle-cell disease. Pediatr Blood Cancer. 2011;56(1):99–102.
86. McCarville MB, Goodin GS, Fortner G, et al. Evaluation of a comprehensive transcranial doppler screening program for children with sickle cell anemia. Pediatr Blood Cancer. 2008;50(4):818–21.
87. El-Serag HB, Talwalkar J, Kim WR. Efficacy, effectiveness, and comparative effectiveness in liver disease. Hepatology. 2010;52(2):403–7.
88. Crosby LE, Joffe NE, Davis B, et al. Implementation of a process for initial transcranial Doppler ultrasonography in children with sickle cell anemia. Am J Prev Med. 2016;51(1 Suppl 1):S10–6.
89. Hussain S, Nichols F, Bowman L, Xu H, Neunert C. Implementation of transcranial Doppler ultrasonography screening and primary stroke prevention in urban and rural sickle cell disease populations. Pediatr Blood Cancer. 2015;62(2):219–23.
90. Muntz DS, Bundy DG, Strouse JJ. Personalized reminders increase screening for stroke risk in children with sickle cell anemia. South Med J. 2016;109(9):506–10.
91. Bundy DG, Strouse JJ, Casella JF, Miller MR. Burden of influenza-related hospitalizations among children with sickle cell disease. Pediatrics. 2010;125(2):234–43.
92. Halasa NB, Shankar SM, Talbot TR, et al. Incidence of invasive pneumococcal disease among individuals with sickle cell disease before and after the introduction of the pneumococcal conjugate vaccine. Clin Infect Dis. 2007;44(11):1428–33.
93. Sobota AE, Kavanagh PL, Adams WG, McClure E, Farrell D, Sprinz PG. Improvement in influenza vaccination rates in a pediatric sickle cell disease clinic. Pediatr Blood Cancer. 2015;62(4):654–7.
94. Peyvandi F, Garagiola I, Young G. The past and future of haemophilia: diagnosis, treatments, and its complications. Lancet. 2016;388(10040):187–97.
95. Mannucci PM, Tuddenham EG. The hemophilias--from royal genes to gene therapy. N Engl J Med. 2001;344(23):1773–9.
96. Rosendaal FR, Briët E. The increasing prevalence of haemophilia. Thromb Haemost. 1990;63(1):145.
97. Srivastava A, Brewer AK, Mauser-Bunschoten EP, et al. Guidelines for the management of hemophilia. Haemophilia. 2013;19(1):e1–47.
98. Guh S, Grosse SD, McAlister S, Kessler CM, Soucie JM. Health care expenditures for Medicaid-covered males with haemophilia in the United States, 2008. Haemophilia. 2012;18(2):276–83.
99. Guh S, Grosse SD, McAlister S, Kessler CM, Soucie JM. Healthcare expenditures for males with haemophilia and employer-sponsored insurance in the United States, 2008. Haemophilia. 2012;18(2):268–75.
100. Colvin BT, Astermark J, Fischer K, et al. European principles of haemophilia care. Haemophilia. 2008;14(2):361–74.
101. Dandoy CE, Hariharan S, Weiss B, et al. Sustained reductions in time to antibiotic delivery in febrile immunocompromised children: results of a quality improvement collaborative. BMJ Qual Saf. 2016;25(2):100–9.
102. Fletcher M, Hodgkiss H, Zhang S, et al. Prompt administration of antibiotics is associated with improved outcomes in febrile neutropenia in children with cancer. Pediatr Blood Cancer. 2013;60(8):1299–306.
103. Volpe D, Harrison S, Damian F, et al. Improving timeliness of antibiotic delivery for patients with fever and suspected neutropenia in a pediatric emergency department. Pediatrics. 2012;130(1):e201–10.
104. Tagliaferri A, Di Perna C, Biasoli C, et al. A web site to improve Management of Patients with inherited bleeding disorders in the emergency department: results at 2 years. Semin Thromb Hemost. 2016;42(5):589–98.

105. Fijnvandraat K, Cnossen MH, Leebeek FW, Peters M. Diagnosis and management of haemophilia. BMJ. 2012;344:e2707.
106. Manco-Johnson MJ, Abshire TC, Shapiro AD, et al. Prophylaxis versus episodic treatment to prevent joint disease in boys with severe hemophilia. N Engl J Med. 2007;357(6):535–44.
107. Schrijvers LH, Uitslager N, Schuurmans MJ, Fischer K. Barriers and motivators of adherence to prophylactic treatment in haemophilia: a systematic review. Haemophilia. 2013;19(3):355–61.
108. Thornburg C. Prophylactic factor infusions for patients with hemophilia: challenges with treatment adherence. J Coagul Disord. 2010;2:9–14.
109. Kyngäs H. Compliance of adolescents with chronic disease. J Clin Nurs. 2000;9(4):549–56.
110. Witkop ML, McLaughlin JM, Anderson TL, Munn JE, Lambing A, Tortella B. Predictors of non-adherence to prescribed prophylactic clotting-factor treatment regimens among adolescent and young adults with a bleeding disorder. Haemophilia. 2016;22(4):e245–50.
111. Carlsson M, Berntorp E, Björkman S, Lethagen S, Ljung R. Improved cost-effectiveness by pharmacokinetic dosing of factor VIII in prophylactic treatment of haemophilia a. Haemophilia. 1997;3(2):96–101.
112. Ar MC, Vaide I, Berntorp E, Björkman S. Methods for individualising factor VIII dosing in prophylaxis. Eur J Haematol Suppl. 2014;76:16–20.
113. Spira J, Plyushch OP, Andreeva TA, Andreev Y. Prolonged bleeding-free period following prophylactic infusion of recombinant factor VIII reconstituted with pegylated liposomes. Blood. 2006;108(12):3668–73.
114. Quon D, Reding M, Guelcher C, et al. Unmet needs in the transition to adulthood: 18- to 30-year-old people with hemophilia. Am J Hematol. 2015;90(Suppl 2):S17–22.
115. Bahr NC, Song J. The effect of structural violence on patients with sickle cell disease. J Health Care Poor Underserved. 2015;26(3):648–61.
116. Porter JS, Matthews CS, Carroll YM, Anderson SM, Smeltzer MP, Hankins JS. Genetic education and sickle cell disease: feasibility and efficacy of a program tailored to adolescents. J Pediatr Hematol Oncol. 2014;36(7):572–7.
117. Frost JR, Cherry RK, Oyeku SO, et al. Improving sickle cell transitions of care through health information technology. Am J Prev Med. 2016;51(1 Suppl 1):S17–23.

Chapter 17
Quality and Safety in Hematopoietic Stem Cell Transplant Patients

Kathy Ruble, Christa Krupski, Allen Chen, and Christopher E. Dandoy

Introduction

The field of hematopoietic stem cell transplant (HSCT) has undergone tremendous advancement in the past 60 years since E. Donnall Thomas et al. first attempted to treat leukemic patients with irradiation and marrow grafting [1]. Advances in antiviral therapies [2], extension of graft selection [3–6], establishment of donor registries, and advanced understanding of human lymphocyte antigen (HLA) matching have all contributed to improved outcomes [6–13]. Today, allogeneic HSCT is a treatment modality offered to pediatric patients with a variety of disorders including hematologic malignancies, bone marrow failure syndromes, immunodeficiencies, and hemoglobinopathies [11]. Autologous HSCT can be used in conjunction with high-dose chemotherapy to treat tumors such as neuroblastoma and CNS malignancy [14].

Patients undergoing HSCT have complex medical courses; they undergo prolonged hospitalizations, often require subspecialty consultations, and are at risk for multiple complications in the posttransplant period. Coordinating care for this

To appear in: Improving Patient Safety and Quality in the Pediatric Hematology Oncology and Hematopoietic Stem Cell Transplant Practice

K. Ruble
Department of Oncology, The Sidney Kimmel Comprehensive Cancer Center, Johns Hopkins University School of Medicine, Baltimore, MD, USA

C. Krupski • C.E. Dandoy (✉)
Department of Bone Marrow Transplantation and Immune Deficiency, Cancer and Blood Disease Institute, Cincinnati Children's Hospital Medical Center, Cincinnati, OH, USA
e-mail: christopher.dandoy@cchmc.org

A. Chen
Department of Pediatric Oncology, The Sidney Kimmel Comprehensive Cancer Center, Johns Hopkins University School of Medicine, Baltimore, MD, USA

group of patients not only necessitates substantial resources but also careful attention in order to ensure patient safety. HSCT patients utilize a substantial amount of resources, as they encounter complications posttransplant (i.e. infection) and utilize measures included in the chronic care model [15, 16]. Both the continuing evolution of clinical care and the diversity of patients and diseases treated with HSCT have led to disagreement regarding the establishment of quality metrics among programs. Additionally, HSCT practices are heterogeneous; substantial variations exist between centers and individual providers.

Although extensive guidelines have been published regarding HSCT, data evaluating barriers to improving delivery of care and adherence to the recommendations is sparse. Despite the lack of published reports, processes at all stages of care should be continuously refined, and strategies for improvement should be shared. As it currently stands, the field of quality and safety in HSCT is in its infancy; extensive opportunities exist to learn and share mechanisms for improving patient care.

Quality can be defined as the best possible science in the context of the patients' wants and needs. Quality improvement describes the process and methods used to assess and implement the best quality care. In this chapter, we will review the following topics:

- HSCT accreditation organizations
- Mechanisms to ensure marrow donor safety
- Strategies to improve coordination of care throughout the HSCT process, including the pre-HSCT evaluation, transplant itself, and the post-HSCT period of survivorship
- Review of selective safety issue opportunities in hospitalized HSCT patients
- Follow-up care, late effects, and improving standardized screening

In our efforts to demonstrate mechanisms for improvement, we will utilize reported data as available from the HSCT literature and, when not available, reports published in relation to the fields of pediatrics and/or oncology. It is important to review briefly the differences between *quality improvement* and *quality assurance*. *Quality assurance* measures compliance against certain necessary standards and is required, and *quality improvement* is a continuous proactive process to improve healthcare delivery systems.

Accreditation: FACT and JACIE

Measurement of quality is critical in the HSCT arena due to the life-threatening nature of the diseases (and, occasionally, the treatment), the opportunity for cure, the intensive resource utilization, and the involvement of healthy donors in HSCT. Standardization of HSCT has been advocated as a way of improving patient care and outcome. Thus, accreditation for transplantation centers has become an accepted standard in the USA and Europe and is required by law in some countries.

The Foundation for the Accreditation of Cellular Therapy (FACT) and JACIE (The Joint Accreditation Committee of the International Society for Cellular Therapy Europe) are advanced quality management systems whose aim is to certify clinical excellence in processes and outcomes within HSCT centers and improve the quality of care in clinical HSCT by the use of well-defined standards and rules and verified through inspections [17, 18].

FACT and JACIE maintain specific standards for accreditation, including: mandating a minimum annual number of transplants centers must perform, guidelines for HSCT center laboratories and clinical oversight, and methodologies for HLA typing and processing. In addition, institutions must maintain adequate nursing and physician staffing, assure institutional standardized policies and procedures, and perform recommended donor evaluations. Centers performing pediatric bone marrow harvests should have appropriate facilities and pediatric anesthesiology specialty care available. Centers performing leukopheresis for peripheral blood stem cell (PBSC) donation should have appropriate equipment and staffing for children [17–25].

In Europe, JACIE implementation has significantly improved patient outcomes, including non-relapse mortality, relapse incidence, and relapse-free survival after allogeneic and autologous HSCT. Gratwohl et al. showed outcomes that were significantly better for patients who received transplantations in accredited centers compared with patients who received transplantation in centers [22]. This was true both in the pre-application baseline, preparation, or application periods and was independent of the year of HSCT [17]. In the USA, after adjusting for patient and center characteristics, FACT centers have shown statistically superior results relative to non-FACT centers, especially for more complex HSCT [18]. Adherence with best practices in evidence-based medicine is likely an underlying driver of the improved outcomes. These examples provide evidence of a quality management system that contributes to the overall survival of patients treated with a highly specific medical procedure and represents significant progress in HSCT quality and safety [26–28].

Although there is significant oversight through accreditation in maintaining minimum standards in HSCT care, there are no specific regulations on clinical care, leading to variation in patient management and supportive care. In 2008, Lee et al. evaluated practice variations in HSCT among transplant centers and countries. A survey administered to 526 adult and pediatric transplant physicians showed wide variation in management approaches to specific clinical scenarios, including chronic myeloid leukemia, acute and chronic graft-versus-host disease, and choice of graft source for patients with aplastic anemia. Among adult transplant physicians, there was little agreement on the patient factors favoring reduced intensity conditioning or myeloablative conditioning [29].

Due to variations in practice and heterogeneity between centers, quality measurements can vary between centers; however, some metrics should be monitored closely (Fig. 17.1) [30]. It is important that institutions have an active and engaged quality assurance team, to measure compliance with the necessary standards that are required. In addition, the committee can mitigate institutional forces impacting the

Fig. 17.1 Quality and
safety metrics in
hematopoietic stem cell
transplantation. Adopted
from Rice and Bailey [31]

- Annual volume (number of patients transplanted)
- Disease-free survival
- Engraftment
- Treatment-related complications
- Infectious complications, bloodstream infection rates
- Treatment-related mortality (100-day and 1-year)
- Donar safety
- Hospital length of stay
- Unplanned re-admissions
- Patient satisfaction

HSCT program [31]. HSCT centers should also maintain and support a quality improvement team, to continuously implement processes to ensure quality care.

Donor Safety

As unrelated hematopoietic cell (HC) donation is only reserved for individuals >18 years of age worldwide, we will only review HC donation for related donors. There is no direct medical benefit from serving as a stem cell donor, though there is a psychosocial benefit of helping a sibling or close family member [32]. There are safety, quality, and ethical implications for both donors and recipients; consequently, various processes have been implemented by registries worldwide to minimize the risk to both parties. HLA-matched siblings are considered to be the best HC donors for both practical and biological purposes [33]. However, when the recipient is a child, potential sibling donors are often also children themselves. Today, more than one third of children undergoing allogeneic HSCT receive HC grafts from siblings under the age of 18 years [34, 35].

All stem cell sources, including bone marrow (BM), peripheral blood stem cells (PBSC), and cord blood (CB), can be obtained from pediatric donors, but BM-derived cells are the preferred source for many reasons such as a decreased risk of graft-versus-host disease (GVHD) [34, 35]. PBSC donation requires the donor to receive granulocyte colony-stimulating factor (G-CSF) and then undergo central venous catheter placement under anesthesia and apheresis. BM harvests are generally regarded as safe, but also require general anesthesia and may lead to pain at the harvest site. Although the BM and PBSC collection procedures differ greatly, the main symptoms experienced by BM and PBSC donors were similar: pain, fatigue, insomnia, local reactions, dizziness, anorexia, emesis, rash, and occasional fever or syncope [36] (Fig. 17.2). It is important to note there is no evidence that patients receiving G-CSF have an increased risk for cancer, autoimmune diseases, and/or stroke [37].

In 2010, the American Academy of Pediatrics (AAP) released a policy statement on the use of children as donors. The statement outlined five conditions that the AAP recommends should be met in order for a minor to serve as a stem cell donor [38].

Fig. 17.2 Symptoms associated with hematopoietic cell collect (bone marrow and peripheral blood collection). Adopted from Styczynski [36]

Bone Marrow Collection
- Pain (62%)
- Hemoglobin concentration below 5 g/dL (10%)

Symptoms After Anesthesia Post Bone Marrow Harvest
- Vomiting (12%)
- Sore throat (7%)
- Decreased blood pressure (6%)
- Tachycardia (4%)
- Laryngospasm (<1%)

Peripheral Blood Stem Cell Collection
- Pain related to Central line placement (21%)
- Symptomatic hypocalcemia (21%)
- Muscle/bone pain from G-CSF (9%)
- Thrombocytopenia (4%)
- Fever while receiving G-CSF (1%)

- There is no medically equivalent HLA adult relative who is willing and able to donate.
- A strong personal and positive relationship exists between the donor and recipient.
- There is some likelihood that the recipient will benefit from transplantation.
- The clinical, emotional, and psychosocial risks to the donor must be minimized and reasonable in relation to the benefits expected for both the donor and the recipient.
- Parental permission and donor assent (when developmentally appropriate) must be obtained.

FACT and JACIE have specific guidelines for the collection of cellular products to protect the safety of donors during the process of HC collection. As donor safety is of utmost importance, checklists should be utilized to verify completion of the pre-procedure steps (e.g., testing for hemoglobinopathy, pregnancy, etc.) [39].

Coordination of Care

HSCT care is complex, involving multiple treatment modalities such as chemotherapy, radiation, and surgery; all need to be coordinated among different medical specialties. Treatment regimens can be time-intensive and debilitating and may result in serious, sometimes long-term, complications. Care coordination involves deliberately organizing patient care activities and sharing information between all of the participants involved in a patient's care in order to provide safe and effective care. Simply put, the patient's needs must be known and communicated to the right people at the right time, and this information must then be used to provide quality patient care [40–42]. There are three periods where comprehensive and effective care coordination is needed in the HSCT period: (a) pre-HSCT referral from the

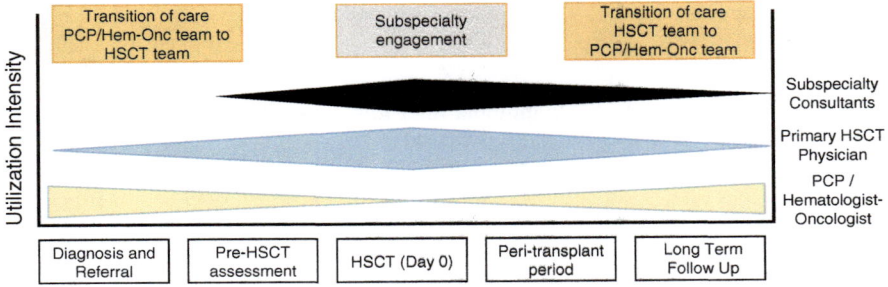

Fig. 17.3 Transitions of care in hematopoietic stem cell transplant (HSCT)

pediatrician or pediatric hematology-oncology physician, (b) during the peri-HSCT period where coordination between the HSCT team and other healthcare providers is needed, (c) in the post-HSCT period when the HSCT survivor is transitioned back to the PCP (Fig. 17.3).

Pre-HSCT Care Coordination

Although the need for care coordination is clear, there are obstacles within our healthcare delivery system that must be overcome in order to provide thorough medical care. The Agency for Healthcare Research and Quality (AHRQ) acknowledges that our healthcare delivery system is often disjointed, and processes vary among primary care and specialty sites. Patients are often not certain of the reasons they are being referred from primary care to a specialist, how to make appointments, and what to do after seeing a specialist. Furthermore, specialists do not consistently receive clear reasons for the referral or adequate information on diagnostic evaluations that have been done prior to the referral [41].

The transfer of care of patients across clinical specialties is a complex process and is made even more challenging by cultural differences, individual expectations, and pressure from patients and families [43]. Oftentimes, referrals fail to meet the needs of either the initiating facility or the receiving provider [40, 43, 44]. Reasons for dissatisfaction include redundancies in the referral process, poor communication between physicians, the time required to write a referral note, and missing information in the referral letter or report [44]. Interestingly, pediatric specialists who received timely patient referral information reported providing optimal care twice as often as specialists who did not [45]. Unfortunately, in pediatric HSCT, there are no published reports relating to the referral process; this leaves opportunity for research and quality improvement in this area.

An effective referral mechanism ensures a close relationship between the initiating facility and the receiving facility. Successful subspecialty referrals require considerable coordination and interaction among the PCP, the subspecialist, and the patient, which may be challenging in the outpatient setting. Hysong et al. conducted a qualitative study to understand coordination breakdowns related to electronic referrals in an integrated healthcare system [46]. The authors examined work-system factors that affect the timely receipt of subspecialty care. Four overarching themes emerged: lack of an institutional referral policy, lack of standardization in certain referral procedures, ambiguity in roles and responsibilities, and inadequate resources to adapt and respond to referral requests effectively. Marked differences in PCPs' and subspecialists' communication styles and individual mental models of the referral processes likely precluded the development of a *shared* mental model to facilitate coordination and successful referral completion [46].

The AHRQ provides guidelines to improve care coordination with referrals. This approach can be utilized both in pre-HSCT referrals (from the PCP or hematologist/oncologist) or post-HSCT care back to the referring physician. AHRQ recommends that the referral process be designed by key stakeholders (e.g., referring oncology and BMT teams) to include all of the pertinent details necessary for effective and safe management of patients. As checklists have been shown to improve transitions of care through referrals [47], stakeholders should create a formalized checklist for patient referrals. These referral forms should include pertinent demographic, social, and medical information. AHRQ recommends that centers should not rely on patients to relay information, but should discuss and coordinate language barriers, verify that the patient understands the reason of the referral, and maintain a means to communicate progress throughout the HSCT process [41].

Currently, there are no metrics to measure referral effectiveness in HSCT. Physician teams should sample the number of referrals made over a specific time period (denominator) and calculate the percentage of referrals that included all relevant information (numerator). This could be tracked in real time, and QI methodology can then be used to close gaps in care.

Care Coordination in the Peri-transplant Period

HSCT recipients are complex, and their care involves individuals from multiple specialties and services (Fig. 17.4). HSCT providers requesting subspecialist input in the hospitalized patient should provide the following information when requesting a consultation: (1) address the question that is asked, (2) whom to call with the response, (3) and the urgency of the consultation [48]. Physician consultation should be collaborative and multidisciplinary, and include patient and family engagement [49].

HSCT nurse coordinators are instrumental in the overall management of HSCT patients. Nurse coordinators are involved throughout the entire HSCT course; they coordinate HLA typing between patients and potential donors, assure completeness of referral forms, verify insurance coverage, participate in the initial consultation with the transplant physician, schedule necessary procedures, and educate patients and families. Finally, nurse coordinators can assure adequate transition of care to the posttransplant setting and arrange for long-term follow-up [50].

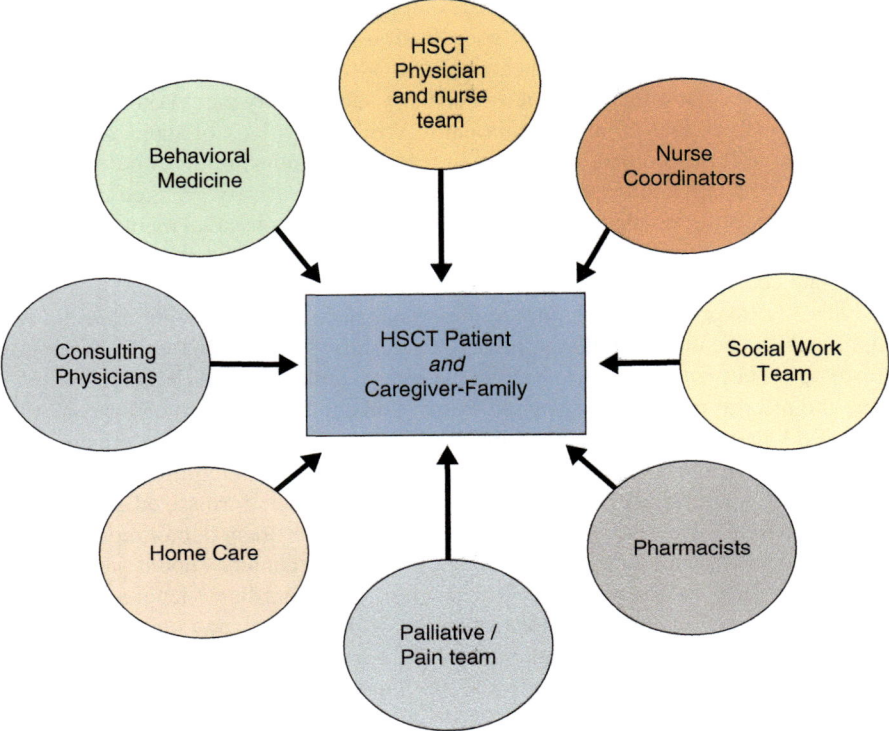

Fig. 17.4 Hematopoietic stem cell transplant (HSCT) care team in the peri-transplant period

Posttransplant Transition

In the absence of relapse and/or active GVHD, most HSCT survivors are eventually able to transition to another set of providers. Ideally, this should be accomplished seamlessly with good communication. However, the vulnerabilities and complexities of such transitions of care have become evident, and medical and/or psychological crises may emerge or resurface among certain groups of patients who are at risk being lost in transition [51]. Oftentimes, HSCT survivors are accustomed to unique living arrangements and receive medical care within a complex healthcare delivery system which includes physicians, social workers, and other pediatric specialists. At times, the transition from the protective environment of the "bone marrow transplant medical home" can be difficult, as pediatric patients may rely on their caregivers well into their 30s and 40s [51–54]. The same requirements and steps described above should be used for the transition of care to the PCP. Cupit et al. recently reviewed the mechanisms to transition care of pediatric and adolescent young adult transition to adult healthcare providers [55]. Important considerations in HSCT transition are reviewed in Fig. 17.5.

Adopted from Cubit et al.[55]

- **Identification of a healthcare provider:** Ensure all HSCT survivors have an identified primary care provider (PCP) who can attend to the challenges of transition and who can assume responsibility for current healthcare, care coordination and future planning.
- **Individualized care plans:** Prepare and maintain a comprehensive medical summary that is accessible and available to both the patient, caregivers/parents, PCP, and subspecialist.
- **Healthcare transition plan:** Create a individualized healthcare transition plan the HSCT survivor and his/her family. Discuss the plan at length with the patient's caregivers/parents to address how their roles may changes. This plan should include the services that need to be provided and who will provide them. This plan should be reviewed at all long term follow up visits.
- **Addressing healthcare coverage:** Ensure affordable, continuous health insurance for all HSCT survivors throughout adolescence and adulthood.
- **Communication:** Engage in regular communication with the patient's PCP prior to, during, and after transition to ensure coordination of care.

Fig. 17.5 Considerations for successful transition of HSCT survivors. Adopted from Cubit et al. [55]

Survivorship and Long-Term Screening

Survivorship of HSCT begins on the day of transplantation [51]. There are few patients who have more complicated survivorship care than those who undergo HSCT in childhood. Quality pediatric HSCT care must include appropriate long-term follow-up to monitor and treat the complications associated with this intensive treatment. Many factors should be considered when determining the risk of long-term complications after HSCT and include the type and intensity of treatments received prior to the transplant, conditioning regimen, type of transplant and product, type and severity of GVHD, early complications, comorbid conditions, genetic factors, and lifestyle. HSCT survivorship tools are available to assist in appropriate screening for complications and include the Children's Oncology Group, Long-Term Follow-Up Guidelines [56], and Pediatric Blood and Marrow Transplant Consortium Consensus Paper [57]. HSCT long-term follow-up teams should include, or have the ability to refer patients to, subspecialists with experience in the care of post-HSCT organ dysfunction (Table 17.1).

Hematologic Complications

Many of the underlying diseases that necessitate HSCT require extensive blood product support prior to transplant, and all patients will require transfusion support in the pre-engraftment period. The cumulative effect of transfusion support is varying degrees of iron overload, which is associated with increased mortality before day 100, acute graft-versus-host disease, and blood stream infections [58–61]. While serum ferritin can be falsely elevated as an acute-phase reactant, elevated levels should serve as an indicator of iron overload and prompt further investigation

Table 17.1 Recommended organ function screening and late-effects multidisciplinary team members

	Screening test	Minimum screening frequency	Multidisciplinary team member
Hematologic	Ferritin Hepatic function	Yearly	Hematologist with experience in chelation therapy
Pulmonary	Pulmonary function tests (PFTs)	Every 6 months for first 2 years	Pulmonologist PFT lab Cardiologist with expertise in pulmonary hypertension
Endocrine	Thyroid function Gonadal function Growth hormone	Yearly	Endocrinologist
Renal	Blood pressure Renal function test Urinalysis Urine protein to creatinine ratio	Blood pressure assessment at each clinic visit Laboratory testing at day +80 and yearly post-HSCT	Nephrologist Pharmacist (to help adjust medications with renal dysfunction)
Ocular	Ophthalmology evaluation	Yearly	Ophthalmologist with experience in the management of cataracts and ocular GVHD
Cardiac	Echocardiography HgA1C Lipid screening	Yearly laboratory testing for metabolic syndrome Echo screening 1 and 5 years post-HSCT	Cardiologist with experience managing heart failure Echocardiography team

Adopted from Dietz et al. [56]

and treatment [58, 62–64]. Multidisciplinary teams should include specialists able to manage chelation therapy if needed.

Pulmonary Complications

Pulmonary complications post BMT vary widely, including both restrictive and obstructive conditions due to acute or chronic GVHD, HSCT preparatory regimens, or infectious sequela. Furthermore, subclinical pulmonary dysfunction may be present in asymptomatic post-HSCT patients [65]. Serial pulmonary function tests (PFTs) are used to monitor survivors post-HSCT. A possible life-threatening pulmonary complication, bronchiolitis obliterans syndrome (BOS), typically occurs within the first few months to years after HSCT and leads to progressive pulmonary fibrosis and obstructive lung disease [66, 67]. In patients who develop BOS, providers should have a low threshold for obtaining echocardiographic screening for pulmonary hypertension [68]. Survivorship multidisciplinary teams should include a pulmonologist, PFT lab, and cardiologist with expertise in pulmonary hypertension.

Endocrine Complications

Endocrinopathies after BMT are common and can result from direct injury to endocrine organs or via disruption of the hypothalamic-pituitary axis. Endocrine dysfunction can include gonadal dysfunction, growth impairment, and thyroid dysfunction; [69–72] and screening for endocrine complications should include monitoring hormone levels and physical exam focusing on appropriate anthropometric and developmental measures including growth velocity and Tanner staging in children [73]. Transplant teams should work closely with endocrinology specialists in the screening and management of endocrine complications after HSCT.

Renal Complications

Three major categories of long-term renal complications are seen in BMT survivors: thrombotic microangiopathy, nephrotic syndrome, and idiopathic chronic kidney disease resulting from nephrotoxic medications used during transplant [74–76]. Screening for renal dysfunction during survivorship involves laboratory monitoring and blood pressure assessment. More comprehensive monitoring with glomerular filtration rate, ultrasonography, or renal biopsy may be warranted for survivors with established or suspected renal disease [56, 77]. Management of CKD during survivorship should focus on mitigating factors; discontinuation of nephrotoxic drugs and aggressive blood pressure control should be prioritized [78].

Ocular Complications

Cataracts are the most common ocular complication and are associated with the preparative regimen and/or a history of GVHD (cumulative steroid dose) [79–81].

Cardiac Complications

Multiple cardiac complications may occur in survivors of HSCT. Echocardiographic findings of elevated right ventricular pressure (pulmonary hypertension) [68, 82], pericardial effusions [83–86], and left ventricular systolic dysfunction [87, 88] have been described in both adult and pediatric patients undergoing HSCT. In addition, HSCT survivors are at risk for early onset metabolic syndrome and coronary artery disease [75, 89–91]. Comprehensive teams should include access to echocardiography and a cardiology subspecialist with experience in the management of heart failure.

Standardized Process for HSCT Survivors

Long-term survivors of HSCT should receive comprehensive routine screening to insure early detection of late effects as it may lessen their long-term consequences. Transplant centers should create a reliable system to adequately screen HSCT survivors including compliance measurements of comprehensive follow-up. These data could be calculated over any specific time.

(a) Multidisciplinary teams should create standard screening protocols that are disease specific, and adaptable to previous treatments and HSCT complications (e.g., GVHD).
(b) Establish a mechanism to identify long-term follow-up patients and measure compliance with screening.
(c) Establish partnerships with subspecialists who have experience managing late HSCT complications.
(d) Barriers to follow-up should be identified. These include inconsistent scheduling of long-term follow-up patients, variability in physician practice with deviations from evidenced-based guidelines, and the lack of accountability and consistent tracking of BMT survivors.
(e) Test and develop intervention and processes to improve long-term follow-up rates. Examples of interventions include creation of a standardized follow-up checklist and processes to identify all survivors, as well as delineated roles and responsibilities for the post-BMT follow-up process.
(f) Establish a standardized mechanism for patients with abnormal post-HSCT screening results including referral to appropriate subspecialty care.
(g) It is important to continuously monitor adherence to the long-term survivor guidelines. Teams should encourage accountability to assure process compliance.

Posttransplant Quality of Life

HSCT is an area rich for the consideration of health-related quality of life (HRQOL) due to the profound impact it has on recipient's physical and emotional well-being [92]. As therapies and associated supportive cares improve and patients experience increased survivorship, the idea of what constitutes a "successful" HSCT continues to evolve. It is not enough to cure the underlying disease; preservation of HRQOL including emotional, social, and physical well-being must also be of utmost importance.

HRQOL is a complex, multifaceted, and dynamic entity influenced by psychological and social functioning [93]. It has been endorsed by the World Health Organization as essential for measuring as a clinical outcome, separate from morbidity and mortality [94, 95]. For the purpose of evaluation, HRQOL is frequently divided into physical, social, and emotional/mental domains [96–101]. HRQOL is compromised even before patients undergo HSCT, likely due to prior treatment, underlying disease, and physical symptoms; it then worsens with the preparative regimen [93, 102, 103]. Although medical factors impact HRQOL, certain demographic factors are also potent predictors of HRQOL [103]. A 2009 review article by Tremolada et al. examined 47 studies on pediatric HSCT recipients relating to psychosocial sequelae and HRQOL; many studies showed that older age at HSCT, late effects, female gender, and more proximal time to transplant were risk factors found to be associated with poor HRQOL [93].

Recent studies show variable effects of age at HSCT on HRQOL [95, 103–107]. Patients who are older at the time of HSCT may experience more disruption to their daily lives; they may also more concretely anticipate future distress and prolonged illness than younger children [103]. Additionally, younger patients may not remember the HSCT experience as vividly as older patients do later in life [95]. Additionally, even after controlling for socioeconomic status, ethnicity impacts HRQOL with African-American children reporting the highest HRQOL, while children of Asian descent report the worst decline in HRQOL [103]. It is thought that the patients' culture, behaviors, and values, in combination with their pre-HSCT experience, impact their expectations related to HSCT. Religion, spirituality, and social support, which are often culturally mediated, also impact HRQOL.

When compared to pediatric patients with hematologic malignancies who have been treated with chemotherapy alone, patients who have undergone HSCT have lower overall HRQOL scores [108]. Several studies have shown that these patients generally do not experience decreased social or emotional functioning post-HSCT; it is physical functioning that is most impaired [108–110]. Pediatric HSCT survivors also report more severe chronic health conditions later in life versus patients who received only chemotherapy [111–113]. As social and emotional functioning is essentially unchanged, they seem to adapt emotionally well to their limitations; it is the severity of physical dysfunction that appears to determine HRQOL in this patient population [114, 115].

In the absence of GVHD and late effects, HRQOL does ultimately improve post-HSCT. Studies have shown the timing of improvement to be variable, around 4–12 months post-HSCT [93, 103]. As early as 6 months post-HSCT, HRQOL can be comparable to, and sometimes better than, population normative data [93, 105]. Due to the lack of data investigating quality improvement in HRQOL, more research and investigation is needed.

Impact of Late Effects and GVHD

Post-HSCT late effects are common; they are well documented in the literature and negatively impact HRQOL [116–121]. Monitoring for late effects in pediatric patients post-HSCT is essential and is reviewed separately. Studies comparing childhood cancer survivors treated with chemotherapy alone versus those treated with HSCT demonstrate a significantly higher risk of late effects in those treated with HSCT [91, 114]. Additionally, physical dysfunction or limitations, psychological stress, and problems with social interactions are common in patients' post-HSCT [91].

QOL in patients with late effects may vary by age, partly because some medical causes of impaired QOL, for example, gonadal failure or other organ damage, may not be fully realized until adulthood [114]. Therefore, QOL may be more preserved in children and adolescents but impaired once the patients reach adulthood.

Additionally, when patients experience GVHD, HRQOL declines. The Chronic GVHD Consortium has extensively studied the impact of chronic GVHD on HRQOL in adult post-HSCT patients [122]. Within HSCT recipients, patients with GVHD have significantly worse HRQOL, both clinically and statistically, versus those without GVHD [123].

Challenges to Measuring HRQOL in Pediatric Patients

The National Institutes of Health (NIH) Consensus Conference on Criteria for Clinical Trials in chronic GVHD recommended the use of health-related QOL (HRQOL) tools in adult patients for a standardized measure of the impact of disease burden and patient outcomes [124–126]. A unidimensional measure of global HRQOL has also been developed as part of the Patient-Reported Outcomes Measurement Information System (PROMIS) project [127]. Despite these efforts, there have been no formal recommendations for a pediatric-specific HRQOL tool.

The use of varying HRQOL surveys for assessment in pediatric patients, along with a wide spectrum of diseases and a limited number of patients, leads to inconsistent results among pediatric HRQOL studies [93, 123]. Another major challenge of measuring HRQOL in pediatric patients is that these patients are dynamic; physical, emotional, social, and cognitive development changes occur with time and must be accounted for in a measurement tool [128].

Parent-Patient Concordance

In addition to the lack of age-appropriate QOL measures, another historic limitation in the evaluation of pediatric HR QOL was the belief that children did not have the ability to reflect on their own QOL, necessitating parents as proxy QOL raters. However, HRQOL ratings differ between patients and parents, perhaps due to information variance, the unequal understanding of and/or access to information, effects of age on processing and interpretation of information, and the child's ability to understand the gravity of both the underlying diagnosis and treatment modalities [92]. Criterion variance, the difference in weight given by each to the available information, also impacts proxy HRQOL scores; parents may compare the child's current health status to his/her potential future status, the health status of siblings or peers [92].

New Tools

Using the Child Health Rating Inventories (CHRIs) tool, Rodday et al. created child, adolescent, and parent surveys to evaluate seven HRQOL modalities in pediatric HSCT recipients: physical health, mental health, family life, friendship, self-confidence, fun, and life enjoyment [129, 130]. Its brevity yields simplicity, ease of use, and decreased responder burden, making it an ideal tool for which to screen patients who may require more in-depth HRQOL evaluation.

Lawitschka et al. developed the PedsQL Stem Cell Transplant module, an HSCT-specific tool for HRQOL assessment in children and adolescents [128]. The instrument was based on the PedsQL Generic Core Scale [131, 132]. It contains the following domains: pain and hurt, fatigue, nausea, worry or anxiety about disease and/or treatment, nutritional problems, thinking and remembering, communication about disease and/or treatment, and chronic GVHD symptoms. A multicenter validation trial is currently underway.

Selected Topics in HSCT Quality and Safety

Bloodstream Infections (BSIs)

HSCT patients are at increased risk for developing bacterial bloodstream infections (BSIs), which are among the most serious infectious complications and a known cause of increased non-relapse mortality (NRM) in this patient population [133–135].

BSIs in the healthcare setting are classified as primary BSI, related to either a central venous line (CVL) or other hospital-acquired source, or secondary BSI, a bacteremia related to another site of infection (e.g., abscess or pneumonia) [136]. Thus, unless an alternative source is identified, all BSIs in patients with a CVL are considered central line-associated bloodstream infections (CLABSIs). CLABSIs are serious complications in HSCT recipients and lead to prolonged hospitalization, intensive care admissions, and antibiotic treatment [133, 134, 137]. Some patients with CVLs experience BSIs that do not arise from the catheter, but rather originate from translocation of bacteria through non-intact oral and gut mucosa [136, 138]. To address this type of BSI, the Centers for Disease Control and Prevention defined a specific CLABSI type known as "mucosal barrier injury laboratory-confirmed bloodstream infection" (MBI-LCBI) on the basis of literature review and expert opinion. In 2013, the MBI-LCBI definition was integrated into the National Healthcare Safety Network (NHSN) methods for primary BSI surveillance to identify a subset of BSIs reported as CLABSIs that were likely related to MBI in the mouth and gut and not the presence of the CVL itself and that occurred most frequently in patients with neutropenia [136]. Currently, primary BSIs in patients with a CVL are defined as "laboratory-confirmed bloodstream infection (LCBI)" and subcategorized as "CLABSI" or "MBI-LCBI" [139]. Inherent to this distinction is emerging evidence showing that improved CVL maintenance is effective at reducing CLABSI rates [140–142], but not in preventing MBI-LCBIs [143].

Catheter Care Bundles

Catheter care bundles, for both CVL insertion and maintenance, consist of a standard combination of evidence-based interventions that have been shown to be effective in preventing CLABSIs and improving patient outcomes [144, 145]. Germane bundle components include performance of hand hygiene, full-barrier precautions including the use of sterile technique and chlorhexidine cleansing during insertion, and proper procedures for CVL access, manipulation, and dressing changes. Standardization of bundle elements coupled with systematic implementation and compliance has been shown to significantly reduce CLABSI rates across multiple studies of pediatric oncology and HSCT patients [146–150]. Best practice bundle implementation with particular focus on maintenance strategies also reduces CLABSI rates in the ambulatory setting [146, 151]. As part of a multicenter quality improvement initiative, 32 pediatric hematology/oncology and bone marrow transplant centers across the USA implemented a standardized bundle of CVL care practices. Average compliance with the CVL care bundle across the institutions was greater than 80% during the study period, and the collaboration demonstrated a decrease in CLABSI rates from 2.85 CLABSI/1000 CVL days to 2.04 CLABSI/1000 CVL days, a reduction of 28% (RR, 0.71; 95% CI, 0.55–0.92) [152]. This multi-institutional collaborative improvement effort succeeded at reducing CLABSI rates through standardized CVL bundle care in immunocompromised patients. In a recent study from Memorial Sloan Kettering Cancer Center (MSKCC), rates of hospital-acquired CLABSI in high-risk adult patients, including HSCT recipients, after implementing the use of a disinfection cap were 2.3/1000 days, representing 34% decrease from previous periods and resulted in substantial cost savings [153].

Microsystem Stress

Microsystem stress can arise from high patient volumes and acuity and is associated with increased mortality, failure-to-rescue rates, and increased nurse burnout [154, 155]. Additionally, increased workload can influence the provider's decision to perform various procedures [156], reduce patient satisfaction [157], decrease communication between nurses and patients [158], and decrease collaboration between providers [159].

Dandoy et al. evaluated the effects of microsystem stress on CLABSI rates. Over a 1-year period of time, their institution saw increased stressors to their healthcare delivery system: the average daily float nurse hours increased nearly 400%, average daily census increased 30%, the number of new relapsed or refractory patients increased 200%, and the percentage of nurses with less than 1 license year increased 100%. Corresponding with these acute stressors, the CLABSI rate increased from 1 to 2 CLABSIs/1000 CVL days. The multidisciplinary team identified key processes to mitigate potential drivers to the increased CLABSI rate and, through small tests of change, implemented a standardized process for daily hygiene, increased awareness of high-risk patients with CLABSI, improved education/assistance for nurses performing high-risk central venous catheter procedures, and developed a system to improve allocation of resources to de-escalate system stress. After implementation of the interventions, the CLABSI rate decreased nearly 70% (0.39 CLABSIs/1000 CVL days).

Microsystem stress, caused by increased census and acuity, can be extended to physicians as well. Neuraz et al. performed a multicenter analysis evaluating workload and mortality in eight adult ICUs. The risk of death was increased by 2.0 (95% CI, 1.3–3.2) when the patient-to-physician ratio exceeded 14. High patient turnover (adjusted relative risk, 5.6 [2.0–15.0]) and the volume of life-sustaining procedures performed by staff (adjusted relative risk, 5.9 [4.3–7.9]) were also associated with increased mortality [160]. Additional studies, including hospitalists, intensivists, and surgeons, report that excessive attending physician workload has a negative impact on patient care [161–163]. These studies suggest that hospitals should provide mechanisms to provide greater staffing assistance and systems responsive to acuity and census fluctuations to improve safety and quality of care.

Cardiac Monitor Alarms and Alarm Fatigue

Alarm fatigue, the lack of response due to excessive numbers of alarms resulting in sensory overload, can create desensitization and result in missed alarms [164, 165]. In addition, high alarm rates can lead to decreased response to alarms, discomfort for patient families, and unnecessary resource utilization [166]. Due to the risk for acute decompensation, cardiac monitor alarms are frequently utilized in pediatric HSCT inpatients.

Dandoy et al. determined the impact of implementation of a standardized cardiac monitor care process on the rate of cardiac monitor alarms, and alarm fatigue in the Bone Marrow Transplant Unit at Cincinnati Children's Hospital Medical Center [166]. The team measured the number of alarms per monitored day on patients. The cardiac monitor care process was developed through evaluation of the existing literature, and through Plan-Do-Study-Act testing. The standardized process included measurement of four components:

(a) Age-appropriate parameters for patients upon placement on a cardiac monitor
(b) Daily electrode changes
(c) Daily evaluation of cardiopulmonary monitor parameters
(d) Timely discontinuation of the monitor once the patient was off patient-controlled analgesia or clinically stable

In addition, customized monitor delays and increased parameter threshold settings were evaluated and utilized. The nursing staff also utilized an "excessive monitor algorithm" when patients or staff felt that alarms were too frequent (Fig. 17.6).

The unit's overall compliance with the process increased to a median of 95% (from 30%). As compliance improved, there was a decrease in the number of alarms, from a median of 180 to 40. During the implementation, the median number of false alarms on the floor fell from 95% to 50%. In addition, the median time that individual nurses spent addressing frequent alarms decreased from 25 min per shift to 10 min per shift, including the time it took each nurse to complete the monitor log.

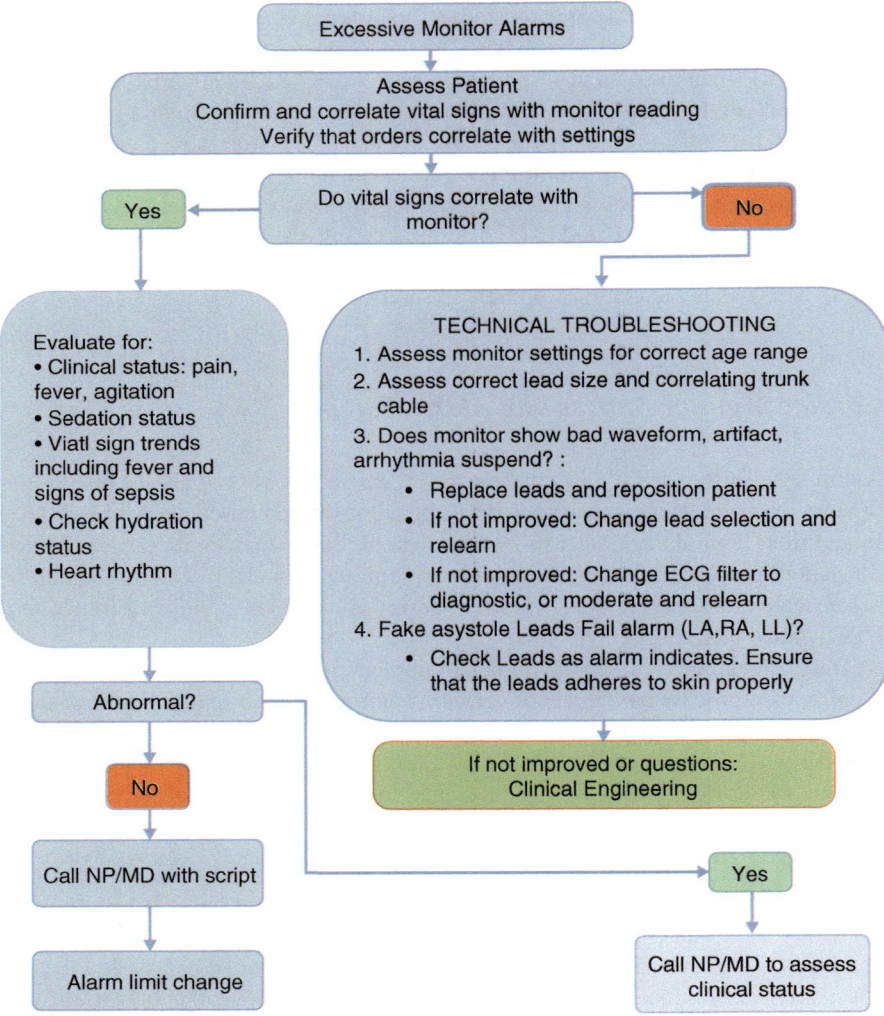

Fig. 17.6 Excessive monitor algorithm. Adopted from Dandoy et al. [166]

Finally, no acute decompensations, code, or staff emergency occurred or were missed because of the cardiac monitor care process.

Hospital Readmission After HSCT

Pediatric HSCT recipients are typically discharged to the outpatient setting shortly after engraftment. However, full immune reconstitution does not occur for many months afterward, especially following an allogeneic transplant [167]. Shulman et al. reviewed the records of pediatric patients who underwent HSCT over a 3- year period of time at Dana-Farber/Boston Children's Hospital Cancer Center to determine the incidence and risk factors for hospital readmission [168]. Their group found 63% of patients had at least on readmission in the first 6 months after transplant (78% of allogeneic, 38% autologous) for mean length of hospital stay of 10.7 days (range of 1–129 days). The majority of patients were readmitted for fever (72% in autologous, 52% in allogeneic) with 30% of allogeneic recipients readmitted for gastrointestinal symptoms. There are no published reports investigating mechanisms to decrease hospital readmission after HSCT, neither in the pediatric nor adult literature. Further investigation could include enhanced predischarge education by nurses and pharmacists and ongoing outpatient education and follow-up [169]. Additional strategies could focus on outpatient management of fever in low-risk patients and early removal of CVLs after HSCT [168].

Future Steps in Pediatric Quality

Long after therapy for a malignancy is over, survivors face ongoing physical, emotional, and practical challenges. Patient-centered research is now focusing more on the development of the best content for, and models of, comprehensive, posttreatment follow-up care. Currently, the only way to determine HSCT success is to evaluate survival at varying time points post-HSCT. We must also focus on outcomes most important to the patients themselves. Through the Patient-Centered Outcomes Research Institute (PCORI), the National Marrow Donor Program (NMDP) is conducting a patient-centered initiative to determine which HSCT outcomes are most important to patients and decide which research questions must be pursued.

References

1. Thomas ED, Lochte HL, Lu WC, Ferrebee JW. Intravenous infusion of bone marrow in patients receiving radiation and chemotherapy. N Engl J Med. 1957;257:491–6.
2. Thomas ED. Landmarks in the development of hematopoietic cell transplantation. World J Surg. 2000;24:815–8.

3. Broxmeyer HE, Douglas GW, Hangoc G, et al. Human umbilical cord blood as a potential source of transplantable hematopoietic stem/progenitor cells. Proc Natl Acad Sci U S A. 1989;86:3828–32.
4. Gluckman E, Broxmeyer HA, Auerbach AD, et al. Hematopoietic reconstitution in a patient with Fanconi's anemia by means of umbilical-cord blood from an HLA-identical sibling. N Engl J Med. 1989;321:1174–8.
5. Broxmeyer HE, Gluckman E, Auerbach A, et al. Human umbilical cord blood: a clinically useful source of transplantable hematopoietic stem/progenitor cells. Int J Cell Cloning. 1990;8 Suppl 1:76–89; discussion 89–91
6. Kohli-Kumar M, Shahidi NT, Broxmeyer HE, et al. Haemopoietic stem/progenitor cell transplant in Fanconi anaemia using HLA-matched sibling umbilical cord blood cells. Br J Haematol. 1993;85:419–22.
7. Malkki M, Single R, Carrington M, Thomson G, Petersdorf E. MHC microsatellite diversity and linkage disequilibrium among common HLA-A, HLA-B, DRB1 haplotypes: implications for unrelated donor hematopoietic transplantation and disease association studies. Tissue Antigens. 2005;66:114–24.
8. Petersdorf EW, Gooley TA, Malkki M, et al. HLA-C expression levels define permissible mismatches in hematopoietic cell transplantation. Blood. 2014;124:3996–4003.
9. Petersdorf EW, Malkki M, O'hUigin C, et al. High HLA-DP expression and graft-versus-host disease. N Engl J Med. 2015;373:599–609.
10. Ruutu T, Barosi G, Benjamin RJ, et al. Diagnostic criteria for hematopoietic stem cell transplant-associated microangiopathy: results of a consensus process by an international working group. Haematologica. 2007;92:95–100.
11. Gratwohl A, Baldomero H, Aljurf M, et al. Hematopoietic stem cell transplantation: a global perspective. JAMA. 2010;303:1617–24.
12. Niederwieser D, Baldomero H, Szer J, et al. Hematopoietic stem cell transplantation activity worldwide in 2012 and a SWOT analysis of the worldwide network for blood and marrow transplantation group including the global survey. Bone Marrow Transplant. 2016;51:778–85.
13. Yoshimi A, Baldomero H, Horowitz M, et al. Global use of peripheral blood vs bone marrow as source of stem cells for allogeneic transplantation in patients with bone marrow failure. JAMA. 2016;315:198–200.
14. Majhail NS, Farnia SH, Carpenter PA, et al. Indications for autologous and allogeneic hematopoietic cell transplantation: guidelines from the American Society for Blood and Marrow Transplantation. Biol Blood Marrow Transplant. 2015;21:1863–9.
15. Afessa B, Tefferi A, Dunn WF, Litzow MR, Peters SG. Intensive care unit support and acute physiology and chronic health evaluation III performance in hematopoietic stem cell transplant recipients. Crit Care Med. 2003;31:1715–21.
16. Glasgow RE, Orleans CT, Wagner EH. Does the chronic care model serve also as a template for improving prevention? Milbank Q. 2001;79:579–612. iv-v
17. Gratwohl A, Brand R, Niederwieser D, et al. Introduction of a quality management system and outcome after hematopoietic stem-cell transplantation. J Clin Oncol. 2011;29:1980–6.
18. Marmor S, Begun JW, Abraham J, Virnig BA. The impact of center accreditation on hematopoietic cell transplantation (HCT). Bone Marrow Transplant. 2015;50:87–94.
19. Warkentin PI, Therapy FAC. Voluntary accreditation of cellular therapies: foundation for the accreditation of cellular therapy (FACT). Cytotherapy. 2003;5:299–305.
20. Cornish JM. JACIE accreditation in paediatric haemopoietic SCT. Bone Marrow Transplant. 2008;42(Suppl 2):S82–6.
21. Pamphilon D, Apperley JF, Samson D, Slaper-Cortenbach I, McGrath E. JACIE accreditation in 2008: demonstrating excellence in stem cell transplantation. Hematol Oncol Stem Cell Ther. 2009;2:311–9.
22. Gratwohl A, Brand R, McGrath E, et al. Use of the quality management system "JACIE" and outcome after hematopoietic stem cell transplantation. Haematologica. 2014;99:908–15.
23. Passweg JR, Baldomero H, Peters C, et al. Hematopoietic SCT in Europe: data and trends in 2012 with special consideration of pediatric transplantation. Bone Marrow Transplant. 2014;49:744–50.

24. Piras A, Aresi P, Angelucci E. Analysis of the accreditation process JACIE transplant program Businco. Prof Inferm. 2015;68:167–73.
25. Anthias C, O'Donnell PV, Kiefer DM, et al. European Group for Blood and Marrow Transplantation Centers with FACT-JACIE accreditation have significantly better compliance with related donor care standards. Biol Blood Marrow Transplant. 2016;22:514–9.
26. Anthias C, Ethell ME, Potter MN, Madrigal A, Shaw BE. The impact of improved JACIE standards on the care of related BM and PBSC donors. Bone Marrow Transplant. 2015;50:244–7.
27. Chabannon C, Pamphilon D, Vermylen C, et al. Ten years after the first inspection of a candidate European Centre, an EBMT registry analysis suggests that clinical outcome is improved when hematopoietic SCT is performed in a JACIE accredited program. Bone Marrow Transplant. 2012;47:15–7.
28. Chabannon C, Pamphilon D, Vermylen C, et al. JACIE celebrates its 10-year anniversary with the demonstration of improved clinical outcome. Cytotherapy. 2011;13:765–6.
29. Lee SJ, Astigarraga CC, Eapen M, et al. Variation in supportive care practices in hematopoietic cell transplantation. Biol Blood Marrow Transplant. 2008;14:1231–8.
30. Rice RD, Bailey G. Management issues in hematopoietic stem cell transplantation. Semin Oncol Nurs. 2009;25:151–8.
31. LeMaistre CF, Loberiza FR. What is quality in a transplant program? Biol Blood Marrow Transplant. 2005;11:241–6.
32. Pulsipher MA, Nagler A, Iannone R, Nelson RM. Weighing the risks of G-CSF administration, leukopheresis, and standard marrow harvest: ethical and safety considerations for normal pediatric hematopoietic cell donors. Pediatr Blood Cancer. 2006;46:422–33.
33. Shaw PJ, Kan F, Woo Ahn K, et al. Outcomes of pediatric bone marrow transplantation for leukemia and myelodysplasia using matched sibling, mismatched related, or matched unrelated donors. Blood. 2010;116:4007–15.
34. Miano M, Labopin M, Hartmann O, et al. Haematopoietic stem cell transplantation trends in children over the last three decades: a survey by the paediatric diseases working party of the European Group for Blood and Marrow Transplantation. Bone Marrow Transplant. 2007;39:89–99.
35. Pasquini MC, Zhu X, Current use and outcome of hematopoietic stem cell transplantation: CIBMTR summary slides. 2015. http://www.cibmtr.org/.
36. Styczynski J, Balduzzi A, Gil L, et al. Risk of complications during hematopoietic stem cell collection in pediatric sibling donors: a prospective European Group for Blood and Marrow Transplantation Pediatric Diseases Working Party study. Blood. 2012;119:2935–42.
37. Pulsipher MA, Chitphakdithai P, Logan BR, et al. Lower risk for serious adverse events and no increased risk for cancer after PBSC vs BM donation. Blood. 2014;123:3655–63.
38. Bioethics AAoPCo. Children as hematopoietic stem cell donors. Pediatrics. 2010;125:392–404.
39. Pronovost PJ, Berenholtz SM, Goeschel CA, et al. Creating high reliability in health care organizations. Health Serv Res. 2006;41:1599–617.
40. Forrest CB, Glade GB, Baker AE, Bocian A, von Schrader S, Starfield B. Coordination of specialty referrals and physician satisfaction with referral care. Arch Pediatr Adolesc Med. 2000;154:499–506.
41. Care Coordination, Quality improvement. 2016. http://www.ahrq.gov/research/findings/evidence-based-reports/caregaptp.html. Accessed 20 Oct 2016
42. Stille CJ, Primack WA, Savageau JA. Generalist-subspecialist communication for children with chronic conditions: a regional physician survey. Pediatrics. 2003;112:1314–20.
43. Beach C, Cheung DS, Apker J, et al. Improving interunit transitions of care between emergency physicians and hospital medicine physicians: a conceptual approach. Acad Emerg Med. 2012;19:1188–95.
44. Gandhi TK, Sittig DF, Franklin M, Sussman AJ, Fairchild DG, Bates DW. Communication breakdown in the outpatient referral process. J Gen Intern Med. 2000;15:626–31.
45. Stille CJ, McLaughlin TJ, Primack WA, Mazor KM, Wasserman RC. Determinants and impact of generalist-specialist communication about pediatric outpatient referrals. Pediatrics. 2006;118:1341–9.

46. Hysong SJ, Esquivel A, Sittig DF, et al. Towards successful coordination of electronic health record based-referrals: a qualitative analysis. Implement Sci. 2011;6:84.
47. Akbari A, Mayhew A, Al-Alawi MA, et al. Interventions to improve outpatient referrals from primary care to secondary care. Cochrane Database Syst Rev. 2008;(3):CD005471
48. Boulware DR, Dekarske AS, Filice GA. Physician preferences for elements of effective consultations. J Gen Intern Med. 2010;25:25–30.
49. Stevens JP, Johansson AC, Schonberg MA, Howell MD. Elements of a high-quality inpatient consultation in the intensive care unit. A qualitative study. Ann Am Thorac Soc. 2013;10:220–7.
50. Thomson B, Gorospe G, Cooke L, Giesie P, Johnson S. Transitions of care: a hematopoietic stem cell transplantation nursing education project across the trajectory. Clin J Oncol Nurs. 2015;19:E74–9.
51. Hashmi S, Carpenter P, Khera N, Tichelli A, Savani BN. Lost in transition: the essential need for long-term follow-up clinic for blood and marrow transplantation survivors. Biol Blood Marrow Transplant. 2015;21:225–32.
52. Ginsberg JP, Hobbie WL, Carlson CA, Meadows AT. Delivering long-term follow-up care to pediatric cancer survivors: transitional care issues. Pediatr Blood Cancer. 2006;46:169–73.
53. Tuchman LK, Slap GB, Britto MT. Transition to adult care: experiences and expectations of adolescents with a chronic illness. Child Care Health Dev. 2008;34:557–63.
54. Wojciechowski EA, Hurtig A, Dorn L. A natural history study of adolescents and young adults with sickle cell disease as they transfer to adult care: a need for case management services. J Pediatr Nurs. 2002;17:18–27.
55. Cupit MC, Duncan C, Savani BN, Hashmi SK. Childhood to adult transition and long-term follow-up after blood and marrow transplantation. Bone Marrow Transplant. 2016;51:176–81.
56. Long-term follow-up guidelines for survivors of childhood, adolescent, and young adult cancer. 2013. http://www.survivorshipguidelines.org/pdf/LTFUGuidelines.
57. Dietz AC, Duncan CN, Alter BP, et al. The Second Pediatric Blood and Marrow Transplant Consortium International Consensus Conference on Late Effects after Pediatric Hematopoietic Cell Transplantation: Defining the Unique Late Effects of Children Undergoing Hematopoietic Cell Transplantation for Immune Deficiencies, Inherited Marrow Failure Disorders, and Hemoglobinopathies. Biol Blood Marrow Transplant. 2017;23(1):24–29.
58. Pullarkat V, Blanchard S, Tegtmeier B, et al. Iron overload adversely affects outcome of allogeneic hematopoietic cell transplantation. Bone Marrow Transplant. 2008;42:799–805.
59. Sivgin S, Baldane S, Kaynar L, et al. Pretransplant serum ferritin level may be a predictive marker for outcomes in patients having undergone allogeneic hematopoietic stem cell transplantation. Neoplasma. 2012;59:183–90.
60. Mahindra A, Sobecks R, Rybicki L, et al. Elevated pretransplant serum ferritin is associated with inferior survival following nonmyeloablative allogeneic transplantation. Bone Marrow Transplant. 2009;44:767–8.
61. Porter JB, Garbowski M. The pathophysiology of transfusional iron overload. Hematol Oncol Clin North Am. 2014;28:683–701. vi
62. Busca A, Falda M, Manzini P, et al. Iron overload in patients receiving allogeneic hematopoietic stem cell transplantation: quantification of iron burden by a superconducting quantum interference device (SQUID) and therapeutic effectiveness of phlebotomy. Biol Blood Marrow Transplant. 2010;16:115–22.
63. Lee JW, Kang HJ, Kim EK, Kim H, Shin HY, Ahn HS. Effect of iron overload and iron-chelating therapy on allogeneic hematopoietic SCT in children. Bone Marrow Transplant. 2009;44:793–7.
64. Kanda J, Kawabata H, Chao NJ. Iron overload and allogeneic hematopoietic stem-cell transplantation. Expert Rev Hematol. 2011;4:71–80.
65. Oh AL, Patel P, Sweiss K, Chowdhery R, Dudek S, Rondelli D. Decreased pulmonary function in asymptomatic long-term survivors after allogeneic hematopoietic stem cell transplant. Bone Marrow Transplant. 2016;51:283–5.

66. Cooke KR, Yanik G. Thomas' hematopoietic cell transplantion. 4th ed. 2009. Wiley-Blackwell: Hoboken, NJ. P. 1456–72.
67. Sengsayadeth SM, Srivastava S, Jagasia M, Savani BN. Time to explore preventive and novel therapies for bronchiolitis obliterans syndrome after allogeneic hematopoietic stem cell transplantation. Biol Blood Marrow Transplant. 2012;18:1479–87.
68. Pate A, Rotz S, Warren M, et al. Pulmonary hypertension associated with bronchiolitis obliterans after hematopoietic stem cell transplantation. Bone Marrow Transplant. 2016;51(2):310–2.
69. Gunn HM, Rinne I, Emilsson H, Gabriel M, Maguire AM, Steinbeck KS. Primary gonadal insufficiency in male and female childhood cancer survivors in a long-term follow-up clinic. J Adolesc Young Adult Oncol. 2016;5(4):344–350.
70. Davis NL, Stewart CE, Moss AD, et al. Growth hormone deficiency after childhood bone marrow transplantation with total body irradiation: interaction with adiposity and age. Clin Endocrinol. 2015;83:508–17.
71. Galletto C, Gliozzi A, Nucera D, et al. Growth impairment after TBI of leukemia survivors children: a model- based investigation. Theor Biol Med Model. 2014;11:44.
72. Sanders JE, Hoffmeister PA, Woolfrey AE, et al. Thyroid function following hematopoietic cell transplantation in children: 30 years' experience. Blood. 2009;113:306–8.
73. Oudin C, Auquier P, Bertrand Y, et al. Metabolic syndrome in adults who received hematopoietic stem cell transplantation for acute childhood leukemia: an LEA study. Bone Marrow Transplant. 2015;50:1438–44.
74. Abboud I, Porcher R, Robin M, et al. Chronic kidney dysfunction in patients alive without relapse 2 years after allogeneic hematopoietic stem cell transplantation. Biol Blood Marrow Transplant. 2009;15:1251–7.
75. Nieder ML, McDonald GB, Kida A, et al. National Cancer Institute-National Heart, lung and blood institute/pediatric blood and marrow transplant consortium first international consensus conference on late effects after pediatric hematopoietic cell transplantation: long-term organ damage and dysfunction. Biol Blood Marrow Transplant. 2011;17:1573–84.
76. Jodele S, Davies SM, Lane A, et al. Diagnostic and risk criteria for HSCT-associated thrombotic microangiopathy: a study in children and young adults. Blood. 2014;124(4):645–53.
77. Abboud I, Peraldi MN, Hingorani S. Chronic kidney diseases in long-term survivors after allogeneic hematopoietic stem cell transplantation: monitoring and management guidelines. Semin Hematol. 2012;49:73–82.
78. Cohen EP, Pais P, Moulder JE. Chronic kidney disease after hematopoietic stem cell transplantation. Semin Nephrol. 2010;30:627–34.
79. Tabbara KF, Al-Ghamdi A, Al-Mohareb F, et al. Ocular findings after allogeneic hematopoietic stem cell transplantation. Ophthalmology. 2009;116:1624–9.
80. Tear Fahnehjelm K, Tornquist AL, Olsson M, Backstrom I, Andersson Gronlund M, Winiarski J. Cataract after allogeneic hematopoietic stem cell transplantation in childhood. Acta Paediatr. 2016;105:82–9.
81. Horwitz M, Auquier P, Barlogis V, et al. Incidence and risk factors for cataract after haematopoietic stem cell transplantation for childhood leukaemia: an LEA study. Br J Haematol. 2015;168:518–25.
82. Dandoy CE, Hirsch R, Chima R, Davies SM, Jodele S. Pulmonary hypertension after hematopoietic stem cell transplantation. Biol Blood Marrow Transplant. 2013;19:1546–56.
83. Neier MJZ, Kleinman C, Baldinger L, Bhatia M, Silver E, van de Ven C, Morris E, Satwani P, George D, Garvin J, Bradley MB, Schwartz J, Cairo MS. Pericardial effusion post-SCT in pediatric recipients with signs and/or symptoms of cardiac disease. Bone Marrow Transplant. 2011;46:529–38.
84. Liu Y-C, Gau J-P, Hong Y-C, et al. Large pericardial effusion as a life-threatening complication after hematopoietic stem cell transplantation—association with chronic GVHD in late-onset adult patients. Ann Hematol. 2012;91:1953–8.
85. Lerner D, Dandoy C, Hirsch R, Laskin B, Davies SM, Jodele S. Pericardial effusion in pediatric SCT recipients with thrombotic microangiopathy. Bone Marrow Transplant. 2014;49(6):862–3.

86. Dandoy CE, Davies SM, Hirsch R, et al. Abnormal echocardiography 7 days after stem cell transplantation may be an early indicator of thrombotic microangiopathy. Biol Blood Marrow Transplant. 2015;21:113–8.

87. Murbraech K, Smeland KB, Holte H, et al. Heart failure and asymptomatic left ventricular systolic dysfunction in lymphoma survivors treated with autologous stem-cell transplantation: a National Cross-Sectional Study. J Clin Oncol. 2015;33(24):2683–2691.

88. Roziakova L, Mistrik M, Batorova A, et al. Can we predict clinical cardiotoxicity with cardiac biomarkers in patients after haematopoietic stem cell transplantation? Cardiovasc Toxicol. 2015;15:210–6.

89. Griffith ML, Savani BN, Boord JB. Dyslipidemia after allogeneic hematopoietic stem cell transplantation: evaluation and management. Blood. 2010;116:1197–204.

90. Martin PJ, Counts GW, Appelbaum FR, et al. Life expectancy in patients surviving more than 5 years after hematopoietic cell transplantation. J Clin Oncol. 2010;28:1011–6.

91. Ishida Y, Honda M, Ozono S, et al. Late effects and quality of life of childhood cancer survivors: part 1. Impact of stem cell transplantation. Int J Hematol. 2010;91:865–76.

92. Parsons SK, Tighiouart H, Terrin N. Assessment of health-related quality of life in pediatric hematopoietic stem cell transplant recipients: progress, challenges and future directions. Expert Rev Pharmacoecon Outcomes Res. 2013;13:217–25.

93. Tremolada M, Bonichini S, Pillon M, Messina C, Carli M. Quality of life and psychosocial sequelae in children undergoing hematopoietic stem-cell transplantation: a review. Pediatr Transplant. 2009;13:955–70.

94. The World Health Organization Quality of Life Assessment (WHOQOL): development and general psychometric properties. Soc Sci Med. 1998;46:1569–85

95. Barrera M, Atenafu E, Hancock K. Longitudinal health-related quality of life outcomes and related factors after pediatric SCT. Bone Marrow Transplant. 2009;44:249–56.

96. Lee S, Cook EF, Soiffer R, Antin JH. Development and validation of a scale to measure symptoms of chronic graft-versus-host disease. Biol Blood Marrow Transplant. 2002;8:444–52.

97. Cella DF, Tulsky DS, Gray G, et al. The functional assessment of cancer therapy scale: development and validation of the general measure. J Clin Oncol. 1993;11:570–9.

98. McQuellon RP, Russell GB, Cella DF, et al. Quality of life measurement in bone marrow transplantation: development of the functional assessment of cancer therapy-bone marrow transplant (FACT-BMT) scale. Bone Marrow Transplant. 1997;19:357–68.

99. McHorney CA, Ware JE, Raczek AE. The MOS 36-item short-form health survey (SF-36): II. Psychometric and clinical tests of validity in measuring physical and mental health constructs. Med Care. 1993;31:247–63.

100. Daughton DM, Fix AJ, Kass I, Bell CW, Patil KD. Maximum oxygen consumption and the ADAPT quality-of-life scale. Arch Phys Med Rehabil. 1982;63:620–2.

101. Herzberg PY, Heussner P, Mumm FH, et al. Validation of the human activity profile questionnaire in patients after allogeneic hematopoietic stem cell transplantation. Biol Blood Marrow Transplant. 2010;16:1707–17.

102. Clarke SA, Eiser C, Skinner R. Health-related quality of life in survivors of BMT for paediatric malignancy: a systematic review of the literature. Bone Marrow Transplant. 2008;42:73–82.

103. Brice L, Weiss R, Wei Y, et al. Health-related quality of life (HRQoL): the impact of medical and demographic variables upon pediatric recipients of hematopoietic stem cell transplantation. Pediatr Blood Cancer. 2011;57:1179–85.

104. Tanzi EM. Health-related quality of life of hematopoietic stem cell transplant childhood survivors: state of the science. J Pediatr Oncol Nurs. 2011;28:191–202.

105. Loiselle KA, Rausch JR, Bidwell S, Drake S, Davies SM, Pai AL. Predictors of health-related quality of life over time among pediatric hematopoietic stem cell transplant recipients. Pediatr Blood Cancer. 2016;63:1834–9.

106. Barrera M, Boyd-Pringle LA, Sumbler K, Saunders F. Quality of life and behavioral adjustment after pediatric bone marrow transplantation. Bone Marrow Transplant. 2000;26:427–35.

107. Parsons SK, Shih MC, Duhamel KN, et al. Maternal perspectives on children's health-related quality of life during the first year after pediatric hematopoietic stem cell transplant. J Pediatr Psychol. 2006;31:1100–15.

108. Sundberg KK, Wettergren L, Frisk P, Arvidson J. Self-reported quality of life in long-term survivors of childhood lymphoblastic malignancy treated with hematopoietic stem cell transplantation versus conventional therapy. Pediatr Blood Cancer. 2013;60:1382–7.
109. Schultz KA, Chen L, Chen Z, et al. Health conditions and quality of life in survivors of childhood acute myeloid leukemia comparing post remission chemotherapy to BMT: a report from the children's oncology group. Pediatr Blood Cancer. 2014;61:729–36.
110. Oberg JA, Bender JG, Morris E, et al. Pediatric Allo-SCT for malignant and non-malignant diseases: impact on health-related quality of life outcomes. Bone Marrow Transplant. 2013;48:787–93.
111. Robison LL, Mertens AC, Boice JD, et al. Study design and cohort characteristics of the childhood cancer survivor study: a multi-institutional collaborative project. Med Pediatr Oncol. 2002;38:229–39.
112. Robison LL. The childhood cancer survivor study: a resource for research of long-term outcomes among adult survivors of childhood cancer. Minn Med. 2005;88:45–9.
113. Robison LL, Green DM, Hudson M, et al. Long-term outcomes of adult survivors of childhood cancer. Cancer. 2005;104:2557–64.
114. Michel G, Bordigoni P, Simeoni MC, et al. Health status and quality of life in long-term survivors of childhood leukaemia: the impact of haematopoietic stem cell transplantation. Bone Marrow Transplant. 2007;40:897–904.
115. Maunsell E, Pogany L, Barrera M, Shaw AK, Speechley KN. Quality of life among long-term adolescent and adult survivors of childhood cancer. J Clin Oncol. 2006;24:2527–35.
116. Löf CM, Winiarski J, Giesecke A, Ljungman P, Forinder U. Health-related quality of life in adult survivors after paediatric Allo-SCT. Bone Marrow Transplant. 2009;43:461–8.
117. Brennan BM, Shalet SM. Endocrine late effects after bone marrow transplant. Br J Haematol. 2002;118:58–66.
118. Leiper AD. Non-endocrine late complications of bone marrow transplantation in childhood: part I. Br J Haematol. 2002;118:3–22.
119. Leiper AD. Non-endocrine late complications of bone marrow transplantation in childhood: part II. Br J Haematol. 2002;118:23–43.
120. Sanders JE. Chronic graft-versus-host disease and late effects after hematopoietic stem cell transplantation. Int J Hematol. 2002;76(Suppl 2):15–28.
121. Socié G, Salooja N, Cohen A, et al. Nonmalignant late effects after allogeneic stem cell transplantation. Blood. 2003;101:3373–85.
122. Krupski C, Jagasia M. Quality of life in the chronic GVHD consortium cohort: lessons learned and the long road ahead. Curr Hematol Malig Rep. 2015;10:183–91.
123. Kurosawa S, Yamaguchi T, Mori T, et al. Patient-reported quality of life after allogeneic hematopoietic cell transplantation or chemotherapy for acute leukemia. Bone Marrow Transplant. 2015;50:1241–9.
124. Filipovich AH, Weisdorf D, Pavletic S, et al. National Institutes of Health consensus development project on criteria for clinical trials in chronic graft-versus-host disease: I. Diagnosis and staging working group report. Biol Blood Marrow Transplant. 2005;11:945–56.
125. Pavletic SZ, Lee SJ, Socie G, Vogelsang G. Chronic graft-versus-host disease: implications of the National Institutes of Health consensus development project on criteria for clinical trials. Bone Marrow Transplant. 2006;38:645–51.
126. Pavletic SZ, Martin P, Lee SJ, et al. Measuring therapeutic response in chronic graft-versus-host disease: National Institutes of Health consensus development project on criteria for clinical trials in chronic graft-versus-host disease: IV. Response criteria working group report. Biol Blood Marrow Transplant. 2006;12:252–66.
127. Hays RD, Bjorner JB, Revicki DA, Spritzer KL, Cella D. Development of physical and mental health summary scores from the patient-reported outcomes measurement information system (PROMIS) global items. Qual Life Res. 2009;18:873–80.
128. Lawitschka A, Güclü ED, Varni JW, et al. Health-related quality of life in pediatric patients after allogeneic SCT: development of the PedsQL stem cell transplant module and results of a pilot study. Bone Marrow Transplant. 2014;49:1093–7.

129. Parsons SK, Shih MC, Mayer DK, et al. Preliminary psychometric evaluation of the child health ratings inventory (CHRIs) and disease-specific impairment inventory-hematopoietic stem cell transplantation (DSII-HSCT) in parents and children. Qual Life Res. 2005;14:1613–25.

130. Rodday AM, Terrin N, Parsons SK, Study JR, Study H-C. Measuring global health-related quality of life in children undergoing hematopoietic stem cell transplant: a longitudinal study. Health Qual Life Outcomes. 2013;11:26.

131. Varni JW, Burwinkle TM, Katz ER, Meeske K, Dickinson P. The PedsQL in pediatric cancer: reliability and validity of the pediatric quality of life inventory generic Core scales, multidimensional fatigue scale, and cancer module. Cancer. 2002;94:2090–106.

132. Varni JW, Burwinkle TM, Seid M, Skarr D. The PedsQL 4.0 as a pediatric population health measure: feasibility, reliability, and validity. Ambul Pediatr. 2003;3:329–41.

133. Poutsiaka DD, Price LL, Ucuzian A, Chan GW, Miller KB, Snydman DR. Blood stream infection after hematopoietic stem cell transplantation is associated with increased mortality. Bone Marrow Transplant. 2007;40:63–70.

134. Wilson MZ, Rafferty C, Deeter D, Comito MA, Hollenbeak CS. Attributable costs of central line-associated bloodstream infections in a pediatric hematology/oncology population. Am J Infect Control. 2014;42:1157–60.

135. Dandoy CE, Haslam D, Lane A, et al. Healthcare burden, risk factors, and outcomes of mucosal barrier injury-laboratory confirmed bloodstream infections after stem cell transplantation. Biol Blood Marrow Transplant. 2016;22(9):1671–7.

136. See I, Iwamoto M, Allen-Bridson K, Horan T, Magill SS, Thompson ND. Mucosal barrier injury laboratory-confirmed bloodstream infection: results from a field test of a new National Healthcare Safety Network definition. Infect Control Hosp Epidemiol. 2013;34:769–76.

137. Cecinati V, Brescia L, Tagliaferri L, Giordano P, Esposito S. Catheter-related infections in pediatric patients with cancer. Eur J Clin Microbiol Infect Dis. 2012;31:2869–77.

138. Freeman JT, Elinder-Camburn A, McClymont C, et al. Central line-associated bloodstream infections in adult hematology patients with febrile neutropenia: an evaluation of surveillance definitions using differential time to blood culture positivity. Infect Control Hosp Epidemiol. 2013;34:89–92.

139. Center for Disease Control and Prevention: bloodstream infection event (central line-associated bloodstream infection and non-central line-associated bloodstream infection). 2016. http://www.cdc.gov/nhsn/PDFs/pscManual/4PSC_CLABScurrent.pdf. Accessed 26 Mar 2016.

140. Bundy DG, Gaur AH, Billett AL, et al. Preventing CLABSIs among pediatric hematology/oncology inpatients: national collaborative results. Pediatrics. 2014;134:e1678–85.

141. Pronovost P, Needham D, Berenholtz S, et al. An intervention to decrease catheter-related bloodstream infections in the ICU. N Engl J Med. 2006;355:2725–32.

142. Miller MR, Griswold M, Harris JM, et al. Decreasing PICU catheter-associated bloodstream infections: NACHRI's quality transformation efforts. Pediatrics. 2010;125:206–13.

143. Metzger KE, Rucker Y, Callaghan M, et al. The burden of mucosal barrier injury laboratory-confirmed bloodstream infection among hematology, oncology, and stem cell transplant patients. Infect Control Hosp Epidemiol. 2015;36:119–24.

144. Schiffer CA, Mangu PB, Wade JC, et al. Central venous catheter care for the patient with cancer: American Society of Clinical Oncology clinical practice guideline. J Clin Oncol. 2013;31:1357–70.

145. O'Grady NP, Alexander M, Burns LA, et al. Guidelines for the prevention of intravascular catheter-related infections. Clin Infect Dis. 2011;52:e162–93.

146. Barrell C, Covington L, Bhatia M, et al. Preventive strategies for central line-associated bloodstream infections in pediatric hematopoietic stem cell transplant recipients. Am J Infect Control. 2012;40:434–9.

147. Rinke ML, Chen AR, Bundy DG, et al. Implementation of a central line maintenance care bundle in hospitalized pediatric oncology patients. Pediatrics. 2012;130:e996–e1004.
148. Chang AK, Foca MD, Jin Z, et al. Bacterial bloodstream infections in pediatric allogeneic hematopoietic stem cell recipients before and after implementation of a central line-associated bloodstream infection protocol: a single-center experience. Am J Infect Control. 2016;44(12):1650–5.
149. Choi SW, Chang L, Hanauer DA, et al. Rapid reduction of central line infections in hospitalized pediatric oncology patients through simple quality improvement methods. Pediatr Blood Cancer. 2013;60:262–9.
150. Wilson MZ, Deeter D, Rafferty C, Comito MM, Hollenbeak CS. Reduction of central line-associated bloodstream infections in a pediatric hematology/oncology population. Am J Med Qual. 2014;29:484–90.
151. Rinke ML, Bundy DG, Chen AR, et al. Central line maintenance bundles and CLABSIs in ambulatory oncology patients. Pediatrics. 2013;132:e1403–12.
152. Bundy DG, Gaur AH, Billett AL, He B, Colantuoni EA, Miller MR. Preventing CLABSIs among pediatric hematology/oncology inpatients: National collaborative results. Pediatrics. 2014;134:e1678–e85.
153. Kamboj M, Sheahan A, Sun J, et al. Transmission of Clostridium Difficile during hospitalization for allogeneic stem cell transplant. Infect Control Hosp Epidemiol. 2016;37:8–15.
154. Aiken LH, Clarke SP, Sloane DM, Sochalski J, Silber JH. Hospital nurse staffing and patient mortality, nurse burnout, and job dissatisfaction. JAMA. 2002;288:1987–93.
155. Aiken LH, Clarke SP, Sloane DM. Hospital staffing, organization, and quality of care: cross-national findings. Nurs Outlook. 2002;50:187–94.
156. Griffith CH, Wilson JF, Desai NS, Rich EC. Housestaff workload and procedure frequency in the neonatal intensive care unit. Crit Care Med. 1999;27:815–20.
157. Anderson FD, Maloney JP, Beard LW. A descriptive, correlational study of patient satisfaction, provider satisfaction, and provider workload at an army medical center. Mil Med. 1998;163:90–4.
158. Llenore E, Ogle KR. Nurse-patient communication in the intensive care unit: a review of the literature. Aust Crit Care. 1999;12:142–5.
159. Baggs JG, Schmitt MH, Mushlin AI, et al. Association between nurse-physician collaboration and patient outcomes in three intensive care units. Crit Care Med. 1999;27:1991–8.
160. Neuraz A, Guérin C, Payet C, et al. Patient mortality is associated with staff resources and workload in the ICU: a multicenter observational study. Crit Care Med 2015;43(8):1587–1594.
161. Michtalik HJ, Yeh HC, Pronovost PJ, Brotman DJ. Impact of attending physician workload on patient care: a survey of hospitalists. JAMA Intern Med. 2013;173:375–7.
162. Thomas M, Allen MS, Wigle DA, et al. Does surgeon workload per day affect outcomes after pulmonary lobectomies? Ann Thorac Surg. 2012;94:966–72.
163. Ward NS, Read R, Afessa B, Kahn JM. Perceived effects of attending physician workload in academic medical intensive care units: a national survey of training program directors. Crit Care Med. 2012;40:400–5.
164. Graham KC, Cvach M. Monitor alarm fatigue: standardizing use of physiological monitors and decreasing nuisance alarms. Am J Crit Care. 2010;19:28–34. quiz 5
165. Cvach M. Monitor alarm fatigue: an integrative review. Biomed Instrum Technol. 2012;46:268–77.
166. Dandoy CE, Davies SM, Flesch L, et al. A team-based approach to reducing cardiac monitor alarms. Pediatrics. 2014;134:e1686–94.
167. Koenig M, Huenecke S, Salzmann-Manrique E, et al. Multivariate analyses of immune reconstitution in children after Allo-SCT: risk-estimation based on age-matched leukocyte sub-populations. Bone Marrow Transplant. 2010;45:613–21.

168. Shulman DS, London WB, Guo D, Duncan CN, Lehmann LE. Incidence and causes of hospital readmission in pediatric patients after hematopoietic cell transplantation. Biol Blood Marrow Transplant. 2015;21:913–9.
169. McKenna DR, Sullivan MR, Hill JM, et al. Hospital readmission following transplantation: identifying risk factors and designing preventive measures. J Community Support Oncol. 2015;13:316–22.

Chapter 18
Quality in Pediatric Palliative Care

**Emma Jones, Rachel Thienprayoon, Michelle Hidalgo,
and Stacie Stapleton**

Palliative Care, Patient- and Family-Centered Care, Team Composition, and Interdisciplinary Team

Palliative care means patient- and family-centered care aimed at optimizing quality of life by anticipating, preventing, and treating suffering. It should be provided throughout the continuum of illness regardless of the age of the patient or stage of disease. Physical, intellectual, emotional, social, and spiritual needs should all be addressed. Many of these elements are already incorporated into interdisciplinary care of children with cancer and hematologic disease. Recognizing and further developing the palliative elements of care should be a focus of improving quality care for this group of patients. The specialty palliative care consultation team is one element of comprehensive palliative care, which must be complemented by population-level standards and institutional policies to ensure that all patients receive optimal benefit. This chapter will describe the palliative care metrics that should be applied to the

E. Jones
Division of Pediatric Palliative Care, Department of Psychosocial Oncology and
Palliative Care, Dana-Farber Cancer Institute and Department of Medicine,
Boston Children's Hosptial, Boston, MA, USA

R. Thienprayoon
Division of Palliative Care, Department of Anesthesia, Cincinnati Children's Hospital
Medical Center, University of Cincinnati College of Medicine, Cincinnati, OH, USA

M. Hidalgo
Johns Hopkins All Children's Hospital, Office of Medical Education, St. Petersburg, FL, USA

S. Stapleton (✉)
Cancer and Blood Disorders Institute,
Johns Hopkins All Children's Hospital, St. Petersburg, FL, USA
e-mail: stacie.stapleton@jhmi.edu

© Springer International Publishing AG 2017
C.E. Dandoy et al. (eds.), *Patient Safety and Quality in Pediatric Hematology/
Oncology and Stem Cell Transplantation*, DOI 10.1007/978-3-319-53790-0_18

entire population of children with cancer or hematologic disease as well as specific guidelines and metrics for ensuring the highest quality care from a specialty palliative care team. Literature in this area is lacking and specific definitions of quality are currently in developmental phases; concepts presented in this chapter should serve as a framework upon which to base further improvement and research efforts.

Evidence for Integration of Palliative Care into Care of Children with Cancer, Blood Disorders, and Undergoing Bone Marrow Transplant

The Standards for Psychosocial Care of Children with Cancer, which were published in *Pediatric Blood and Cancer* in 2015 [1], outline elements of whole person care which could all be considered elements of quality palliative care.

- Youth with cancer and their families should be introduced to palliative care concepts to reduce suffering throughout the disease process regardless of disease status. When necessary youth and families should receive developmentally appropriate end-of-life care.
- A member of the healthcare team should contact the family after a child's death to assess family needs, to identify those for negative psychosocial sequelae, to continue care, and to provide resources for bereavement support.
- Open, respectful communication and collaboration among medical and psychosocial providers, patients, and families is essential to effective patient- and family-centered care. Psychosocial professionals should be integrated into pediatric oncology care settings as integral team members and be participants in patient care rounds/meetings.

The National Comprehensive Cancer Network (NCCN) has published guidelines [2] for palliative care in oncology patients, which recommend screening all patients at every visit to identify unmet palliative care needs. All patients who screen positively require a care plan developed by an interdisciplinary team. Additionally, NCCN gives specific guidance on elements of a palliative care assessment as well as the interventions that should be provided.

Palliative Care Is, at Its Core, Patient- and Family-Centered Care

Patient- and family-centered care maintains the focus on the patient with close involvement of all of the helpful individuals involved in decision-making and support at any level. This includes the immediate family including parents and siblings, extended family, close friends that the family has identified as faith-based support systems, and the primary hematology/oncology/BMT team, pertinent additional subspecialists, and other support personnel from the palliative care team (these roles are defined more clearly elsewhere in this chapter). Patient- and family-centered care is ideal for all diagnoses, but this model is even more essential for diagnoses which are potentially complex, chronic, or life limiting, such as cancer or blood disorders, and is critical at the end of life.

Quality of Patient-/Family-Centered Care, End of Life, and Death Experience

Humans have tried to defy the universal problem of guaranteed death since the beginning of time. It is the goal of palliative and hospice care to maintain high quality of care during the curative treatment phase of the child's treatment, as goals change, at the end of life, and attend to a death that is patient centered.

The involvement of the patient in the patient-centered care seems obvious, but deserves special mention, as sometimes the patient is the last one to be involved, especially in pediatrics. As the patient is the expert in her own needs, the quality of her care can be improved significantly when she is involved in decision-making alongside her physician, parents, and team. The age of the patient should drive her level of involvement in her own care. This can be a difficult balance to strike depending on a child's social development, mental health, psychosocial complexity, and any disease- or treatment-related neurocognitive deficits. However, even a young or developmentally delayed child can find ways to communicate. Additionally important is the involvement of the patient in her care during the entire disease course and what her understanding of her illness has been to date. A teenager who has never been informed of the criticalness of her disease will not be able to bear the whole burden of information in one meeting at the time of relapse, while a younger child who has been informed at age-appropriate levels along the course may be able to be more involved in her own end-of-life care.

Incorporating the Palliative Care Team

Palliative care is about improving the patient's life. But who needs palliative care? We do not advocate palliative care for every person admitted to the hospital, although perhaps this should be entertained, as palliative care teams spend significant time addressing and managing symptoms and alleviating suffering. However, given limited resources, the quality of care is likely to be maximally impacted when palliative care teams are focused on the situations and patients that need them the most. Whether certain triggers that should be considered for a palliative care consult continues to be a topic of debate in pediatric hematology-oncology and bone marrow transplant, and to date no consensus guidelines have been recommended by the Children's Oncology Group, the American Society of Pediatric Hematology-Oncology, or other pediatric hematology-oncology organizations. Many experts feel that certain diagnoses, such as bone marrow transplant, high-grade brain tumor, or relapsed cancer with poor likelihood of salvage, should automatically evoke a palliative care consult. Others feel certain criteria need to be met that would trigger a palliative care consult, while still yet others might require a combination. Table 18.1 provides a list of potential criteria for which to consider consulting a palliative care team.

Table 18.1 Examples of palliative care referral criteria

Presence of complex chronic or life-limiting condition
Difficult pain or physical symptom management
Emotional or social distress
Unable to perform activities of daily living resulting in poor quality of life
Patient, family, or healthcare team with differing views and/or understanding regarding prognosis
Family/staff moral distress
Ethical conflicts
Conflicts regarding use of medical interventions in cognitively impaired, seriously ill, or dying patients
Disrupted or fragmented communication resulting in challenges delivering quality medical care
Frequent hospitalizations
Prolonged hospitalization
Need for end-of-life care coordination
Need for hospice resource utilization

Early Integration of Palliative Care into the Care of Children with Cancer, Blood Disorders, and Undergoing Bone Marrow Transplant

Palliative care is appropriate at any age and at any stage in a serious illness and can be provided together with curative treatment [3]. In a remarkable phase III random controlled study published in 2010, Temel et al. describe the benefits of early integration of palliative care into the treatment of patients with metastatic non-small cell lung cancer (NSCLC) [4]. Patients had significant improvement in mood and even survival in the group that received support by palliative care from the beginning. For children with cancer, early integration of palliative care allows for improved symptom control, parental adjustment, and preparation for the end-of-life period [5]. Additionally, integrating palliative care as early as at the time of diagnosis for children with high-risk malignancies has been found to be feasible and acceptable to families [6].

Two major barriers remain to early palliative care for all pediatric cancer patients. One is the medical culture and attitudes that create a false dichotomy between curative therapy and palliative care [7]. The other is the lack of access to palliative care teams and/or the inability of a specialty team to fully meet the patient care demands. Currently only 58% of Children's Oncology Group institutions report having a pediatric palliative care team [8]. A combination of generalist or primary palliative care together with specialty consultation when needed is the most sustainable model [9]. A dedicated palliative care team is still essential, but innovative models of integration will allow for the most efficient use of those resources. A significant proportion of palliative cancer care can be provided by the primary cancer care team; and consultation with palliative care specialists may range from a single consultation about a specific issue to several encounters or ongoing involvement until death and into the period of bereavement [10]. Further study is needed to better understand the proportion of pediatric oncology patients who require this level of specialty palliative care consultation, and this figure will vary between institutions based on the primary team composition, competencies, number of clinicians, burden of clinical demand, and clinician skills in advanced symptom control [11].

Team Approach to Integrated Individualized Care Planning

There are vast differences in the size and composition of palliative care teams across the country. Teams are largely dependent upon the size of the institution, as well as its staff, resources, monetary constraints, and culture.

In 2013, the American Academy of Pediatrics (AAP) published guidelines [12] recommending that all hospitals and large healthcare organizations that frequently provide care to children with life-threatening conditions should have dedicated interdisciplinary specialty pediatric palliative care teams. Per these guidelines, the team should have "sufficient collective expertise to address the physical, psychosocial, emotional, practical, and spiritual needs of the child and family." [12]

The AAP further recommends that in order to ensure quality and safety, teams must have an adequate number of dedicated staff who are ideally trained in palliative care and who must be paid specifically to provide pediatric palliative care [12]. This team should be available for consultation at any time, 24 h a day, and 7 days a week. Establishing this minimum capacity should be the focus of initial improvement efforts in any center that does not yet have a dedicated palliative care team.

With such a broad spectrum of expertise required, the AAP suggests that a mature team should include physicians, nurses, social workers, case managers, spiritual care providers, bereavement specialists, and child life specialists. Table 18.2

Table 18.2 Distinctions in expertise between palliative care providers

Medicine/physician	Address medical needs such as pain and symptom management
	Explain the implications of these medical interventions
	Take the lead on framing the illness trajectory and prognosis
	Take on special role interacting with other medical specialties
Nursing	Clinical support and hands-on care
	Teaching families how to best provide care for their children
	Support other staff at bedside
Social work	Address broad spectrum of factors that influence families, such as housing, transportation, and family dynamics
	Provide psychosocial/emotional and bereavement supports
Child life	Provide psychosocially driven intervention that promote coping through play, preparation, education, and self-expression activities for both patient and siblings
Pastoral care	Support spiritual needs of child and family
	Access supports specific to a family's religious belief and values
	Communicate spiritual needs of family to care team for considerations in care plan

Adapted from Ogelby and Goldstein [13]

distinguishes between the responsibilities and roles of these various palliative care providers. As illustrated in the table, each provider on the team provides distinct expertise and patient support. Although there are inherent differences in these roles, overlap and collaboration among these services is essential for unified, interdisciplinary care [4].

Typically, a palliative care team is led by a physician who is board certified in Hospice and Palliative Medicine. The American Board of Pediatrics is only one of ten boards which participate in subspecialty certification in Hospice and Palliative Medicine. However, unlike the majority of medical subspecialties, leadership can shift between the various professionals involved. The palliative care team is encouraged to be truly interdisciplinary, allowing for shifts in the prominence of each discipline as they become more or less relevant to the patient and family's goals of care [14].

As pediatric palliative care is a new and growing field, it is understood that teams may incorporate a variety of disciplines, changing as needs evolve. The team should have access to high-quality adjunct services including psychology, pharmacology, nutrition, expressive therapy (such as music and art), and rehabilitation—including speech, occupational, and physical therapy.

As the members of a palliative care team are interdisciplinary and come from an array of backgrounds, it is important to be aware of the training that is offered for each discipline. It is not unusual for a new team to be composed of members without specialization in palliative and hospice care; however, furthering education should be encouraged for all members and available certification should ideally be acquired. In order to improve the quality of service provided, teams should set goals enabling members to pursue further certification within their respective fields, ideally on an annual basis as additional certification becomes available [15]. Some teams may choose to include ongoing CME/CEU training efforts, and/or educational efforts they provide within their hospital regarding palliative care, as quality metrics.

The Institute for Healthcare Improvement has demonstrated that a patient-centered approach that places an emphasis on coordinated care and communication has been shown to lead to improved patient outcomes, satisfaction, and associated reductions in healthcare costs [6]. We recommend that palliative care teams monitor these outcomes on a regular basis to serve as quality metric tools driving further change and continual improvement.

Care Coordination and Integrated Team Planning

Assessing and establishing goals of care are the primary tasks of the palliative care team. Included in the discussion should be the patient, when appropriate, and their family (who, when appropriate, should be determined by the patient). Prior to addressing goals of care, palliative care teams should first provide a realistic appraisal of prognosis including anticipatory guidance about likelihood of future symptoms, impairments, and mortality, as well as the timeframe in which these outcomes are likely to occur [12]. The assessment should include patient and family expectations of treatment, goals for care, quality of life, and preferences for type and site of care [16].

Interdisciplinary Team Meetings

Per the AAP Guidelines, collaboration between all involved members of the primary as well as specialty healthcare teams is essential in order to meet needs of patients most effectively. This requires that the care is integrated and not only is cure seeking and life prolonging—when in best interest of the patient—but is also comfort enhancing and prioritizes quality of life [12]. Providing this level of care therefore requires close and direct communication between all involved team members, frequently in the form of an interdisciplinary team meeting. When communication between interdisciplinary care providers is unified, "treatment decisions have a greater likelihood of being framed in common terms and delicate decision making is less likely to be abruptly undermined by an uncoordinated caregiver's opinion." [13] In order to facilitate harmonization of goals, there should be clear documentation of the discussions and decisions relating to advanced care planning in the electronic medical record [17].

Who should attend interdisciplinary team meetings? [13]
Attending medical team
Continuing subspecialty providers
Bedside nurse
Case manager
Rehabilitation therapies
Palliative care team
May consist of physician, nurse practitioner, palliative care nurse, social worker, pastoral care, and child life specialist

Interdisciplinary Team Sample Agenda
Process:
Once weekly, 1 h meeting.
Each patient will be discussed: new patients, readmitted/reconsulted patients, continuing patients, discharged patients with any updates.
Facilitator and time keeper assigned.
Each discipline presents their field followed by brief team discussion:
Medical (physician/nurse practitioner)
Pain management
Rehab
Child life
Pastoral care
Social work
Each discipline will document their goals and objectives in the medical record.

How often should these interdisciplinary meetings occur? The frequency of these meetings is not officially established and depends upon the nature and progression of the course of illness. Ideally, these discussions should not take place during times of crisis; we recommend establishing a meeting prior to discharge when the patient's health is relatively stable. However, the patient's health status should not preclude an interdisciplinary team meeting when issues in communication among medical teams and the family arise or in times when difficult decisions surrounding goals of care need to be discussed.

Defining and Measuring Quality in Palliative Care

In 2014, the Institute of Medicine published *Dying in America*, a consensus report which found that improving the quality and availability of medical and social services for patients and their families at the end of life could not only enhance quality of life through the end of life but could also contribute to a more sustainable healthcare system [18]. This report discusses the factors which hamper delivery of high-quality end-of-life care, but also discusses opportunities for improvement within the healthcare system and palliative care teams. Yet the benefit derived from involvement of a palliative care team can only be demonstrated when the team evaluates and measures its performance. In many centers, palliative care teams are in developmental stages and may struggle to identify the best ways to evaluate performance. A vision and/or mission statement paired with program goals is often the starting place of structural assessment. Figure 18.1 provides a sample mission and vision statement with program goals for a typical palliative care team.

The initial efforts toward defining quality in the field of palliative care began in 2001 at a meeting of the National Consensus Project [16]. This collaboration of six major hospice and palliative care organizations, including the AAHPM (American

---

Mission: Provide high quality, compassionate, and expert care to patients with life-limiting or life-threatening illness, utilizing a multidisciplinary and family centered approach to enhance quality of life

Vision: Become a recognized program for pediatric palliative care.

Program Goals:
1. Support the medical, emotional, social, and spiritual needs of the patient and their families across the continuum.
2. Assist in communication and coordination of care both in the hospital and community/home setting.
3. Provide guidance to patients and families during medical decision making.
4. Help patients and families define and meet their goals thereby enhancing the quality of life.
5. Develop a teaching program for multiple skill levels of health care providers and interdisciplinary team members.
6. Design a quality improvement system to monitor the program.
7. Participate in research endeavors related to advancing the field of palliative medicine.

Fig. 18.1 Example of a mission and vision statement with program goals

Academy of Hospice and Palliative Medicine), CAPC (Center to Advance Palliative Care), HPNA (Hospice and Palliative Nurses Association), NHPCO (National Hospice and Palliative Care Organization), NASW (National Association of Social Workers), and NPCRC (National Palliative Care Research Center), resulted in the Clinical Guidelines for Quality Palliative Care, which described the core concepts and structures for quality palliative care, including eight domains of practice. "Domains" of practice are broadly defined as areas within which to develop outcome and process measures for palliative care and hospice programs. The 2009 revision of these guidelines further described the domains and reflected ongoing collaboration between major organizations. The third edition of these guidelines, released in 2013, explicitly includes neonates, children, and adolescents (see Table 18.3) [16].

Following the development of the NCP domains, the National Quality Forum (NQF) endorsed a set of 14 quality indicators for palliative and hospice care with the dual aim of ensuring provision of high-quality care as well as generating ideas for future research [19]. "Indicators" are specific tools that quantitatively assess specific healthcare structures, processes, or outcomes. Finally, the eight domains of care identified by the NCP were utilized by the Measuring What Matters Campaign [20], a consensus project of the AAHPM and HPNA, which aimed to recommend a concise portfolio of valid, clinically relevant, cross-cutting indicators for internal measurement of hospice and palliative care. The MWM campaign identified ten indicators that mapped to five of the domains of care identified in the NCP guidelines. These indicators were published in 2015 [20]. Of note, these domains and indicators have not been evaluated specifically in pediatric palliative and hospice care or the care of children with cancer. NCP domains and MWM indicators mapping to each domain, with suggested measurement sources, are summarized in Table 18.4.

To date, although the National Consensus Project did take pediatric palliative care into account in their most recent update, there are no consensus recommendations for measures to be applied specifically to the care of children. It is also important to note that the domains and indicators listed here are primarily process driven or measures of how the team functions. Beyond pain and symptom management, and satisfaction surveys, metrics that map directly to patient outcomes remain scarce. As the field matures, we anticipate that patient- and family-level outcomes will be defined, benchmarked, and measured across pediatric palliative care programs.

A 2013 survey documented that parents and clinicians highly value many of the elements described in the NCP framework, but also described that these elements are far from universally available. Although this was a single institution study, it represents some of the gaps in care and opportunities for improvement. Highly valued elements from this survey, along with frequency of patients receiving the elements, are listed in Table 18.5 [27].

Table 18.3 National Consensus Project domains of care

National Consensus Project domains of care for palliative care	
1. Structure and processes of care	Guidelines within this domain detail the meaning of interdisciplinary teams and family-centered care. All families should have access to palliative care expertise and staff 24 h a day, 7 days a week, and respite services should be available
2. Physical aspects of care	The interdisciplinary team should assess and manage pain and other symptoms based on best available evidence within the context of disease status. This includes the use of validated measurement tools appropriate for the age of the child. Treatment of distressing symptoms and side effects should include a broad spectrum of pharmacologic, behavioral, and complementary or integrative therapies including referral to appropriate specialists as needed
3. Psychological and psychiatric aspects of care	Care should include regular, ongoing assessment of psychological reactions related to illness including stress, coping strategies, and anticipatory grieving as well as evaluation for psychiatric conditions, especially anxiety and depression. Grief and bereavement support should be provided to all families
4. Social aspects of care	The interdisciplinary team should perform a comprehensive social assessment to identify the social strengths, needs, and goals of each patient and family
5. Spiritual, religious, and existential aspects of care	Communication with the patient and family should be respectful of religious and spiritual beliefs, rituals, and practices. All members of the care team should recognize spiritual distress when present and attend to this distress within their scope of practice. All patients should have access to spiritual care professionals
6. Cultural aspects of care	Each patient receives care in a culturally and linguistically appropriate manner. Professional interpreter services should be utilized and written materials should be available in the patient/family's preferred language
7. Care of the patient at the end of life	Care of any patient at the end of life is time and detail intensive. This is especially true for pediatric patients. The interdisciplinary team should assess the patient for symptoms and proactively prepare the family on the recognition and management of potential symptoms and concerns. Care planning at this stage may include a hospice referral if this option is congruent with the patient and family's goals of care
8. Ethical and legal aspects of care	The interdisciplinary team should educate the patient and family about advanced care planning documents to promote clear communication of care preferences across the continuum of care. These documents may include designation of a healthcare proxy, inpatient and/or outpatient orders for limited resuscitation, and advance directives. Knowledge of state-specific documentation as well as guidelines for the use of such documents by minors is imperative. Ethical clinical issues should be documented and appropriate ethics consultation utilized to assist in conflict resolution as well as policy development. All care should be provided in accordance with professional, state, and federal laws, regulations, and current accepted standards of care

Table 18.4 Measuring what matters quality indicators mapping to NCP domains, with validated sources for measurement

National Consensus Project domain	Measuring what matters indicator	Source
1. Structure and processes of care	Comprehensive assessment Hospice: % of patients enrolled for more than 7 days for whom a comprehensive assessment was completed within 5 days of admission (documentation of prognosis, functional assessment, screening for physical and psychological symptoms, and assessment of social and spiritual concerns) Seriously ill patients receiving specialty palliative care in an acute hospital setting: % of patients admitted for more than 1 day who had a comprehensive assessment (screening for physical symptoms and discussion of patient/family's emotional or psychological needs) completed within 24 h of admission	PEACE Set [21–23]
2. Physical aspects of care	Screening for physical symptoms % of seriously ill patients receiving specialty PC in an acute hospital setting for more than 1 day or patients enrolled in hospice for more than 7 days who had a screening for physical symptoms (pain, dyspnea, nausea, constipation) during admission visit	PEACE Set [21–23]
	Pain treatment % of seriously ill patients receiving specialty PC in an acute hospital setting for more than 1 day or patients enrolled in hospice for more than 7 days who screened positive for moderate to severe pain on admission, % with medication or non-medication treatment within 24 h of screening	PEACE Set [21–23]
	Dyspnea screening and management % of patients with advanced chronic or serious life-threatening illnesses who are screened for dyspnea. For those who are diagnosed with moderate or severe dyspnea, % with a documented plan of care to manage dyspnea	AMA-PCPI/NCQA [24]
3. Psychological and psychiatric aspects of care	Discussion of emotional or psychological needs % of seriously ill patients receiving specialty PC in an acute hospital setting for more than 1 day or patients enrolled in hospice for more than 7 days with chart documentation of a discussion of emotional or psychological needs	PEACE Set [21–23]
4. Social aspects of care	No indicators	

(continued)

Table 18.4 (continued)

National Consensus Project domain	Measuring what matters indicator	Source
5. Spiritual, religious, and existential aspects of care	Discussion of spiritual/religious concerns % of hospice patients with documentation of a discussion of spiritual/religious concerns or documentation that patient/caregiver/family did not want to discuss	Deyta, LLC/ NQF#1647
6. Cultural aspects of care	No indicators	
7. Care of the patient at the end of life	No indicators	
8. Ethical and legal aspects of care	Documentation of surrogate % of seriously ill patients receiving specialty PC in an acute hospital setting for more than 1 day or patients enrolled in hospice for more than 7 days with name and contact information for surrogate decision-maker in the chart or documentation that there is no surrogate	PEACE Set [21–23]
	Treatment preferences % of seriously ill patients receiving specialty PC in an acute hospital setting for more than 1 day or patients enrolled in hospice for more than 7 days with chart documentation of preferences for life sustaining treatments	PEACE Set [21–23]/ NQF#1641
	Care consistency with documented care preferences If a vulnerable elder has specific treatment preferences documented in a medical record, then these treatment preferences should be followed	ACOVE PC and EOL Care [25, 26]
Global measure	No specific measure endorsed, but committee, panels, membership, and stakeholders agreed that patient and/ or family assessments of quality of are a key part of measuring quality for any setting caring for palliative or hospice care patients	

Future Directions for Quality Improvement in Palliative Care

To demonstrate why the patients and families need palliative care and to show how they benefit, it is imperative that the team establishes process measures to monitor and measure various parameters based on their goals. Further research is needed to establish consensus guidelines regarding domains of quality in pediatric palliative care and to identify specific indicators to measure patient- and family-centered outcomes in pediatric palliative care. However, in the meantime, all palliative care teams can study their own processes and patient outcomes, apply quality improvement methodology, and see meaningful improvement. The following patient-level outcomes and team-driven process measures may be considered as quality continues to be defined in this field:

Table 18.5 Elements of palliative care delivery highly valued by parents and clinicians and likelihood of receiving the element [27]

Highly valued element	Patients that received the element (%)
Structure of care	
Involvement of palliative care specialist	56
Access to 24/7 telephone advice from palliative clinician	50
Access to dedicated palliative inpatient bed	36.8
Access to direct admission policy to hospital	16.2
Emotional, social, and spiritual aspects of care	
Involvement of a social worker for parent	55.4
Involvement of a social worker for child when appropriate	63.1
Sibling support	44.4
Communication	
Discussion of death and dying with parents by healthcare team	67.6
Discussion of death and dying with child by the healthcare team when appropriate	33.3
Provide parents with guidance on how to talk to their child about death and dying	37.3
Discussion of resuscitation status with parents by healthcare team	82.2
End-of-life care	
Prepare parents for medical aspects surrounding death	59.5
Home death	54.7
Parent control over the location of death	59.5
Contact with family after death	90.7

Palliative care patient- and family-level outcomes	
Outcome	**Potential measurement tool or data source**
Health-related quality of life	Peds-QL
Serious adverse event rate	EMR, safety team
Patient and family have accurate understanding of prognosis and treatment options	Family satisfaction survey
Death occurs at location of preference	EMR
Patient feels supported throughout trajectory of illness	Patient/family satisfaction survey
Family feels supported throughout trajectory of illness and in bereavement	Patient/family satisfaction survey
Family feels prepared for medical issues and circumstances at time of death	Patient/family satisfaction survey
Process measures for oncology and palliative care teams	
Process measure	**Potential measurement tool or data source**
Assessment and timely treatment of distressing symptoms	MSAS at time of consult/hospice enrollment and at established frequency thereafter FACES, FLACC scales for pain

Completion and documentation of new patient consults within 24 h	EMR
Institutional educational efforts regarding palliative care	Frequency of talks locally, regionally, nationally by team members
Documentation of goals of care, advance directive, DNR orders	EMR
Documentation of preferred location of death	EMR

Teams may consider tracking their quality improvement efforts in a "dashboard" or spreadsheet to document team quality priorities and whether these goals are being met. Teams may wish to focus on broad categories such as professionalism, safety, patient satisfaction, and patient care. Specific measures within each broad category can then be identified; for example, within patient care, a palliative care team may focus on pain management and then, specifically, the % of patients screened for pain at the time of the consult or the % of patients with improvement in pain scores within a certain time period of the consult. For each specific measure, the team must know their baseline level of success to set a reasonable goal for the next four quarters or fiscal year. Key driver diagrams may be developed outside of the dashboard for each specific measure that is being tracked. Results are then followed quarterly with clear identification of whether goals are being met and an action plan for the future. See below for an example of a palliative care team quality "dashboard":

Patient care quality measure	Specific measure	FY2015 goal	Q1 results	Meeting goal?	Action plan
Pain	% of patients screened for pain at time of consult	100%	89%	No	Failure mode and effects analysis
Pain	% of patients with improvement in pain scores within 24 h of consult	80%	85%	Yes	Continue current process Increase goal to 90% for Q2
Constipation	% of patients on opioids with a bowel regimen in place	100%	100%	Yes	Start measuring % of patients on opioids without constipation
Clinical care	% of patients with DIPG or GBM seen within 1 month of diagnosis	100%	50%	No	Outreach to neuro-oncology team, failure mode, and effects analysis
Team education	# of national conferences attended by team members	3 (1 per quarter)	2	Yes	Continue current processes

Quality Improvement in Pediatric Palliative Care: A Case-Based Example

Step 1: Identify Leaders and Create the Team

The pediatric palliative care team at Blue Ribbon Children's Hospital has been asked to incorporate quality improvement (QI) into their team workflow. Nancy, a nurse practitioner on the team, recently participated in a quality improvement workshop and knows some basics about QI methodology. She volunteers to lead the project and several of her co-workers volunteer to be part of the "QI Team."

Step 2: Define the Problem

After some discussion, consultation with other palliative care teams, and a literature review, the team decides that they would like to start with a small project designed to help them all learn QI methodology. They choose to work on improving their efficiency in completing new inpatient consults. Since they are working on improving the function of their system, they recognize that this is a process measure.

Step 3: Identify Global Aim and SMART Aim

The team defines the global aim for this project as "Improved palliative care team efficiency" and the SMART aim as "Between March 1, 2016 and July 1, 2016 the palliative care team will increase the percentage of new inpatient consults completed within 24 h from x% to >90%."

Step 4: Observe the Current Process, Obtain Baseline Data, and Identify Failures and Their Causes

As a first step, because the team does not closely track time to consult completion, Nancy suggests that they do a chart review to obtain baseline data to understand how long it takes the team, on average, to complete a new consult. Bob volunteers for this job. He creates a data collection sheet (see below) to track patient information, date and time of consult, the consulting team, the reason for consult, and date and time that the consult was completed. For these purposes, he defines "completion" as the date that the consult note is signed by the attending physician or nurse practitioner in the electronic medical record. The source of data for this project was the electronic medical record. To obtain enough data to learn from meaningfully,

Bob reviews 6 months of inpatient consults. He is confident that the way the team functioned was stable during this time (i.e., no turnover of employees, no major holidays, etc.).

An example of his data collection sheet with the first week of data is below:

Patient MRN	Date and time of consult order	Team ordering consult	Reason for consult	Date consult completed	Time to completion in hours
12345678	1/1/2016 0830	Oncology	Difficulty coping with new diagnosis of DIPG	1/4/2016 1500	78.5
23456789	1/3/2016 1150	NICU	Withdrawal of care, same day	1/3/2016 1720	5.5
11223345	1/3/2016 1400	PICU	Parents considering tracheostomy placement	1/4/2016 1000	20
22222222	1/4/2016 0930	Oncology	Stage IV neuroblastoma with relapse	1/6/2016 1830	57
67676767	1/5/2016 0800	Cardiology	Heart failure, anxiety after VAD placement	1/5/2016 1200	4

Bob finds that the average time to completion of new consults is 50 h. Additionally, only 20% of consults are completed within 24 h. Thus the SMART aim becomes "Between March 1, 2016 and July 1, 2016 the palliative care team will increase the percentage of new inpatient consults completed within 24 h from 20% to >90%." Nancy creates a run chart and plots this baseline data. The title of the run chart is "Average percentage of new inpatient consults completed by the palliative care team, by week." The x axis is time and the y axis is average percentage of new inpatient consults completed per week. Bob recognizes that he is collecting counts or classifications or *attribute data* (see Chap. 6, Fig. 6.4 "Selection of Shewhart Chart"). He is counting passes or failures or classification/nonconforming, and from week to week the subgroup size may be different. Thus he utilizes a P Chart to display his data. *(Operationalize the measure and plot it on a run chart to display change over time.)*

Bob and Nancy then examine the data further to understand reasons for "failures" or times that they have not been able to complete consults within 24 business hours. He finds that there are three main categories of reasons for failing to complete consults:

1. There is an unclear process for others to contact the team and let them know a consult order has been placed (40%).
2. The team is aware of the consult but another more emergent consult (such as withdrawal of care) takes priority (30%).

3. The team has less staffing (only one provider) on Tuesdays and Thursdays which makes consult completion difficult (10%), and the patient has been seen, but the physician or nurse practitioner has not documented the consult note by the day's end (20%).

Bob creates a Pareto diagram based on these results. The team creates a failure mode effects analysis to gain additional insight into the barriers to consult completion in a timely manner. For more details on creating a Pareto diagram, see Chap. 6. (Create Pareto Diagram.)

Step 5: Create a Key Driver Diagram

Based on the results of their Pareto diagram, the team created the following key driver diagram (Fig. 18.2).

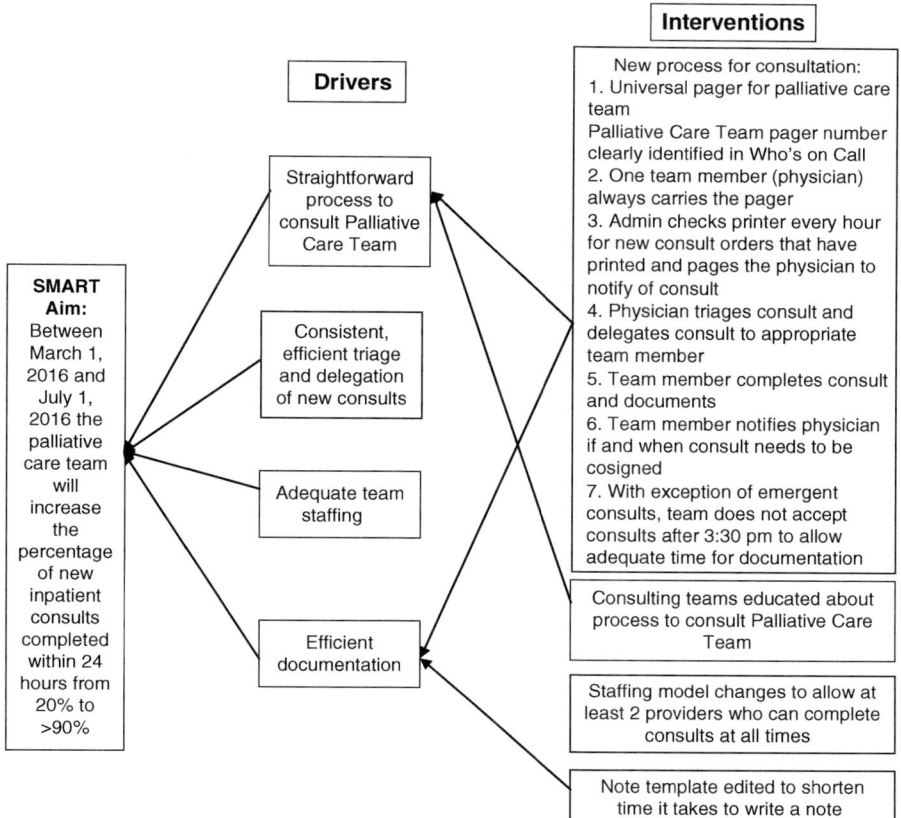

Fig. 18.2 Key driver diagram

Step 6: Design and Execute PDSA Cycles

The team designs and executes multiple PDSA cycles around each intervention, ramping up appropriately. The key driver diagram is edited as they learn which interventions lead to improvement. They continue to track their average percentage of consults completed within 24 h, by week, on their run chart. If an intervention does not result in expected improvement, additional PDSA cycles are run to study what will improve their process instead. Over the next 6 months, they find that the interventions in their key driver diagram result in improvement and their average percentage of consults completed within 24 h improves to >90% and remains there for >3 months.

Step 7: Implement Successful Interventions

When the team is confident that they have reached a new "steady state" in their process, they cease testing (running PDSA cycles) and implement all interventions in their key driver diagram.

What Should Centers Without Palliative Care Program Do?

We recommend that centers without a dedicated palliative care program advocate establishing one. Although expanding workforce may be difficult to advocate for in this cost-conscious environment, the proven ability of palliative care to simultaneously improve quality and save money makes it a critical part of the care plan for the most seriously ill (and expensive) patients [9].

However, there are actions that hospitals can take to promote palliative care until a formal team is incorporated. Hospital clinicians are positioned to provide "primary" palliative care, such as prioritizing honest, clear, and compassionate communication to discuss goals of care or medical decisions with families or promoting comfort and quality of life [28]. A palliative care approach to communication begins with eliciting family values and hopes for the child. This allows families and providers to integrate relevant information and make the best decisions for their child. This approach can be used by hospital-based palliative care "generalists" and palliative care specialists alike [28].

A few core elements of palliative care should routinely be delivered by all practitioners, such as aligning treatment with a patient's goals and basic symptom management. Other skills are more complex and require years of training to learn and apply, such as negotiating a difficult family meeting, addressing veiled existential distress, and managing refractory symptoms. Quill and Abernathy provide a table (Table 18.6) on the distinctions of care that should be provided by primary and specialist palliative care physicians [9].

Table 18.6 Representative skill sets for primary and specialty palliative care [9]

Primary palliative care
Basic management of pain and symptoms
Basic management of depression and anxiety
Basic discussions about
Prognosis
Goals of treatment
Suffering
Resuscitation status
Specialty palliative care
Management of refractory pain or other symptoms
Management of more complex depression, anxiety, grief, and existential distress
Assistance with conflict resolution regarding goals or methods of treatment
Within families
Between staff and families
Among treatment teams
Assistance in addressing cases of near futility

We recommend that every health system should delineate basic expectations regarding primary palliative care skills to be learned and practiced by its members, which includes triage system for calling on palliative care specialists whenever necessary [9]. The primary palliative care curriculum must be taught—even to mid-career clinicians—and reinforced by performance measurement and remediation as needed.

There are a few resources available to improve provider communication concerning palliative and end-of-life topics. The Oncotalk Teach program aims to provide faculty development for oncology faculty involved in teaching communication skills at their home institutions [29]. It provides free modules and videos on improving provider communication for a variety of difficult conversation topics. Courses such as Education in Palliative and End-of-Life Care and End-of-Life Nursing Education Consortium should be encouraged by healthcare systems. Apart from the Board of Hospice and Palliative Medicine for physicians, there are also certification courses available for nurse practitioners, nurses, social workers, and chaplains.

Ultimately, we recommend that hospital centers without a dedicated palliative care team work to get one. However, in the absence of a specialist program, palliative care concepts should still be fostered by the healthcare system by delineating basic expectations for providers and promoting an educational environment.

Hospice Care

Hospice is both a philosophy and a system of care and, in the United States, represents a preference for home care and family support as opposed to institutional care and hospital-based intervention [30, 31]. In the United States, "hospice" also refers to a Medicare insurance benefit that requires a life expectancy of 6 months or less, with additional specific criterion required to be met for the primary diagnosis which led to hospice care. The majority of hospice care is delivered in the patient's home, although many care agencies also have a hospice facility to which patients may be admitted for short periods of time.

According to the Centers for Disease Control, in 2013, children aged 0–19 years accounted for 42,328 total deaths in the United States [32]. Approximately three-quarters of these deaths are classified as non-preventable, comprising about 30,000 children annually [33]. Hospice care is considered to be the model for quality compassionate care for people facing a life-limiting illness, and many children who die are eligible for hospice care. But a white paper produced by the Children's International Project on Palliative/Hospice Services (ChiPPS) for the National Hospice and Palliative Care Organization (NHPCO) reported that less than 10% of eligible children receive hospice care [34]. This may be related to the fact that, because children represent less than 1% of hospice enrollees, most children who are enrolled in hospice are cared for in traditional adult-centered hospice programs [35]. A 2007 survey of member hospices by the NHPCO found that 78% of respondent hospices reported caring for children, but only 36.6% offered formal pediatric programs [33]. In contrast, Lindley et al. found that the percentage of hospices caring for children in California declined from 40% in 2002 to 28% in 2012 [36] and a similar study from North Carolina found that, in 2012, only 43% of hospices provided hospice care at home to children [37]. Some counties in this study offered no hospice agencies at all. Thus, low pediatric hospice enrollment may be driven in part by poor access to, and low availability of, pediatric hospice care.

The largest review of children enrolled in hospice care, based on data from the Coalition of Hospices Organize to Investigate Comparative Effectiveness (CHOICE) network of hospices, found that the most common diagnoses for children include neoplasms, complex chronic conditions such as neurological disorders, chromosomal abnormalities, congenital malformations, and inherited orders of metabolism [35]. In that study, remarkably, 42.6% of hospice enrollment diagnoses for children were encountered only once during the 4-year interval studied. Several studies have found that children on hospice are more likely to be older, generally between the ages of 15 and 20 years, though the mean age of children in the CHOICE data set was only 4.6 years [35, 38, 39]. Finally, pediatric minorities are significantly more likely to be represented in hospice use than are adult minorities [35, 40, 41]. Therefore, the cohort of children in hospice care represents a highly diverse sample of diagnoses, ages, races, and ethnicities.

Hospices perceive several barriers in providing care to children. The most important barrier recognized by hospice agencies, regardless of whether current services were offered to children, was a lack of pediatric referrals, thought to be due in part to inflexible hospices services [37]. The second most important barrier was a desire by families to continue pursuing curative therapies for children while in hospice care [37]. Family and provider difficulty with accepting a child's prognosis has been separately cited as a possible reason for low hospice utilization, as have state and federal reimbursement policies [42–44]. The Patient Protection and Affordable Care Act (ACA), passed in 2010, specifies that children enrolled in Medicaid or the Children's Health Insurance Program can concurrently receive both hospice services and life-extending disease-directed therapy [45]. Ultimately, implementation of the ACA will improve pediatric referrals to hospice care, hospice reimbursement for care provided to children, and families' willingness to enroll on hospice services earlier in the course of pediatric life-limiting illness.

Hospices also perceive the high complexity of children's care needs, lack of pediatric trained personnel, poor access to pediatric consultations, language barriers, and difficulty in certifying that a child has less than 6 months to live as barriers in the provision of pediatric hospice care [37]. Agencies that do not serve children are significantly more likely to denote a lack of pediatric trained staff as a "very important" issue [37]. Inconsistent hospice plans of care by pediatricians, lack of pediatric pharmacy services, and lack of pediatric consultation if needed were also cited as "very important" or "important" barriers by hospices in this group.

These concerns become even more amplified when considered in the context of the meaningful differences between pediatric and adult hospice care. Children who are admitted to hospice are significantly less likely to have a diagnosis of cancer than adults and are more likely to carry rare diagnoses, presenting unique challenges to hospice agencies which already lack access to pediatric specialists [35]. Children are more likely to leave hospice care, perhaps due to earlier enrollment and a changing course of illness, but among those who remain on hospice, children are more likely to die at home [35, 46]. One study found that children with cancer frequently revoked hospice care due to poor pain and symptom control [47]. Finally, children have significantly longer lengths of stay on hospice than adults and are significantly less likely to die within 1 week of hospice enrollment [35, 46]. This longer length of stay may be related to the unpredictable nature of life-limiting conditions in children, again highlighting that the adult definition of hospice care, based on specific prognostic factors, can be inappropriate when applied to pediatric conditions.

Data regarding parental perceptions of hospice care are limited. One study of bereaved parents of children with cancer who enrolled on hospice revealed that, while many families perceived a high quality in hospice care, some families expressed frustration with hospice care when compared to prior experiences with aging family members [47]. This study did find meaningful differences in how families described hospice care based on primary language; Spanish-speaking families were overall more positive in describing their experiences with hospice than were English-speaking families. Poor pain and symptom control led 6 of 20 families, all English-speaking, to leave hospice and experience their child's death in the hospital rather than at home. Revocation due to poor symptom control may again indicate a higher complexity of care for children receiving hospice care, which traditional hospice agencies lacking dedicated pediatric personnel are unprepared to manage.

Thus, the decision to enroll a child into a hospice program should be approached with care and planning. The ACA established concurrent care for children, ensuring that they do not need forgo disease-directed therapies, physician visits, or even hospitalization to be enrolled in hospice. Unfortunately, concurrent care is not yet fully integrated in all states, and many traditional hospice groups find it difficult to impossible to be refunded appropriately for providing concurrent hospice and cure-based care for children. This issue is compounded by the timing of hospice enrollment for children. Ideally, children nearing the end of life should be referred to hospice programs as early as possible to allow ample time for the hospice team to build rapport and determine the plan of care. Families will experience a period of transition in enrolling in a hospice program, in which the psychosocial burden on the family may increase as they meet a new care team, and receive equipment and supplies delivered to the home, and a sense of "normalcy" is reestablished. This investment is worthwhile, and careful planning and close collaboration can minimize the burden to the family. For oncologists and palliative care providers, it is essential to establish strong relationships with area hospice agencies to ease this transition for the family. Closer consultation with a pediatric palliative care team should be considered particularly if the hospice has little experience with children.

Patient Quality and Safety in the Home

Many palliative care teams provide continuity of care with their patients in the hospital, in ambulatory clinics, in hospice inpatient units, and in the patient home. For any palliative care team entering a child's home, it is appropriate to include safety and quality of care in the home as part of the patient's overall care plan. Additionally some children's hospitals offer homecare divisions that provide private duty nursing, durable medical equipment, home-based physical and/or occupational therapies, and home-based pharmacotherapy. Those pediatric institutions that offer dedicated pediatric hospice groups often do so through existing homecare divisions. Thus, there may be overlap between quality assurance/performance improvement efforts within a pediatric hospital's homecare division and within their hospice group.

For palliative care teams providing home-based care, patient outcomes and team performance measures may overlap between inpatient, clinic, and the home. Children receiving hospice care are significantly less likely to have cancer than adults, and a recent review of data from the CHOICE (Coalition of Hospices Organize to Investigate Comparative Effectiveness) network found that over 40% of hospice enrollment diagnoses for children were encountered only once for the time period studied [35]. As medical and surgical advances have improved length of survival for children with complex chronic conditions, the complexity of caring for such children has also increased [48]. Thus, pediatric palliative care teams and homecare divisions may find that they care for children who are dependent on tracheostomies, ventilators, enteral feedings through gastrostomy tubes, and/or indwelling central venous catheters in the home. This complexity must be taken into account when considering how to provide safe, high-quality home-based care throughout the trajectory of illness and should be reflected in those patient-level outcomes and performance measures chosen in quality assurance/performance improvement efforts.

The following table provides an example of a home-based quality "dashboard" for palliative care teams or homecare divisions to consider:

Home-based palliative care patient- and family-level outcomes	
Outcome	Potential measurement tool or data source
Patient and family have accurate understanding of prognosis and treatment options	Family satisfaction survey
Patient/family satisfaction with care	Patient/family satisfaction survey
Death occurs at location of preference	EMR
Home-based palliative care process measures	
Process measure	Potential measurement tool or data source
Risk assessment for falls (% of patients with falls management plan if patient is at risk for falls)	EMR
Infections: # of patients with central line blood stream infections related to central venous catheter	EMR
Medication safety (% of medications ordered with clear indication for PRN use)	EMR, home-based pharmacy tracking system
Assessment and treatment of distressing symptoms (% of patients assessed for pain, dyspnea, constipation at time of enrollment)	MSAS
Patient/family preference: (% of patients with documentation of goals of care, advance directive, DNR orders at time of enrollment)	EMR
Patient/family preference: (% of documentation of preferred location of death at time of enrollment)	EMR
Spiritual care (% of patients screened for spiritual needs/ issues on initial visit)	EMR

Safe Prescribing of Schedule II Medications

The United States has experienced an epidemic of prescription drug abuse, frequently leading to heroin abuse. As opioids are the cornerstone of treatment for cancer-related pain, potential patient misuse of prescription medications and national regulatory responses should be of particular concern to palliative care physicians and oncologists [49]. An emerging body of literature has focused on screening for drug misuse in adult patients with cancer or who are receiving palliative care [49–52]. A recent retrospective review of adults with cancer followed by a palliative care team found that 43% of patients were classified as medium- or high-risk of opioid misuse [49]. To our knowledge, only one retrospective chart review study from St. Jude's Children's Research Hospital has focused on the question of opioid misuse in children, adolescents, and young adults. The medical records of nearly 400 adolescents and young adults were examined for "aberrant opioid-associated behavior." Of the nearly 400 patients included, researchers found that 94 received opioids, and 11.7% of these exhibited aberrant opioid-associated behaviors [53].

Prospective studies among pediatricians evaluating patients for risk of opioid abuse or diversion, and consensus recommendations for management, are not available to our knowledge. However, in 2009, the American Pain Society and American Academy of Pain Medicine (APS-AAPM) formulated recommendations for the use of chronic opioid therapy in chronic non-cancer pain, which include guidelines for obtaining informed consent for opioids, monitoring patients, and caring for high-risk patients [54]. Routine pill counts, urine drug screening, family or caregiver interviews, and use of prescription drug monitoring program data are noted to be helpful supplements in monitoring for potential misuse [54]. Thus, using these recommendations, it is feasible for palliative care programs to establish a process to screen all patients receiving opioid therapy for their potential for opioid misuse. All patients who receive opioids should be contracted for behaviors surrounding these prescriptions. Patients who are found to at moderate- or high-risk of opioid misuse through urine drug screens, pill counts, and other means can be monitored more closely in the home or ambulatory setting, given prescriptions for shorter supplies of medications, transitioned to long-acting opioids more quickly, and screened more frequently to ensure safer opioid prescribing. A "heightened awareness" of these patients may also lead to detection of misuse, discontinuation of opioid therapy, and/or referral to addiction specialists at an earlier time than would have otherwise been accomplished.

References

1. Kearney JA, Salley CG, Muriel AC. Standards of psychosocial care for parents of children with cancer. Pediatr Blood Cancer. 2015;62(Suppl 5):S632–83.
2. Levy MH, Smith T, Alvarez-Perez A, et al. Palliative care, version 1. 2014. Featured updates to the NCCN guidelines. J Natl Compr Cancer Network. 2014;12:1379–88.
3. Meier DE, Brawley OW. Palliative care and the quality of life. J Clin Oncol Off J Am Soc Clin Oncol. 2011;29:2750–2.
4. Temel JS, Greer JA, Muzikansky A, et al. Early palliative care for patients with metastatic non-small-cell lung cancer. N Engl J Med. 2010;363:733–42.
5. Mack JW, Wolfe J. Early integration of pediatric palliative care: for some children, palliative care starts at diagnosis. Curr Opin Pediatr. 2006;18:10–4.
6. Mahmood LA, Casey D, Dolan JG, Dozier AM, Korones DN. Feasibility of early palliative care consultation for children with high-risk malignancies. Pediatr Blood Cancer. 2016;63:1419–22.

7. Dalberg T, Jacob-Files E, Carney PA, Meyrowitz J, Fromme EK, Thomas G. Pediatric oncology providers' perceptions of barriers and facilitators to early integration of pediatric palliative care. Pediatr Blood Cancer. 2013;60:1875–81.

8. Johnston DL, Nagel K, Friedman DL, Meza JL, Hurwitz CA, Friebert S. Availability and use of palliative care and end-of-life services for pediatric oncology patients. J Clin Oncol Off J Am Soc Clin Oncol. 2008;26:4646–50.

9. Quill TE, Abernethy AP. Generalist plus specialist palliative care–creating a more sustainable model. N Engl J Med. 2013;368:1173–5.

10. Kaye EC, Friebert S, Baker JN. Early integration of palliative care for children with high-risk cancer and their families. Pediatr Blood Cancer. 2016;63:593–7.

11. Johnston DL, Vadeboncoeur C. Palliative care consultation in pediatric oncology. Support Care Cancer. 2012;20:799–803.

12. Medicine AAoPSoHaP. Pediatric palliative care and hospice care commitments, guidelines and recommendations. Pediatrics. 2013;132:966–72.

13. Ogelby M, Goldstein RD. Interdisciplinary care: using your team. Pediatr Clin North Am. 2014;61:823–34.

14. Wolfe J, Hinds PS, Sourkes BM. Textbook of interdisciplinary pediatric palliative care. Philadelphia: Elsevier/Saunders; 2011.

15. CME/CEU Courses. 2016. https://www.capc.org/providers/courses/. Accessed 9 Aug 2016.

16. National Consensus Project Guidelines for Quality Palliative Care. Clinical practice guidelines for quality palliative care. 3rd ed. 2013. http://www.nationalconsensusproject.org/. Accessed 19 Aug 2015.

17. Levine D, Lam CG, Cunningham MJ, et al. Best practices for pediatric palliative cancer care: a primer for clinical providers. J Support Oncol. 2013;11:114–25.

18. Dying in America: improving quality and honoring individual preferences near the end of life. Washington, DC: National Academies Press; 2015.

19. Palliative and end of life care performance measures. 2012. http://www.qualityforum.org/. Accessed 19 Aug 2015.

20. Dy SM, Kiley KB, Ast K, et al. Measuring what matters: top-ranked quality indicators for hospice and palliative care from the American academy of hospice and palliative medicine and hospice and palliative nurses association. J Pain Symptom Manage. 2015;49:773–81.

21. Schenck AP, Rokoske FS, Durham DD, Cagle JG, Hanson LC. The PEACE project: identification of quality measures for hospice and palliative care. J Palliat Med. 2010;13:1451–9.

22. Hanson LC, Scheunemann LP, Zimmerman S, Rokoske FS, Schenck AP. The PEACE project review of clinical instruments for hospice and palliative care. J Palliat Med. 2010;13:1253–60.

23. Schenck AP, Rokoske FS, Durham D, Cagle JG, Hanson LC. Quality measures for hospice and palliative care: piloting the PEACE measures. J Palliat Med. 2014;17:769–75.

24. American Medical Association. Physician consortium on performance improvement palliative and end of life care physician performance measurement set 2008. 2008. http://www.amaassn.org/ama/pub/physician-resources/physician-consortiumperformance-improvement/pcpi-measures.page. Accessed 9 Aug 2016.

25. Lorenz KA, Rosenfeld K, Wenger N. Quality indicators for palliative and end-of-life care in vulnerable elders. J Am Geriatr Soc. 2007;55(Suppl 2):S318–26.

26. Walling AM, Asch SM, Lorenz KA, et al. The quality of care provided to hospitalized patients at the end of life. Arch Intern Med. 2010;170:1057–63.

27. Kassam A, Skiadaresis J, Habib S, Alexander S, Wolfe J. Moving toward quality palliative cancer care: parent and clinician perspectives on gaps between what matters and what is accessible. J Clin Oncol Off J Am Soc Clin Oncol. 2013;31:910–5.

28. Ullrich CK, Wolfe J. Caring for children living with life-threatening illness: a growing relationship between pediatric hospital medicine and pediatric palliative care. Pediatr Clin North Am. 2014;61:xxi–ii.

29. Back AL, Arnold RM, Baile WF, et al. Faculty development to change the paradigm of communication skills teaching in oncology. J Clin Oncol Off J Am Soc Clin Oncol. 2009;27:1137–41.

30. DuBois PM. The hospice way of death. New York: Human Sciences Press; 1980.
31. Smith DH, Granbois JA. The American way of hospice. Hastings Cent Rep. 1982;12:8–10.
32. Osterman MJ, Kochanek KD, MacDorman MF, Strobino DM, Guyer B. Annual summary of vital statistics: 2012–2013. Pediatrics. 2015;135:1115–25.
33. National Hospice and Palliative Care Organization. NHPCO's facts and figures: pediatric palliative and hospice care in America 2015 edition. 2015. http://www.nhpco.org/sites/default//files/public/quality/Pediatric_Facts-Figures.pdf. Accessed 11 Aug 2015.
34. ChiPPS: a call for change: recommendations to improve the care of children living with life-threatening conditions. Alexandria. National Hospice and Palliative Care Organization; 2001.
35. Dingfield L, Bender L, Harris P, et al. Comparison of pediatric and adult hospice patients using electronic medical record data from nine hospices in the United States, 2008-2012. J Palliat Med. 2015;18:120–6.
36. Lindley LC, Mark BA, Daniel Lee SY, Domino M, Song MK, Jacobson VJ. Factors associated with the provision of hospice care for children. J Pain Symptom Manage. 2013;45:701–11.
37. Varela AM, Deal AM, Hanson LC, Blatt J, Gold S, Dellon EP. Barriers to hospice for children as perceived by hospice organizations in North Carolina. Am J Hosp Palliat Care. 2012;29:171–6.
38. National Hospice and Palliative Care Organization. NHPCO's pediatric standards: a key step in advancing care for America's children. 2009. http://www.nhpco.org/sites/default/files/public/quality/Peds-Standards_article_NL-0209.pdf. Accessed 11 Aug 2015
39. Knapp CA, Shenkman EA, Marcu MI, Madden VL, Terza JV. Pediatric palliative care: describing hospice users and identifying factors that affect hospice expenditures. J Palliat Med. 2009;12:223–9.
40. Lindley LC, Shaw SL. Who are the children using hospice care? J Spec Pediatr Nurs. 2014;19:308–15.
41. Thienprayoon R, Lee SC, Leonard D, Winick N. Racial and ethnic differences in hospice enrollment among children with cancer. Pediatr Blood Cancer. 2013;60:1662–6.
42. Dabbs D, Butterworth L, Hall E. Tender mercies: increasing access to hospice services for children with life-threatening conditions. MCN Am J Matern Child Nurs. 2007;32:311–9.
43. Davies B, Sehring SA, Partridge JC, et al. Barriers to palliative care for children: perceptions of pediatric health care providers. Pediatrics. 2008;121:282–8.
44. Lindley LC, Lyon ME. A profile of children with complex chronic conditions at end of life among medicaid beneficiaries: implications for health care reform. J Palliat Med. 2013;16:1388–93.
45. The Patient Protection and Affordable Care Act. 2 U.S.C. § 18001 (2010). 2010.
46. Thienprayoon R, Lee SC, Leonard D, Winick N. Hospice care for children with cancer: where do these children die? J Pediatr Hematol Oncol. 2015;37:373–7.
47. Thienprayoon R, Marks E, Funes M, Martinez-Puente LM, Winick N, Lee SC. Perceptions of the pediatric hospice experience among English- and Spanish-speaking families. J Palliat Med. 2015;19:30–41.
48. Simon TD, Berry J, Feudtner C, et al. Children with complex chronic conditions in inpatient hospital settings in the United States. Pediatrics. 2010;126:647–55.
49. Barclay JS, Owens JE, Blackhall LJ. Screening for substance abuse risk in cancer patients using the opioid risk tool and urine drug screen. Support Care Cancer. 2014;22:1883–8.
50. Blackhall LJ, Alfson ED, Barclay JS. Screening for substance abuse and diversion in Virginia hospices. J Palliat Med. 2013;16:237–42.
51. Childers JW, Arnold RM. "I feel uncomfortable 'calling a patient out'": educational needs of palliative medicine fellows in managing opioid misuse. J Pain Symptom Manage. 2012;43:253–60.
52. Tan PD, Barclay JS, Blackhall LJ. Do palliative care clinics screen for substance abuse and diversion? Results of a national survey. J Palliat Med. 2015;18:752–7.
53. Ehrentraut JH, Kern KD, Long SA, An AQ, Faughnan LG, Anghelescu DL. Opioid misuse behaviors in adolescents and young adults in a hematology/oncology setting. J Pediatr Psychol. 2014;39:1149–60.
54. Chou R, Fanciullo GJ, Fine PG, et al. Clinical guidelines for the use of chronic opioid therapy in chronic noncancer pain. J Pain. 2009;10:113–30.

Chapter 19
Careers in Quality Improvement and Patient Safety

Jeff Hord, Allyson Hays, and Roland Chu

Quality Improvement Education for Physicians

During the early part of this century, two *Institute of Medicine* reports were published and initiated significant changes in our health-care system and medical education. *To Err Is Human* highlighted the frequency and human cost of medical errors, while *Crossing the Quality Chasm* offered a plan for improvement of the health-care system which included quality improvement (QI) education for both physicians-in-training and practicing physicians [1, 2]. Soon after, thought leaders and professional organizations in medicine and nursing endorsed teaching quality improvement to clinicians [3–6].

In 2002, the Accreditation Council on Graduate Medical Education (ACGME) Outcome Project was launched and defined core competencies to guide curriculum development and performance assessment for postgraduate medical education training programs. Two of these competencies are related to quality improvement: (1) practice-based learning and improvement and (2) system-based practices. The ACGME expects that residents and fellows will develop skills and habits to be able

J. Hord (✉)
Division of Pediatric Hematology/Oncology,
Akron Children's Hospital, Akron, 44308 Ohio, USA
e-mail: jhord@chmca.org

A. Hays
Division of Pediatric Hematology/Oncology,
Children's Mercy Hospital, Kansas City, MO, USA
e-mail: jahays@cmh.edu

R. Chu
Division of Pediatric Hematology/Oncology,
Children's Hospital of Michigan, Detroit, MI, USA
e-mail: rchu@med.wayne.edu

© Springer International Publishing AG 2017
C.E. Dandoy et al. (eds.), *Patient Safety and Quality in Pediatric Hematology/ Oncology and Stem Cell Transplantation*, DOI 10.1007/978-3-319-53790-0_19

to systematically analyze practice using quality improvement methods and implement changes with the goal of practice improvement [7].

There is great variability in the design of QI education curricula, and best practices in QI education have not been solidly established. Common barriers to QI education success include the lack of faculty expertise, lack of institutional support, lack of trainee interest, and lack of educational opportunities as hospital-based QI projects are often conducted without resident or fellow involvement [8].

There is growing evidence that longitudinal training leads to better QI education for residents. Simasek and Patel have described longitudinal quality improvement rotations which were incorporated into their institutions' respective residency training programs and were found to be feasible and efficacious [9, 10]. Scales and colleagues incorporated team-based game mechanics into an evidence-based online learning platform which increased resident participation in a QI curriculum [11].

The American Board of Pediatrics (ABP) Maintenance of Certification (MOC) program assesses the six core competencies established by ACGME. Part 4 of the ABP's MOC process, Improving Professional Practice, requires pediatricians and pediatric subspecialists to demonstrate competence in *systematic measurement and improvement* in patient care. Pediatricians participate in a range of ABP-approved QI projects designed to assess and improve the quality of patient care including collaborative quality improvement projects, QI projects initiated in the workplace, web-based improvement activities, and QI articles or posters [12]. The effectiveness of these Part 4 activities has yet to be widely demonstrated, but there are isolated reports of QI CME activities leading to improved compliance with quality measures [13].

What Kind of Investigation Qualifies as Quality Improvement Versus Research?

As hospital systems are guided by pressure from private and public sectors to improve patient safety and efficiency in an effort to contain health-care costs and improve outcomes, it can be difficult to differentiate what investigations are classified as QI versus research investigation. It is the similarities in the definitions of QI versus research that lends itself to some confusion. The US Dept. of Health Resources and Services Administration (HRSA) defines quality improvement as a group of "systematic and continuous actions that lead to measurable improvement in health care services and the health status of targeted patient groups" [14]. Research is defined as a "systematic investigation (research design, testing and evaluation) that develops or contributes to generalized knowledge" [15]. As QI work and research in health care involves human subjects and both types of work may lead to publications, clinicians can struggle with determining if QI work falls under the regulations of the Dept. of Health and Human Services policy protecting the rights of human subjects in research. The role of Institutional Review Boards (IRBs) in aiding in the determination if QI work needs to be reviewed with the same scrutiny as research is also unclear. Because of this overlap between quality improvement initiatives and research, the Agency for Healthcare Research and Quality (AHRQ) provided a grant to the Hastings Center to provide guidance on this matter.

The Hastings Center is an independent, nonpartisan, and nonprofit bioethics research institute whose mission is to address fundamental and ethical issues in the areas of health, medicine, and the environment that may affect individuals, communities, and societies. The summary of their work, "The Ethics of Using QI Methods to Improve Health Care Quality and Safety," was published in 2006 and is frequently referenced in QI publications [16].

To understand how QI differs, principles of research (clinical investigation) need to be understood. All research is designed to contribute to the advancement of generalized knowledge, not necessarily in the implementation of that knowledge. To ensure the results are without bias, research requires the methods to be strictly followed to ensure that the outcome achieves a statistical difference over a set period of time. To ensure the accuracy of this research, it may be years before the results of the study are disseminated. The design of the research project may involve a randomization and only a subset of patients. As it is unclear if the hypothesis is beneficial to an individual, human subjects must provide voluntary consent to participate. Despite the uncertainty of any benefit, subjects are allowed to participate based on the principle that there is an expectation of a social benefit (directly or indirectly) from this new knowledge. Methodology is generally not changed even if it results in a negative impact to the study. Publication of this knowledge is an important aspect of research, to allow others downstream to use this knowledge that may benefit their patients. An important distinction is that research can happen *outside* routine medical care. Research and its results may not have necessarily been done at the local system and thus does not take into account what steps are needed to change the process for patients to ensure the patients see the benefit of the research. Lastly, funding for research may be from outside the system and may only be used to run that research project, for that given period of time. Lastly, one motivation for research is that it may benefit the individual physician's professional goals leading to promotion, tenure, and prestige within the academic community.

Quality improvement in health care has become part of the process to continually improve the system to deliver care to its patients and to ensure that an institution meets national benchmarks. It is usually mandated by the institution or the clinic as part of its operations. It can use knowledge gained from research but may need to adapt to the local systems and processes to use this knowledge. The role of QI is to bring about immediate improvement in care through the use of QI methodology (PDSA, Six Sigma, FADE, etc.) and to continuously and systematically analyze changes in processes and their impact on care and its delivery. Unlike research, QI methods continuously adapt to bring about rapid improvement as quickly as possible. It generally does not involve a randomization. If the risk is minimal and does not exceed routine medical care, patients' participation in QI may not be voluntary as it is the responsibility for the organization to continually improve and deliver optimal cost-efficient care within the community it serves. It is important that QI activities be limited to the patients that are associated with the health-care team involved in the QI activity to ensure protection of Protected Health Information (PHI). Attached is a table (Table 19.1) outlining the differences between research and QI work. It is important to consider these distinctions when designing QI activities as it will help determine if the QI activity will need IRB review and if consent is required.

Table 19.1 Differences Between Research and Quality Improvement Projects

	Research investigation	Quality improvement
Purpose	To develop or contribute to generalizable knowledge	Designed to implement knowledge, assess a process or program as judged by established/accepted standards
Motivation for the project	Independent of routine care. To answer a question or hypothesis. Project occurs in part as a result to further an individuals' professional goal	Result of knowledge is integral to ongoing management of local health-care system. May not be initiated by people involved in the project. May not benefit the evaluator professionally
Project design	Rigid protocol that is unchanged through a period of time. May involve a randomization Activity is *not* mandated by institution or program	Adaptive, design changes in response to data gathered, no fixed time period. Generally does *not* involve a randomization to different processes Activity mandated by the institution or clinic as part of its operations
Benefits	May not benefit current subjects, intended to benefit future patients	System or program may see direct benefit; patients may or may not benefit
Risks	May put subjects at risk	Should not increase risk to patients, with exception of potential breech of confidential patient information
Participant obligation	No obligation to participate	Responsibility to participate as a part of their care
Endpoint	To answer a research question	Improve current program, process, or system
Analysis	Statistically to prove/disprove hypothesis	To compare local program, process, or system to established standards
Adoption of results	Low priority to disseminate results quickly	Adopt results rapidly into local care system
Publication/presentation	Investigator obliged to share results	QI group encouraged to share systematic reporting of insights

When Is IRB Review Needed of QI Work?

As both QI projects and research can involve human subjects, it can be difficult to determine if QI projects require IRB review. Since research can be independent of clinical work and routine operations of the institution, research is usually outside the institution's supervisory and management structure and thus requires IRB review to ensure the safety of human subjects. QI projects are directly linked to the clinical operations of the institution and thus are under the surveillance of the institution's safety and quality supervision. Furthermore, the improvement cycles involved in QI projects make it difficult for IRB review as the time frame for review may hamper the ability of QI projects to benefit the patients being treated within the institution.

IRB review should be considered when there is uncertainty by the team, when the QI activity poses increased risk to the patient, or may consume substantial resources. External funding usually requires IRB involvement to ensure that the parties are complying with DHHS for human subject research. As QI activity continues to grow at local institutions, many local IRBs have developed worksheets to help local investigators determine if the IRB needs to review the QI project. Review of information from institutions' IRBs shows there are common considerations as to what requires IRB review [17–19]. Some of the factors which appear to universally indicate the need for IRB review include testing of new treatments, inclusion of randomization, involvement of personnel who have no direct interest in improving the institution's quality of care, delay in reporting data for feedback, and outside funding from organizations with an interest in the use of the results. The Office of Human Research Protections has provided guidance on when QI activities may infringe upon research on human subjects [20]. Publication of QI activities can also be viewed differently by local IRBs based as the dissemination of the results from the QI work may be considered contributing to general knowledge, similar to research.

Considerations When Publishing QI Work

Although QI projects focus on making improvements at local sites rather than on generating new scientific knowledge, publishing the work has several benefits. Publishing a QI activity makes one ensure the reason for the activity along with verifying the observations seen at the institution. It can help other facilities determine if their system can benefit from these improvements. Improvements seen in multi-institution collaborative QI work may prevent outside systems from wasting resources on verifying the results. Many health-care journals now include areas for publication of QI projects. However, due to the nature of improvement cycles in QI work, it can be difficult to know how to publish QI work in a meaningful way to disseminate the methods in how the results were achieved. In 2008, the Standards for Quality Improvement Reporting Excellence (SQUIRE 1.0) guidelines were developed to help with improving completeness, precision, and transparency of published QI work so others might learn from it. As experience in QI work grew in health care, the SQUIRE guidelines were updated and published in 2015 [21, 22]. Although broken down into topics similar to a research article, it gives suggestions as to how to prepare the manuscript to ensure that QI work is described in a consistent manner. Increasingly, manuscripts detailing the results of QI work are being published in traditional medical journals.

Using Quality Improvement to Advance a Career

Quality Improvement efforts have involved every category of personnel in medicine, but perhaps the most challenging group to engage is the physician group. From resident trainees to attending physicians, there is reluctance to participate in QI and safety efforts [23]. Many reasons are given, from lack of reimbursement for this time to lack of training to punitive measures [24, 25]. However, it is well documented that QI and safety efforts are more successful with physician engagement and support. Involvement of physicians may signify to all those involved that this effort is important and gain credibility with patients and families [26]. Some institutions are moving toward a physician quality officer of chief safety officer to help spearhead QI and safety efforts and communicate with peers on their importance [27].

Pediatric hematology and oncology lends itself to ongoing practice improvement. Safety mechanisms are inherent in chemotherapy administration guidelines and incorporate safety efforts for patients and staff. Due to more medically complex pediatric patients requiring central venous access, efforts to reduce venous thromboembolism with mechanical or pharmacological means have been introduced [28]. In hemophilia, national registries exist to measure specific outcome measures including compliance with factor preparations. Palliative care is an area of pediatric hematology, oncology, and stem cell transplant that has filled a need for formal education with a train-the-trainer method of teaching and is performing periodic evaluations to examine its impact [29].

Within the field of pediatric hematology and oncology, there are numerous opportunities for physicians to become involved in QI and safety [30]. Most hospitals have organized efforts to improve chemotherapy safety with involvement of information technology and pharmacy staff. In the 15 years since publication of *To Err is Human*, there has been tremendous emphasis on health-care-associated conditions, and collaborative efforts have formed to address many of them including catheter-related central line bloodstream infections (CLABSI), other hospital-acquired infections, deep vein thromboses, and readmissions [31–34].

Quality improvement work has been ongoing for decades, and those who have participated in this work extensively have unique and valuable perspectives for those considering such a career path. In a brief, anonymous survey of general academic pediatricians and pediatric academic subspecialists recognized as QI experts by their peers (unpublished data), the respondents shared that they reached this career path in various ways over varying amounts of time. Of the 12 respondents, five had participated in QI work for over a decade, while three had been involved in QI efforts between 6 and 10 years. The remaining quarter had been involved in QI work for less than 6 years. Time spent in QI efforts ranged from greater than 75% of their professional time in about one fourth of those surveyed to between 10 and 25 % of time for half of the respondents.

Eight of 12 reported that they had intentionally focused on QI work, while the remaining quarter were split between continuation of work started in residency or fellowship and the evolution of a small QI project into larger efforts. Nearly all respondents indicated that they feel QI and safety efforts within pediatrics, and pediatric subspecialties will increase in the coming years and will have a positive impact on the field. The pediatric subspecialties represented included allergy/immunology, infectious disease, and critical care. All surveyed indicated that they either have further certification or degrees that pertain to QI and safety efforts, ranging from Lean Six Sigma Green Belt certification, Institute for Healthcare Improvement (IHI) certification, High Reliability Trainer, Baldrige Examiner, Masters in Medical Management, Advanced Training Program (ATP) Intermountain program, Masters in Business Organizational Excellence, and Masters of Science in Clinical Information.

Leaders in QI and safety efforts within pediatrics indicated the QI work being done should be valued by insurance companies/payers, leadership, and fellow physicians. Such work should be taken into account when deciding academic promotion. One respondent encouraged physicians in our subspecialty to "be open to change and remember that all healthcare workers are striving to make things better for patients." Another expert encouraged those within hematology/oncology to embrace quality and safety work and to seek leaders outside of hematology/oncology to guide publishing of QI work as the process differs from the publication of research results. Another wise respondent recommended that "[quality and safety] has to *become part of who we are and not an additional thing to do*—when improving care is as natural as examining a patient we will have achieved a lot!" These lessons indicate that while improvements have been made regarding acceptance of QI and safety work as integral to the success of medicine, there is still more work to be done.

Current and Future Opportunities in Quality Improvement and Safety

In an effort to offer more formal education and training in quality improvement and safety efforts, there are more opportunities for learners at all levels to receive further education. A growing number of universities are offering educational programs leading to a master's degree in the area of health-care QI/operational excellence [35–38].

Nationwide Children's Hospital offers a Clinical Fellowship in Quality and Safety Leadership, which consists of 5 months of immersion into quality and safety efforts at the institution, and coursework to complete the MBOE at The Ohio State University Fisher College of Business. After obtaining the degree, there is another 6 months of work compiling a portfolio of work and manuscript submission. At the completion of the 2-year fellowship, the graduate receives an MBOE and Six Sigma Black Belt certification, training in risk management and scientific writing among other topics [39].

Intermountain Healthcare System and Cincinnati Children's Hospital Medical Center offer training programs in Health Care Delivery Improvement that provide training in QI development, implementation, and investigation. The training includes expert faculty consultation on a QI project completed during the course. This program was developed and designed around health-care workers and offers the opportunity to interact with national leaders, drawing from lessons in the airline industry among others [40, 41].

There is an increasing number of QI and safety educational offerings available to physicians like online training modules from the IHI and educational meetings sponsored by organizations like the IHI, Solutions for Patient Safety, and the National Quality Colloquium. Participation in associations created to promote QI work such as the Council on Quality Improvement, and Patient Safety of the American Academy of Pediatrics can also enhance physicians' QI knowledge. Acting as a grant reviewer for a QI organization, such as AHRQ, provides additional experience and expertise in the field.

While there have been pockets of improvement in quality and safety in medicine overall, there is still significant work to be done. The field of pediatric hematology/oncology offers many opportunities to find a specific area and make important contributions. As the field of QI and safety grows, so too do the opportunities for further training, publication, and leadership.

References

1. Institute of Medicine (US) Committee on Quality of Health Care in America. Kohn LT, Corrigan JM, Donaldson MS, editors. To err is human: building a safer health system. Washington, DC: National Academies Press (US); 2000.
2. Institute of Medicine (US) Committee on Quality of Health Care in America. Crossing the quality chasm: a new health system for the 21st century. Washington, DC: National Academies Press (US); 2001.
3. American Association of Colleges of Nursing. The essentials of master's education for advanced practice nursing. Washington, DC: American Association of Colleges of Nursing; 1996. http://www.aacn.nche.edu/publications/order-form/masters-essentials. Accessed 19 July 2016.
4. Berwick DM. Continuous improvement as an ideal in health care. N Engl J Med. 1989;320(1):53–6.
5. Headrick LA, Neuhauser D, Schwab P, Stevens DP. Continuous quality improvement and the education of the generalist physician. Acad Med. 1995;70(1):S104–9.
6. Institute of Medicine (US) Committee on Health Professions Education Summit. Health professions education: a bridge to quality. Washington, DC: National Academies Press (US); 2003.
7. Accreditation Council on Graduate Medical Education [Internet]. 2016. http://www.acgme.org/What-We-Do/Accreditation/Common-Program-Requirements. Accessed 18 July 2016.
8. Mann KJ, Craig MS, Moses JM. Quality improvement educational practices in pediatric residency programs: survey of pediatric program directors. Acad Pediatr. 2014;14:23–8.
9. Patel N, Brennan PJ, Metlay J, Bellini L, Shannon RP, Myers JS. Building the pipeline: the creation of a residency training pathway for future physician leaders in health care quality. Acad Med. 2015;90(2):185–90.

10. Simasek M, Ballard SL, Phelps P, Pingul-Ravano R, Kolb NR, Finkelstein A, et al. Meeting resident scholarly activity requirements through a longitudinal quality improvement curriculum. J Grad Med Educ. 2015;7(1):86–90.

11. Scales Jr CD, Moin T, Fink A, Berry SH, Afsar-Manesh N, Mangione CM, Kerfoot BP. A randomized, controlled trial of team-based competition to increase learner participation in quality-improvement education. Int J Qual Health Care. 2016;28(2):227–32.

12. American Board of Pediatrics [Internet]. https://www.abp.org/content/improving-professional-practice-part-4. Accessed 18 July 2016.

13. Sapir T, Moreo K, Carter JD, Greene L, Patel B, Higgins PD. Continuing medical education improves gastroenterologists' compliance with inflammatory bowel disease quality measures. Dig Dis Sci. 2016;61(7):1862–9.

14. Health Resources and Services Administration [Internet]. http://www.hrsa.gov/quality/toolbox/methodology/qualityimprovement/. Accessed 18 July 2016.

15. Office for Human Research Protections, 45 CFR 46.46.102 [Internet]. http://www.hhs.gov/ohrp/regulations-and-policy/regulations/45-cfr-46/. Accessed 18 July 2016.

16. Baily MA, Bottrell M, Lynn J, Jennings B. Hastings center. The ethics of using QI methods to improve health care quality and safety. Hast Cent Rep. 2006;36(4):S1–40.

17. The Children's Hospital of Philadelphia Institutional Review Board [Internet]. Quality Improvement vs Research. 2015. https://irb.research.chop.edu/quality-improvement-vs-research. Accessed 22 May 2016.

18. Stanford University Research Compliance Office, S. U. Quality Assessment and Quality Improvement (QA/QI) FAQs [Internet]. http://humansubjects.stanford.edu/research/documents/qa_qi_faqs_AID03H16.pdf. Accessed 22 May 2016.

19. University of Wiscosin KnowledgeBase. Guidance on Research vs. Quality Improvement and Program Evaluation [Internet]. https://kb.wisc.edu/hsirbs/33386. Accessed 22 May 2016.

20. Office for Human Research Protections. Quality Improvement Activities FAQs. [Internet]. http://www.hhs.gov/ohrp/regulations-and-policy/guidance/faq/quality-improvement-activities/index.html#. Accessed 22 May 2016.

21. Davidoff F, Batalden P, Stevens D, Ogrinc G, Mooney S. Publication guidelines for quality improvement studies in health care: Evolution of the SQUIRE project. J Gen Intern Med. 2008;23(12):2125–30. doi:10.1007/s11606-008-0797-4.

22. Ogrinc G, Davies L, Goodman D, Bataldan P, Davidoff F, Stevens D. SQUIRE 2.0 (Standards for QUality Improvement Reporting Excellence): revised publication guidelines from a detailed consensus process. Am J Crit Care. 2015;24(6):466–73.

23. Johnson Faherty L, Mate KS, Moses JM. Leveraging trainees to improve quality and safety at the point of care: three models for engagement. Acad Med. 2016;91(4):503–9.

24. Altman DE, Clancy C, Blendon RJ. Improving patient safety--five years after the IOM report. New Engl J Med. 2004;351(20):2041–3.

25. Vonnegut M. Is quality improvement improving quality? A view from the doctor's office. New Engl J Med. 2007;357(26):2652–3.

26. Reinertsen JL, Gosfield AG, Rupp W, Whittington JW. Engaging Physicians in a Shared Quality Agenda. IHI Innovation Series white paper [Internet]. www.IHI.org. Accessed 25 Apr 2016

27. Walsh KE, Ettinger WH, Klugman RA. Physician quality officer: a new model for engaging physicians in quality improvement. Am J Med Qual. 2009;24(4):295–301.

28. Mahajerin A, Webber EC, Morris J, Taylor K, Saysana M. Development and implementation results of a venous thromboembolism prophylaxis guideline in a tertiary care pediatric hospital. Hosp Pediatr. 2015;5(12):630–6.

29. Widger K, Friedrichsdorf S, Wolfe J, Liben S, Pole JD, Bouffet E, et al. Protocol: evaluating the impact of a nation-wide train-the-trainer educational initiative to enhance the quality of palliative care for children with cancer. BMC Palliat Care. 2016;15(1):12.

30. Zweidler-McKay PA, Hogan MS, Jubran R, Black V, Casillas J, Harper J, et al. Navigating your career path in pediatric hematology/oncology: on and off the beaten track. Pediatr Blood Cancer. 2016;63(10):1723–30. doi:10.1002/pbc.26094.

31. Bundy DG, Gaur AH, Billett AL, He B, Colantuoni EA, Miller MR, et al. Preventing CLABSIs among pediatric hematology/oncology inpatients: national collaborative results. Pediatrics. 2014 Dec;134(6):e1678–85.
32. Children's Hospital's Solutions for Patient Safety [Internet]. http://www.solutionsforpatient-safety.org/about-us/. Accessed 19 July 2016.
33. Dandoy CE, Hausfeld J, Flesch L, Hawkins D, Demmel K, Best D, et al. Rapid cycle development of a multifactorial intervention achieved sustained reductions in central line-associated bloodstream infections in haematology oncology units at a children's hospital: a time series analysis. BMJ Qual Saf. 2015;25(8):633–43. doi:10.1136/bmjqs-2015-004450.
34. Pronovost PJ, Cleeman JI, Wright D, Srinivasan A. Fifteen years after to err is human: a success story to learn from. BMJ Qual Saf. 2016;25(6):396–9.
35. The George Washington University Healthcare Quality Program [Internet]. http://smhs.gwu.edu/health-care-quality/. Accessed 20 July 2016.
36. Northwestern University Feinberg School of Medicine Center for Education in Health Sciences [Internet].   http://www.feinberg.northwestern.edu/sites/cehs/masters-programs/healthcare-quality-patient-safety/. Accessed 29 June 2016.
37. The Ohio State University Fisher College of Business [Internet]. http://fisher.osu.edu/mboe. Accessed 29 Feb 2016.
38. Thomas Jefferson University Jefferson College of Population Health [Internet]. http://www.jefferson.edu/university/population-health/degrees-programs/healthcare-quality-safety.html. Accessed 22 July 2016.
39. Nationwide Children's Clinical Fellowship in Quality and Safety Leadership Program Overview [Internet]. http://www.nationwidechildrens.org/quality-fellowship-mboe. Accessed 22 July 2016
40. Cincinnati Children's Hospital Medical Center [Internet]. http://www.cincinnatichildrens.org/education/clinical/graduate/grad/scholars/default/. Accessed 19 July 2016.
41. Intermountain Healthcare Advanced Training Program: 20-day course for executives and quality improvement leaders [Internet]. https://intermountainhealthcare.org/about/transforming-healthcare/intermountain-healthcare-leadership-institute/courses/advanced-training-program/. Accessed 4 Mar 2016.

Chapter 20
Quality Improvement and Patient Safety Resources

Christopher E. Dandoy, Joanne M. Hilden, Amy L. Billett, and Brigitta U. Mueller

Overview

Pediatric hematology/oncology/hematopoietic stem cell transplant patients are highly susceptible to preventable harm. They usually have central venous catheters exposing them to infectious or thrombotic complications, receive toxic medications, are highly susceptible to healthcare-acquired infection, and are at high risk of home medication errors and nonadherence. The Institute of Medicine defines patient safety as the prevention of harm to patients, and workers in healthcare delivery systems have an obligation to prevent harm through cultivation of a culture of safety that prevents errors and learns from the errors that do occur.

The goal of this chapter is to provide a useful reference of resources to assist individuals and organizations in its quality improvement and safety efforts. It provides a concise summary of selected patient safety and quality manuscripts and books.

C.E. Dandoy (✉)
Department of Bone Marrow Transplant and Immune Deficiency, Cincinnati Children's Hospital Medical Center, University of Cincinnati, Cincinnati, OH, USA
e-mail: christopher.dandoy@cchmc.org

J.M. Hilden
Center for Cancer and Blood Disorders, Children's Hospital Colorado, University of Colorado School of Medicine, Aurora, CO, USA

A.L. Billett
Dana-Farber/Boston Children's Cancer and Blood Disorders Center, Harvard Medical School, Boston, MA, USA

B.U. Mueller
Johns Hopkins All Children's Hospital, Johns Hopkins University School of Medicine, Baltimore, MD, USA

© Springer International Publishing AG 2017
C.E. Dandoy et al. (eds.), *Patient Safety and Quality in Pediatric Hematology/Oncology and Stem Cell Transplantation*, DOI 10.1007/978-3-319-53790-0_20

361

Quality Improvement Resources

Books

Crossing the Quality Chasm: A New Health System for the 21st Century. 2001. 1st Edition. Institute of Medicine Committee on Quality of Health Care in America (Author).

- *A follow-up to the Institute of Medicine (IOM) patient safety report, To Err is Human: Building a Safer Health System, Crossing the Quality Chasm encourages and advocates for a redesign of the healthcare system.*

The Improvement Guide: A Practical Approach to Enhancing Organizational Performance. 2009. 2nd Edition. Gerald J. Langley, Ronald D. Moen, Kevin M. Nolan, Thomas W. Nolan, Clifford L. Norman, and Lloyd P. Provost (Authors).

- *The Improvement Guide offers and integrated approach to process improvement with step-by-step instruction on the Model for Improvement. The book provides a practical set of examples and applications for the implementation and acceleration of improvement.*

Quality Improvement Through Planned Experimentation. 2012. 3rd Edition. Ronald M. Moen, Thomas W. Nolan, Lloyd P. Provost (Authors).

- *This book discusses the principles and methodologies for planned experimentation to improve processes and systems. The book incorporates case studies sequentially to provide the reader the knowledge needed to test and implement improvement strategies.*

A Lean Guide to Transforming Healthcare: How to Implement Lean Principles in Hospitals, Medical Offices, Clinics, and Other Healthcare Organizations. 2006. 1st Edition. Thomas Zidel (Author).

- *A Lean Guide to Transforming Healthcare provides a practical review of the concepts of Lean and Six Sigma.*

Basics of Health Care Performance Improvement: A Lean Six Sigma Approach. 2011. 1st Edition. Donald Lighter (Author).

- *Basics of Health Care Performance Improvement provides an overview of the principles and procedures of Lean Six Sigma. In addition, the book provides in-depth information on planning and implementing a "Define-Measure-Analyze-Improve-Control" initiative to reduce errors and improve performance.*

The Lean Six Sigma Pocket Toolbook: A Quick Reference Guide to 100 Tools for Improving Quality and Speed. 2004. 1st Edition. Michael L. George, John Maxey, David Rowlands and, Mark Price (Authors).

- *Through summaries and examples, the Lean Six Sigma Pocket Toolbook assists the reader to determine which quality improvement tool is best suited for specific purposes.*

Lean Hospitals: Improving Quality, Patient Safety, and Employee Engagement. 2011. 2nd Edition. Mark Graban (Author).

- *Lean Hospitals: Improving Quality, Patient Safety, and Employee Engagement explains how to use the Lean philosophy and management system to improve safety, quality, access, and morale while reducing costs in healthcare delivery.*

Lean Six Sigma for Hospitals: Simple Steps to Fast, Affordable, and Flawless Healthcare. 2011. 1st Edition. Jay Arthur.

- *The purpose of Lean Six Sigma for Hospitals is to provide simple steps to help hospitals get faster, better, and cheaper in 5 days.*

Why Hospitals Should Fly: The Ultimate Flight Plan to Patient Safety and Quality Care.
2008. 1st Edition. John J. Nance (Author).

- *Written as a novel, touches upon all the tenets of quality and safety in hospitals.*

Beyond Heroes: A Lean Management System for Healthcare. 2014. 1st Edition. Kim Barnas (Author).

- *Beyond Heroes outlines the leadership system necessary to achieve improvements in healthcare and explores the essential components of the lean system.*

Manuscripts and White Papers

Mueller BU. Quality and Safety in Pediatric Hematology/Oncology. Pediatric Blood and Cancer. 2014;61(6):966-9.

- *This review describes healthcare gaps and opportunities for improved healthcare quality and safety in pediatric hematology/oncology patients.*

Scoville R, Little K. Comparing Lean and Quality Improvement. Institute for Healthcare Improvement white paper. 2014.

- *This IHI white paper details Lean and the IHI approach to quality improvement, including the basic concepts and principles of each approach, and for what purposes each approach is the most appropriate.*

Resar R, Griffin FA, Haraden C, Nolan TW. Using Care Bundles to Improve Health Care Quality. Institute for Healthcare Improvement Innovation Series white paper. 2012.

- *This white paper reviews the theory, design, and outcomes associated with the development and use of bundled care.*

Going Lean in Health Care. Institute for Healthcare Improvement Innovation Series white paper. 2005.

- *Lean management principles have been used effectively in manufacturing companies for decades; this white paper reviews the mechanisms Lean principles can be applied into healthcare.*

Margolis P, Provost LP, Schoettker PJ, Britto MT. Quality improvement, clinical research, and quality improvement research–opportunities for integration. Pediatric Clinics of North America. 2009;56(4):831-41.

- *This article describes opportunities to integrate quality improvement and clinical research.*

Campbell M, Fitzpatrick M, Fitzpatrick R, Haines A, Kinmonth AL, Sandercodk P, Spiegelhalter D, Tyrer P. Framework for design and evaluation of complex interventions to improve health. British Medical Journal. 2000; 321: 694-696.

- *This article describes the importance and practicality of a phased approach to the development and evaluation of complex interventions in healthcare.*

Organizational Patient Safety Resources

Books

To Err is Human: Building a Safer Health System. 2000. 1st Edition. Institute of Medicine Committee on Quality of Health Care in America (Author).

- *Through this report, the Institute of Medicine presents a comprehensive strategy to reduce medical errors.*

Patient Safety. 2010. 1st Edition. Charles Vincent (Author).

- *Patient Safety reviews the evidence behind the issues directly related to patient safety issues and provides practical guidance on implementing safer practices.*

Error Reduction in Health Care: A Systems Approach to Improving Patient Safety. 2011. 2nd Edition. Patrice L Spath (Author).

- *Error Reduction in Healthcare provides case series examples of incidences associated with patient safety and provides mechanisms to provide improved care.*

Safe Patients, Smart Hospitals: How One Doctor's Checklist Can Help Us Change Health Care from the Inside Out. 2011. 1st Edition. Peter Pronovost and Eric Vohr (Authors).

- *Written by a leader in patient safety who revolutionized bloodstream infection prevention by creating a simple checklist.*

Manuscripts and White Papers

Gandhi TK, Berwick DM, Shojania KG. Patient Safety at the Crossroads. JAMA. 2016;315(17):1829-30.

- *The report makes recommendations necessary to achieve total systems safety. This viewpoint focuses on the mechanisms and recommendations for healthcare leaders to maintain a safety culture.*

Birk S. Lists that work: The healthcare leader's role in implementation. Healthcare Executive. 2013;28(2):28-37.

- *The article reviews the experiences of several organizations in implementing checklists to improve patient safety.*

Sadler BL, Joseph A, Keller A, Rostenberg B. Using evidence-based environmental design to enhance safety and quality. IHI Innovation Series white paper. Institute for Healthcare Improvement; 2009.

- *This paper shows healthcare leaders how evidence-based environmental design interventions can measurably enhance the care they provide.*

Botwinick L, Bisognano M, Haraden C. Leadership guide to patient safety. IHI Innovation Series white paper. Institute for Healthcare Improvement; 2006.

- *The IHI White Paper presents eight steps recommended to follow to achieve high reliability in the healthcare organization.*

Gandhi TK, Berwick DM, Shojania KG. Patient safety at the crossroads. Journal of the American Medical Association. 2016;315(17):1829-1830.

- *The authors reevaluate the status of patient safety 15 years after "To Err Is Human" was published and proposes a course for future patient safety work.*

Medical Errors

Manuscripts and White Papers

Leape LL. Reporting of adverse events. New England Journal of Medicine. 2002;347(20):1633-1638.

- *The article reviews medical error reporting and explores options for improved reporting systems.*

Federico F. An overview of error-reduction options. Nursing Management IT Solutions. 2010 Sep:14-16.

- *This article provides a brief overview of low-tech approaches to decrease medication administration errors.*

Hannisdal E, Arianson H, Braut GS, Schlichting E, Vinnem JE. A risk analysis of cancer care in Norway: the top 16 patient safety hazards. The Joint Commission Journal on Quality and Patient Safety. 2013 Nov;39(11):511-6.

- *Through retrospective analysis and interviews with key personnel, the Norwegian Board of Health Supervision reviewed the top hazards associated with cancer care in their country.*

Kullberg A, Larsen J, Sharp L. 'Why is there another person's name on my infusion bag?' Patient safety in chemotherapy care - a review of the literature. European Journal of Oncology Nursing. 2013;17(2):228–35.

- *This review article identified and discussed evidence-based practices to improve the safety of chemotherapy administration.*

Human Factors

Books

Human Error. 1990. 2nd Edition. James Reason (Author).

- *Considered the "Bible" of error theory, Human Error reviews the framework for understanding error.*

Human Error in Medicine. 1994. 2nd Edition. Marilyn Sue Bogner (Author).

- *Human error reviews many aspects of healthcare topics and provides solutions through improved healthcare delivery system design.*

Human Factors and Ergonomics in Health Care and Patient Safety. 2012. 2nd Edition. Pascale Carayon (Editor).

- *This book discusses the contributions of human factors and ergonomics to the improvement of patient safety and quality. The book argues that in order to take the next steps in quality of care and patient safety, of care, collaboration between human factor professionals and healthcare providers must occur.*

The Checklist Manifesto: How to Get Things Right. 2011. Reprint Edition. Atul Gawande (Author).

- *Through examples, the Checklist Manifesto demonstrates how the use of checklists can improve care.*

Measurement of Improvement

Books

The Health Care Data Guide: Learning from Data for Improvement. 2011. 1st Edition. Lloyd p. Provost and Sandra K. Murray (Authors).

- *The Health Care Data Guide provides a practical step-by-step guide to statistical process control (SPC), including Shewhart charts, run charts, frequency plots, scatter diagrams, and Pareto analysis.*

  Measuring Quality Improvement in Healthcare. 2001. 1st Edition. Robert C. Lloyd and Raymond G. Carey (Authors).

- *This book addresses the effectiveness of quality improvement efforts and covers practical applications of the tools and techniques of statistical process control (SPC), including run charts and control charts.*

  Improving Healthcare with Control Charts: Basic and Advanced SPC Methods and Case Studies. 2003. 1st Edition. Raymond G. Carey and Larry V. Stake (Authors).

- *Improving Healthcare with Control Charts provides a comprehensive review of statistical process control (SPC). In addition, the authors utilize case studies to demonstrate applicability of SPC in the healthcare setting.*

Manuscripts and White Papers

Berwick DM. Controlling Variation in Health Care: A Consultation from Walter Shewhart. Medical Care. 1991;29(12):1212–25.

Sustainability

Books

Managing the Unexpected: Sustained Performance in a Complex World. 2015. 3rd Edition. Karl E. Weick and Kathleen M. Sutcliffe (Authors).

- *Explaining the need for hospitals to become high-reliability organizations.*

Manuscripts and White Papers

Scoville R, Little K, Rakover J, Luther K, Mate K. Sustaining Improvement. Institute for Healthcare Improvement White Paper. 2016.

- *This white paper presents the framework of healthcare delivery systems that can be used to sustain improvements in the safety, effectiveness, and efficiency of patient care.*

Nolan T, Resar R, Haraden C, Griffin FA. Improving the Reliability of Health Care. Institute for Healthcare Improvement Innovation Series white paper. 2004.

- *This white paper describes the principles and strategies used to evaluate, calculate, and improve the reliability of complex systems.*

Spread

Manuscripts and White Papers

Massoud MR, Nielsen GA, Nolan K, Schall MW, Sevin C. A Framework for Spread: From Local Improvements to System-Wide Change. Institute for Healthcare Improvement White Paper. 2016.

- *This white paper delineates the steps successful organizations have taken to spread successful improvement. These include mechanisms to prepare for spread, establish an aim for spread, and develop a spread plan.*

Leadership

Books

Leading Change. 2012. 1st Edition. John P. Kotter (Author).

- *In this business manual, John P. Kotter provides an eight-step framework to manage change with positive results.*

ADKAR: A Model for Change in Business, Government and our Community. 2006. 1st Edition. Jeffrey M. Hiatt (Author)

- *The ADKAR model (Awareness, Desire, Knowledge, Ability, Reinforcement) has emerged as a holistic approach that brings together the collection of change management work into a simple, results-oriented model. This model ties together all aspects of change management including readiness assessments, sponsorship, communications, coaching, training, and resistance management.*

Index

© Springer International Publishing AG 2017
C.E. Dandoy et al. (eds.), *Patient Safety and Quality in Pediatric Hematology/Oncology and Stem Cell Transplantation*, DOI 10.1007/978-3-319-53790-0

PGSTL 07/14/2017